Praise for

"I believe Dr. Rediger is the perfect ... and timely book, which shows us a ... physical illness. His unique docume ... ... strategies of individuals who have manifested their own medical recoveries, against all odds, will offer not only hope but also genuine insight to anyone facing a medical crisis."

—Jill Bolte Taylor, Ph.D., neuroanatomist, spokesperson
for the Harvard Brain Bank, and author of the
New York Times bestseller *My Stroke of Insight*

"Dr. Rediger's work adds enormously to the growing body of work willing to take on the medical establishment and show that we may have far more control over our health than most physicians, researchers, and the lay public realize."

—Ellen Langer, Ph.D., professor of psychology,
Harvard University, and author of *Counterclockwise*

"*Cured* is a book for everyone. This new pathway to healing is potentially life changing, both for those with a terminal diagnosis and those who simply want to live the healthiest life possible. In these illuminating pages, Dr. Rediger gives medicine a much-needed push toward a science of health and hope."

—Daniel Friedland, M.D., former chair of the
Academy of Integrative Health and Medicine
and author of *Leading Well from Within*

"*Cured* is packed with cutting-edge science and powerful, eye-opening real-life case studies. Dr. Jeff Rediger offers groundbreaking and scientifically backed evidence of how trauma can have long-lasting effects on our bodies. This is a hopeful tale of how through resilience and meaningful lifestyle adjustments even the most serious of cases can be redeemed. Timely and beautifully written. Everyone should read this book."   —Bessel van der Kolk, author of the
#1 *New York Times* bestseller *The Body Keeps the Score*

"Packed with pearls of wisdom gleaned from Dr. Rediger's intensive immersion in the field of remarkable recoveries and from his thoughtful reflections about his own personal journey, *Cured* will touch the hearts and souls of everyone who reads this book and will inspire them to take charge of their health—and their mind-set. This exciting book is bound to be a page-turner for anyone who wants to die from old age—and not before then."

—Martha Stark, M.D., and faculty at Harvard Medical School

"Seasoned with the author's penetrating insights about healing, clearly articulated science, and illuminating case histories, *Cured* opens genuine vistas of transforming illness into health even in the face of diagnoses conventional medical thinking habitually dismisses as hopeless."

—Gabor Maté, M.D.,
author of *When the Body Says No*

"Have you ever wondered why some people 'miraculously' heal from disease, while others don't? This question can seem so mysterious that we often think there's simply no way to understand it. But there are answers, and *Cured* presents them in a beautifully written and deeply personal way. Dr. Rediger's brilliance and wisdom are profound and eminently practical. But it's his humility and humanity that make this book the masterpiece that it is."

—John Robbins, president, Food Revolution Network

"*Cured* is one of the most important books I've ever read. Dr. Rediger presents dozens of case studies of people who defied the odds, many making complete recoveries even after being told to go home and get their affairs in order. In this book, he shows us why they recovered and gives us insights into how we, too, can tap into this amazing curative and regenerative power of the human body. This is a deeply inspiring book. I could hardly put it down."

—David R. Hamilton, Ph.D., author of
How Your Mind Can Heal Your Body

"Fascinating bioscience on the phenomenon of spontaneous healing . . . [*Cured*] doubles as a pragmatic guide to improving general health . . . [and the author's] expert analysis drives much of this intriguing volume. . . . Arrestingly written and chockablock with practical, empowering medical information, this thought-provoking and convincing chronicle of disease avoidance and 'remarkable recovery' will give even skeptics something to ponder." —*Kirkus Reviews*

"Rediger makes a compelling argument. . . . [He] adds to spontaneous-healing research by presenting case studies of terminal patients, and includes engaging lessons about pathophysiology and the history of medicine. . . . As a leading voice challenging current healthcare systems and treatment models, Rediger makes a convincing case to study spontaneous remissions. By doing so, we may become closer to learning why some survive, despite their odds." —*Library Journal*

"An experienced physician who is also a skilled, driven, and compassionate writer is a winning combination. This pioneering book by psychiatrist Jeffrey Rediger analyzes unexplained spontaneous recoveries from potentially fatal medical conditions. . . . Rediger concludes that each recovery was 'unique' and only partially explicable, but that all provide evidence of 'a powerful link' between our identities and our immune systems." —*Nature*

CURED

STRENGTHEN YOUR IMMUNE SYSTEM
AND HEAL YOUR LIFE

JEFFREY REDIGER, M.D.

FLATIRON
BOOKS
NEW YORK

CURED. Copyright © 2020 by Jeffrey Rediger. All rights reserved. Printed in the United States of America. For information, address Flatiron Books, 120 Broadway, New York, NY 10271.

www.flatironbooks.com

Designed by Omar Chapa

The Library of Congress has cataloged the hardcover edition as follows:

Names: Rediger, Jeffrey, author.
Title: Cured : the life-changing science of spontaneous healing / Jeffrey Rediger, M.D.
Description: First edition. | New York : Flatiron Books, 2020. | Includes bibliographical references. |
Identifiers: LCCN 2019045269 | ISBN 9781250193193 (hardcover) |
    ISBN 9781250193209 (ebook)
Subjects: LCSH: Medicine, Psychosomatic. | Healing—Psychological aspects.
Classification: LCC RC49 .R44 2020 | DDC 616.08—dc23
LC record available at https://lccn.loc.gov/2019045269

ISBN 978-1-250-19321-6 (trade paperback)

Our books may be purchased in bulk for promotional, educational, or business use. Please contact your local bookseller or the Macmillan Corporate and Premium Sales Department at 1-800-221-7945, extension 5442, or by email at MacmillanSpecialMarkets@macmillan.com.

First Flatiron Books Paperback Edition: 2021

10 9 8 7 6 5

I dedicate this book to Rachael Ann Donalds,
a magnificent source of color in my life,
and to those whose stories don't yet have a voice.

CONTENTS

CURED

INTRODUCTION

Unpacking the Black Box of Medical Miracles

There are two ways to be fooled. One is to believe what isn't true. The other is to refuse to believe what *is* true.

—*Søren Kierkegaard*

In 2008, the road ahead looked smooth for Claire Haser. At sixty-three, she'd settled into the rhythm of her life, easily weathering its ups and downs. The map she had sketched out for her future was unfolding just the way she'd drawn it: she and her husband were a couple of years away from retirement. Their kids were grown and doing well, and they had a posse of healthy grandchildren. For most of their adult lives, they'd lived in Portland, Oregon, with its soft rain, vibrant green parks, and red brick. And for most of her career, Claire had been a health-care administrator, sitting at a desk all day in a fluorescent-lit room, buried under paperwork.

Claire and her husband adored Portland, but their dream was to retire to Hawaii. They'd been saving and planning for it for years, and now it was just around the corner. And then, the axis on which Claire's contented, ordinary life was spinning started to tilt. Worrisome but vague symptoms—increasingly frequent nausea, a stabbing pain that ricocheted through her abdomen—sent her to the doctor. Concerned, her doctor recommended a CT scan. Claire lay on the slab of the CT machine, arms over her head, trying to breathe normally, hoping that the powerful magnetic field her body was passing through would find nothing. But the scan revealed a mass on her pancreas, about two centimeters in diameter. A biopsy dashed her last hopes; the mass was malignant, meaning cancerous. Claire was diagnosed with adenocarcinoma of the pancreas, a brutal and incurable form of pancreatic cancer.

Cancer is a loaded word in our culture, a modern bogeyman, associated more than many illnesses with damage and death. However, the truth is that every cancer varies in regard to the possibilities of a cure and the likelihood of remission. Some cancers are not fatal, and in those instances, one dies not *from* the cancer but *with* the cancer, which can live quietly and unobtrusively in the body for many years, until the person passes away from other causes. Some cancers grow slowly but steadily; others wax and wane for a number of years. Many cancers are deadly when left alone but are highly responsive to treatment—whether that be surgery, chemotherapy, or radiation. Certain cancers will even go away by themselves, while others are not responsive to treatment at all, so any treatment the patient receives is palliative and provided only with the hope of slowing down symptoms. And there are many cancers that live between all these categories, in varying degrees of severity.

Here's what we know about Claire's cancer, pancreatic adenocarcinoma: it is the most lethal form of pancreatic cancer that exists. It is rapidly progressive and leads to a brutal death. Approximately forty-five thousand people are diagnosed each year in the United States, and twice as many in Europe. Most are dead by the end of the first year. It is the fourth-leading cause of cancer death in both men and women and is projected to soon be the third.

A diagnosis of pancreatic adenocarcinoma is a death sentence. The question is not *if* you will die from the disease but *when*. Why is pancreatic cancer so deadly? In the early stages of the disease, there are no symptoms. The cancer progresses silently, stealthily. By the time the first signs emerge—loss of appetite, weight loss, back pain, sometimes mild jaundice, a faint yellowing of the skin and eyes—it's already too late. At that point, the cancer has typically metastasized to other parts of the body. Treatment can prolong a life but not save it—the vast majority of pancreatic cancer patients (96 percent) die from the disease within five years. Most succumb much sooner; the typical post-diagnosis survival estimate is three to six months, with treatment. By that standard, Claire was lucky; her doctors gave her one year.

The future Claire had seen laid out before her—her garden, Hawaii, a quiet retirement with her husband—vanished overnight. Cancer swept through like a hurricane and ripped it all away.

Claire had to wait two weeks after her diagnosis to meet with a surgeon. Her family and friends were aghast when they heard she had to wait that long—she had *aggressive pancreatic cancer!* Didn't she need to get it out as soon as possible? How could she go on like this for weeks, knowing that it was inside of her, possibly getting worse, possibly spreading? But she was glad for the pause. She needed to get her feet under her. Receiving a terminal diagnosis had made everything seem like a bizarre dream; her life suddenly had an end point, train tracks running off a cliff right before her eyes. It was unreal. Adding to that was the way she was treated by her doctors: as a box to be checked, a body to be shuffled along to the next procedure. As a patient in the medical system, Claire had a sense of being trapped in a kind of machine, an assembly line that moved her relentlessly from one station to the next. It felt predetermined, impersonal, routine.

At home, she dove headlong into researching her illness. She devoured books, articles, and websites, searching for a glimmer of hope, something her doctors had left out. But everything she read reinforced what they had told her already: nobody survived this type of cancer. Claire scoured the internet for any story of remission or survival—even just one. She found nothing.

Her one chance for survival was a surgical procedure called "the Whipple." A drastic surgery, it would remove part of her pancreas along with her gallbladder, areas of the small intestine (the duodenum and the jejunum), and possibly parts of the stomach and spleen as well. There were serious side effects and complications; after all, the pancreas has important jobs to do—including blood sugar regulation and the breakdown of food—and they wanted to remove a chunk of it. Pancreatic enzymes are particularly strong, and the leakage of those enzymes—which is common after the Whipple procedure—can cause debilitating pain. After the surgery, she would likely experience pain-inducing enzyme leakage, along with fluid retention, stomach spasms, and excruciating gas. Long term, she risked developing diabetes, anemia, and digestive issues leading to weakness and fatigue, along with vitamin and mineral deficiencies.

Unable to sleep, Claire stayed up late into the night, writing down questions to bring to the meeting with her surgeon.

Is the Whipple my only choice? If I have the Whipple, will I get diabetes or stomach paralysis? Will I ever be able to eat normally again? Will I have pain? If so, for how long? How long will the recovery be? Will this fatigue I read about ever go away? How many times have you done this surgery? What were the outcomes? How often is this surgery done in this hospital? What are the outcomes?

The outcomes, her surgeon said at their meeting, were not great. He was blunt and honest, which she appreciated. She asked him to be straight with her, and he was. He told her that at two centimeters, her adenocarcinoma was resectable, which meant it could be operated on with the Whipple surgery. It was her one chance at a cure. But it was a risky procedure—long, imperfect, and with dubious results. He brought out his surgical atlas and opened it up to the section on Whipple closures: a veritable encyclopedia of various techniques for putting you back together after they've taken you apart.

"See how many different ways there are to close this surgery? You know what that means?" He looked at her steadily. "It means there aren't any good ways to do it."

He told her that the procedure could take up to eight hours. He told her if she was going to have a heart attack or a stroke, she'd have it on the table. Statistics were all over the map—some resources told her she had only a 2 percent chance of dying during the surgery, but others said 15 percent. Her surgeon told her that even if she did have the surgery, her chance of living another five years was only about 5 percent—the vast majority of people with her type of cancer would die from the disease within that time, even with the Whipple. Here, her oncologist interjected that five-year survival rates were closer to 20 percent. Her surgeon insisted on 5 percent, and they argued.

"Look," her surgeon finally said. "Some doctors would try to sell this surgery to you. But I don't have anything to prove anymore. I've done enough of these surgeries. I don't need the money. I have my boat."

He wanted to cure her, she could tell; he was a surgeon, trained to fix things, to perform the magic of precision and science. But he was also giving her, as she had requested, the unvarnished truth.

At home, she watched YouTube videos in which Whipple patients writhed in pain, describing the terrible side effects of the surgery. She searched for stats on survival rates, she cried, she prayed. She asked herself hard questions: *How much pain can I stand? How much pain am I willing to live with for the rest of my life? How many limitations am I willing to live with? Can I live without hiking in the mountains again?*

Claire finally decided to decline the surgery. She didn't want to spend the time she had left chasing an elusive, unlikely cure, sitting in doctors' offices and waiting rooms. "I decided to just let nature take its course," she says. "I decided to live with as much zest and happiness as I could for however long I had left."

In 2013, five years after her diagnosis and dismal prognosis, Claire was hospitalized for an illness unrelated to her cancer and required a CT scan of her abdomen. It was the first time since her diagnosis that she'd had any kind of imaging done. She'd expected to die and had simply focused on living, and time just went by. Though the doctors weren't looking for it specifically, her pancreas was visualized on the scan, and it was clean. Where there had once been a tumor, there was none.

Baffled, Claire's doctors convened a diagnosis review and ordered her biopsy slides, convinced that a mistake must have been made. But the diagnosis had been correct. Without treatment or surgery, Claire's pancreatic adenocarcinoma had—impossibly—vanished.

How did it happen? Nobody knew exactly, not even Claire herself. Her doctors only knew what she hadn't done: surgery, chemo, radiation. When I spoke with her, Claire had in fact made important changes after her diagnosis, but none of her doctors were interested in hearing about them. They told her that her experience "didn't have any medical value." It was just one of those things, a one-in-a-million fluke that meant nothing.

Plenty of people would call a case like Claire's a miracle. In the medical profession, we refer to these as cases of *spontaneous remission.* Whatever term you use, recoveries like these remain largely unexamined, black boxes that haven't been unpacked by medical science.

Spontaneous means *without cause,* but the truth is that we mostly haven't looked for the cause. In the history of medicine, we have almost never used the tools of a rigorous science to investigate remarkable recoveries from incurable illnesses. Common sense would suggest that these are the cases we would most want to study, that perhaps these people have stumbled upon profound pathways to healing that we would want to understand. And yet the study of spontaneous remission (SR) is almost completely unexplored terrain. We classify people like Claire as "flukes" and "outliers" and simply accept the narrative that they are unexplainable. But I don't see remarkable recoveries in health as flukes or outliers any more than I see extraordinary performers in other arenas as flukes and outliers. Serena Williams and Michael Jordan are outliers, sure, but they are also luminous examples of human capacities, and by studying their techniques and their methods, we can understand how to improve our own.

In 1968, at the Olympic games in Mexico City, American long jumper Bob Beamon sprinted down the track toward the sandpit and launched himself into the air. In tape from the event, he seems to fly, birdlike, chest-first, before reaching forward with his feet to grab the sand. He broke the existing record by over two feet, shocking the crowd and effectively ending the competition. Observers said the jump was "beyond belief." It was also beyond the limit of the measuring equipment. It became known as "the Leap of the Century."

Athletes and scientists immediately tried to figure out how he did it and how to beat it, even though breaking that new record took almost twenty-three years. Yet when something similar happens in health care—when someone who has been essentially condemned to death by the medical system suddenly gets better—it's as if we're embarrassed. These remarkable cases are seen as threats to the system rather than inspirations, and they are dismissed without examination. *Mystery. Miracle. Fluke. Outlier.* We're heavy on labels, light on explanations.

Throughout human history, we've held a host of ideas about where illness and disease come from. Until fairly recently—within the last couple of hundred years, roughly—most cultures thought of illness as something that came from the spirit world: it was the will of God, perhaps a punishment, or the curse of an evil spirit. If you lived in ancient Egypt, for example, you might carry an amulet to protect yourself from disease and dress your cuts and scrapes with honey (a natural antibiotic). If you were very ill, your doctor might decide to induce vomiting—the theory being that as your body was full of passageways, your illness could indicate a blockage that should be cleared. If you happened to be born in ancient Greece, you would have believed that the human body was made up of elements that must always be in balance; sickness was an indication that they were out of balance and must be corrected. In that instance, you might visit one of the ancient Greek asclepeions, a healing temple where you would undergo Katharsis (purification), dream therapy, and medical care—a blend of physical and spiritual treatments under the watchful eye of Asclepius, the god of healing.

Though the practice of medicine in many ancient cultures relied heavily on magic, religion, and superstition, there were also some important advances: deep knowledge of anatomy, theories of disease and health developed through observation and trial and error, and repeatable methods of treating injuries and illnesses, often with medicinal plants, which were the precursors of modern pharmaceuticals. However, the origin of disease itself continued to elude us. Where did it come from? Why did it choose this person and not another? While we relied on remedies such as bloodletting and astrology, we increasingly observed that many illnesses sprang from dirty water and sewage, and that keeping our bodies, cities, and water sources clean was important, even though we didn't quite understand why.

In 36 B.C., a Roman scholar Marcus Terrentius Varro published his book *On Agriculture,* a practical guide for farmers. In a section on keeping livestock, he warned against raising animals near swamps, due to his theory that "certain minute animals, invisible to the eye, breed there and, borne by the air, reach inside the body by way of the mouth and nose and cause diseases that are difficult to get rid of." An interesting theory, but one that was impossible to prove at the time.

On Contagion and Contagious Disease, by Italian physician Girolamo Fracastoro, appeared in 1546. It detailed his own theory that tiny, rapidly multiplying, disease-causing creatures— microorganisms—spread from person to person through touch, or were carried on the wind. His theory was well received at the time, but again, without any real evidence to back up the concept, it eventually fell by the wayside and was mostly forgotten. It was Louis Pasteur, the French chemist who came up with the pathogen-elimination process that still bears his name, *pasteurization,* who definitively proved germ theory in the 1860s. While it was a huge leap forward for medicine, it also locked us into a certain philosophy toward health and disease, one that was based on this ethos: *kill the pathogen.* Is it possible that today, we've become so focused on that mission that we miss out on important avenues to health?

Doctors are taught to ignore the story, the personal life of the person in order to penetrate through to the underlying signs and symptoms of disease that are present in those with that particular illness. We have been limited by a focus on pathology, on what is missing or diseased, instead of seeing and galvanizing all that is right, special, and great within each individual human life—within your life. As a result, we routinely commit deadly errors even as we seek to heal. We treat the disease instead of the person, missing the larger story of the patient's life, which is rife with clues and revelations about how best to guide them toward health. We focus on symptoms instead of root causes, prescribing medications that often simply mask the symptoms instead of attempting the longer, harder work of building immunity and vitality. We insist on sorting illnesses into those rooted in either the mind or the body, instead of understanding and embracing the connection between them, where most of our illnesses reside.

And finally, we push aside stories of remarkable recovery, which don't fit into our paradigm of one cause, one cure. I'm willing to bet, based on experience, that most of us in the medical profession have seen instances of remarkable recovery. We don't know how to think about them, and so, since they don't fit into our frame of reference, we pigeonhole and forget them, perhaps considering them occasionally only late at night while musing with a cup of coffee at the nursing station, or quietly in the space of our own private thoughts. We don't know how to explain them, we shy away from publishing them for fear of professional ridicule, and we don't repeat them to the patients we see who are suffering from those very same diseases. We don't want to give "false hope."

I first encountered remarkable recoveries seventeen years ago, when I was fresh out of residency and just beginning my career as a psychiatrist. At the time, I'd just accepted a dual appointment to McLean Hospital and Harvard Medical School and had opened a small private practice. The pressure was on. I felt driven to prove myself as both a doctor and a professor.

I met Nikki, an oncology nurse who worked down the road at Mass General, when she came in for a joint session with her adult son. She'd been diagnosed with pancreatic cancer, and she wanted support in breaking the news to him.

Shortly thereafter, she told me she was taking an indefinite leave of absence from Mass General; her health had declined to the point where she could no longer work. She was exhausted, having difficulty eating, losing weight. She planned to travel to Brazil, to a tiny town in the countryside called Abadiânia, to visit a Brazilian healer. She'd tried everything that Western medicine had to offer to fight her disease, and she'd decided she had nothing to lose.

About two weeks after she left, the phone in my office rang. It was Nikki, calling from Brazil.

"You have to come down here," she told me. "I'm getting better. I'm seeing things you wouldn't believe."

She related story after story of people she'd met and healings she'd witnessed, classic tales of the lame beginning to walk and the blind regaining their sight. A woman with breast cancer who felt a "black cloud" go out of her chest when she was touched by the healer, and then saw her tumor shrink. Nikki called and wrote to me from Brazil for months, but I didn't go. The hospital was busy, I had classes to teach, and besides, I was deeply skeptical. I chalked it all up to explainable phenomena. Temporary improvements, misdiagnoses, people who would have gotten better anyway.

When Nikki returned, she did seem revitalized. In fact, her

health had dramatically improved. She was enjoying life, eating steak (one of her favorite foods) and salads. Her time in Brazil had buoyed her. She told me that she felt newly able to both give and receive love. Control issues that had plagued her melted away. She felt energetic and joyful. Her quality of life had skyrocketed compared to her condition before she'd left. But sadly, her story doesn't end like Claire's. To be honest, most stories don't. Nikki did eventually relapse, and she succumbed to her cancer less than a year later. But before she did, she urged me again to investigate what was happening in Brazil.

I'd read in scientific journals that true instances of spontaneous remission are rare, occurring at a rate of about 1 in 100,000 cases. That statistic was repeated over and over in journal articles, always with the patina of absolute truth. So I decided to trace it back, to see where it came from. As it turned out, it had been made up out of the blue and then taken as true, repeated over and over in subsequent articles.

When I dug into the research some more, looking for both current and historical examples of spontaneous healing, I was shocked at what I found. Over the past century, reports of spontaneous remission have slowly increased in both number and frequency, typically with a spike after significant conferences, books, or major media stories. In the early 1990s, the Institute of Noetic Sciences began gathering together all the instances of spontaneous remission that had been described anywhere in medical literature. In the database they published in 1993, *Spontaneous Remission: An Annotated Bibliography*,[1] they documented 3,500 references to spontaneous healing across eight hundred journals. And the cases that actually *were* reported were only the tip of the iceberg. At the first talk I gave where I brought up spontaneous remission and what we, as doctors, might learn from it, I asked the audience of physicians how many of them had witnessed a story of recovery that made no sense from a medical perspective. Hands shot up all around the room. When I asked how many people had written those cases up and published their observations, all hands dropped.

It wasn't that spontaneous remission was rare—it was that a culture of fear and judgment was holding us back from seeing the scope of it. How many cases were out there that never made it into the medical literature for fear of professional ridicule? As a new medical director at McLean, one of the oldest and most venerable psychiatric institutions, I felt it keenly. I was hesitant to publish my observations or seek support in the medical world. And yet each day, I saw how cases of spontaneous remission dovetailed with the problems cropping up with my patients, whether in the medical, psychiatric, or ER setting. Every day, I was seeing patients with the most common yet deadly diseases out there: cancer, diabetes, heart disease, autoimmune illness, and lung disease—the top assassins of the Western world. Many of them are increasingly known to have significant lifestyle components. I was starting to believe that if my patients could try *half* of the strategies that I was seeing people embrace in cases of remarkable recovery, there would be a stark improvement in general health, not only for suffering individuals but also for society. But the pressure to remain within the dogmatic confines of my profession was strong, and I had a difficult time shaking it.

Growing up, I lived on a small family farm in rural Indiana, among the wide, flat corn and soybean fields, under the vast dome of the midwestern sky. I am from an Amish background. My parents left the Amish community when I was two, but we continued to live by its principles. We raised animals and grew much of our own food, including meat and wheat flour. My mother made our clothes by hand. TV, radio, and most modern conveniences and activities were regarded as evil, to be feared and avoided. For me, it was an isolating, difficult world, and I broke out of it as soon as I could, leaving for college at Wheaton in Chicago, followed by seminary at Princeton, medical school at Indiana University School of Medicine, and then residency at Harvard. I still remember how the world seemed to open—a door that had always been closed swung wide to reveal hallways of possibility. I entered seminary full of questions, seeking answers, trying to reconcile the fundamentalist beliefs of my childhood with new knowledge and experiences. I didn't get any answers at Princeton—I got more questions. But I also learned from my mentor there that questions are just as important as answers.

"The goal," he told me, "is not necessarily to arrive at an absolute answer. The goal is to improve the quality of your questions. The quality of your question determines the quality of your answer."

The questions we ask are the guiding light that moves us forward. If we're asking good questions, we very well might be moving in a good direction.

When I got to medical school, the philosophy was so different it felt like whiplash. I still remember where I was standing when I realized that the culture of the medical world was not at all what I had hoped or expected. I was at the front of a recently emptied amphitheater classroom, asking the professor a follow-up question to that day's lecture.

"Just memorize the material," the professor told me. "Don't ask questions."

It was a phrase that would be repeated to me over and over throughout medical school: *Don't ask questions. Don't ask questions. Don't ask questions.* Certainly, medical students need to learn the material; it takes an enormous amount of time and effort to establish the base of knowledge necessary to be a physician. But for me, this phrase was an uncomfortable echo of the philosophy I'd been raised on: that dogma should never be questioned.

Memorizing and not having the freedom to ask questions socializes doctors into keeping their heads down and not rocking the boat. We end up complicit in a system that, while it yields some incredible advances in research and technology, is failing patients on a day-to-day basis, missing important opportunities to heal. After two decades of working within the medical system, I've seen my fair share of lost opportunities—moments where we had the chance to change the trajectory of someone's life and missed it—and it's time to rock the boat. I've finally reached the point where I have the courage to ask the questions that need to be asked and to follow them where they lead, as far as the current science can take us—and then to push a little farther.

There are no clinical trials on spontaneous remissions; no double-blind studies, which are the gold standard by which the medical world operates. It would be impossible to do so, as there currently is no way to control for the conditions under which spontaneous remission might occur, and it would be unethical to test out theories on terminally ill patients. With spontaneous remission, we have to be anthropologists, detectives, and medical investigators, digging through personal accounts, medical records, and the science currently available to put together the pieces of the puzzle. This book is my attempt to do so.

Since 2003, I've been interviewing survivors of incurable illnesses and examining their medical records, and what I've observed is a pattern of principles and behavior. I am no longer surprised about the unexpected disappearance of illness. I've traveled to Brazil, to healing centers where thousands flock with the belief that they can be healed—and more often than makes sense with our existing medical paradigm, they are. I've shadowed a so-called faith healer in the heartland of America, and I've watched my own patients experience unexpected reversals of illness while in my care. I've grappled with my own doubts, and even as I move forward, I still do.

This book is not an argument for patients to stop taking their medicine or turn down medical intervention. The pharmacopoeia and medical technology that we have developed are innovative, necessary, and often lifesaving, and, as the stories featured in this book will show, there are many instances of spontaneous remission that occur in concert with the extraordinary efforts of dedicated physicians working at the tops of their fields. Remarkable recoveries simply tell us that these interventions are not always enough and that they do not hold all the answers to healing.

What I've learned over the course of my investigations, and have put into practice with my own patients, is that we must go deeper, beyond the long-term medication of symptoms, to the roots of illness. It's important and compassionate to treat symptoms in the short term, but in the long term, you have to treat the cause of disease, which is often more hidden. Spontaneous healing offers us a rare window into those root causes. We have a responsibility to study these cases and learn everything we can from them. We can then fold that knowledge into the way we treat chronic and incurable illnesses, using both the tools of modern medicine and the wisdom of these remarkable recoveries.

This book traces my investigative journey into the phenomenon of spontaneous remission over the course of seventeen years. In part 1, we'll begin where I began: by looking at the very building blocks of health. In cases of spontaneous remission, something changes the expected disease course—and changes it radically. The logical place to start was with the immune system, the body's first and most important line of defense against infection and disease, and the factors that impact it: diet, lifestyle, and stress. Over and over, I'd seen survivors of incurable diseases make seismic changes in these areas (which are often passed over in routine medical care), and I knew I needed to begin with a deeper dive into the specifics of what happened and why. This led me not only to some surprising discoveries about exactly how powerful such changes can be when it comes to healing but further into the intricacies of the mind-body connection and the mysteries of the human heart.

I wasn't surprised to discover that the link between our minds and bodies holds a well of potential when it came to radical healing—even mainstream medicine accepts that our stress levels and thought patterns, for example, can impact our physical health. But what did surprise me was the depth of it, which was more profound than my medical training had ever prepared me for. In part 2, I'll take you along with me as I investigate just how interconnected radical healing is with our thoughts, beliefs, and even our most fundamental, often unexamined sense of self. I found myself asking the question: Can my *identity*, in some way, determine my ability to heal? The answer is both revelatory and complex.

Throughout the book, I'll profile, in depth, survivors of incurable diseases who decided to open both their medical files and their lives to me as I searched for answers. I've tried to capture the richness and uniqueness of each of their stories, because I believe that the secrets of spontaneous healing are illuminated not only in the similarities between them but in the differences as well. As the renowned psychologist Carl Rogers once said, "What is most personal is most universal."

What these cases teach us is that we must create a biological environment in the body and mind that sets the stage for healing. The body wants to heal, after all. And there's a lot more to creating the conditions for that than we are taught. My goal is to share the process with you, to take you with me through the journey of investigating these cases one by one, exploring the groundbreaking new science of the mind and body, and following the pathway to healing that is illuminated by these stories. What it eventually led me to was the foundation of a new model of medicine, one that's based around what I now call "the four pillars" of health: healing your immune system, healing your nutrition, healing your stress response, and healing your identity.

This is still very much a developing field of research, and I certainly don't have all the answers. But I do have some preliminary answers and many important questions, and together, they've taken me a long way down the road to understanding what might be happening with these medical "miracles." So often, we use *miracle* as a catchall word to describe something we can't explain. But even miracles have explanations—we just haven't figured them out yet. I think sometimes we shy away from trying to explain them, believing somehow that finding the real-world mechanism behind a "miracle" will diminish it, make it lesser somehow. But to me, understanding the inner workings of these kinds of surprising events doesn't make them any less amazing. To crack the lid, look inside, and see the mechanism of a previously unexplained phenomenon, intricate as the gears of a clock, seems to me even more miraculous.

Long ago, I made a promise to myself that I wouldn't write unless

I had something that absolutely had to be said. The nineteenth-century philosopher Kierkegaard wrote piercingly about what it meant to live as an individual in the noise and din of modern life. In contrast to other writers, he sought not to be one more voice among others in the public square, or the loudest voice—but instead to take something away so that the reader could find the truth they need and once again begin to live.

It is my hope that this book does the same. I'm adding my voice now because I believe it is urgently necessary to talk about these cases. The stories revealed in this book pull back the curtain and show that there are things we know about what creates a healthy, vital, even miraculous life, but also how we have forgotten what we know. The only way to recover this knowledge is to eliminate the noise and opinions from both within and without and get back to something more basic, raw, and true—that buried but inextinguishable light of knowledge that burns within each of us.

While the science is new and we will learn much more in the decades ahead, the research we have now and the potential it holds for millions is too important not to share more widely. It is my hope that this book will illuminate a clear path to recovery for those who are struggling with chronic or even incurable illnesses, those who love someone who is, or those who simply want to live with as much health and vitality as they can.

Modern medicine typically tells you what the situation is and what you will be living with, but it does not help you understand what's possible or what *could be*. Whether the diagnosis is diabetes, heart disease, depression, cancer, an autoimmune illness, or something else, you may not be receiving the hope or tools of recovery that you need to truly heal. We need to place the extraordinary on the operating table so that we can dissect and learn from it, so that the possibilities for the extraordinary that exist within all of us are illuminated for everyone.

•   •   •

Claire lives in Hawaii now, just as she'd planned before she got sick.

"After my diagnosis, I didn't think I'd make it," she says. "But we're right on time."

She and her husband live on O'ahu with their daughter and son-in-law, who are musicians. She spends evenings on her lanai—the type of open, covered porch that is found throughout Hawaii—enjoying the view. She can see the lights of Honolulu and the sky changing with the weather. A hurricane went through recently, threatening to do a lot of damage, but it wasn't nearly as bad as everyone had expected. I thought of how cancer had once threatened to destroy her world like a devastating hurricane.

"We're a little windblown, but fine," she tells me now about the recent storm. "We were lucky. It passed us by."

How do we get the hurricane to pass us by? The answer to that isn't simple, and this is not a book for those seeking easy answers. This is a book about a long journey to discovering the secrets of spontaneous remission—and, perhaps locked inside those, the secrets of lasting health and vitality. There were no easy answers for me as I did this work. Each stone I turned over, looking for an answer, seemed to reveal yet another question. I had to remind myself that the goal wasn't to come to a conclusion as soon as I stumbled upon an apparent "answer." The goal was to improve the quality of my questions. And the first question was: *What was really happening in Brazil?*

PART ONE

INCREDIBLE IMMUNITY

1

Into the Impossible

I believe there is no source of deception in the investigation of nature which can compare with a fixed belief that certain kinds of phenomena are impossible.

—*William James*

The very first surgery I ever performed by myself was a leg amputation.

It was 2:00 in the morning, and I'd already been on the floor for hours. They paged me to the operating room (OR) and briefed me on the patient, an elderly diabetic man who had come in with extreme pain in his left leg. When the nurses examined him, they found multiple gangrenous wounds on his lower leg and foot. Advanced, poorly managed diabetes like his can cause serious circulation issues, slowing blood flow to the limbs and extremities. By the time this man arrived in the ER in the middle of the night, he had extensive tissue damage and a dangerous infection. The leg wasn't salvageable.

I scrubbed in for the required five minutes, between every finger and up to my elbows. I held my arms up to let them air-dry and backed my way through the door into the vestibule that opened onto the OR. The surgical tech draped me in the gown, looped my face mask on, reached up to put the cap on—but couldn't. I'm pretty tall. She went up on tiptoe just as I tried to squat down a bit—we both laughed, and I realized how nervous I was. As an intern just out of medical school, this was my first time in charge in the OR.

My anxiety lifted the moment I made the first cut. As the scalpel slid cleanly around the leg, making a deep, thin line, a sort of meditative calm swept through me, a feeling of utter and complete focus. I'm not sure how many minutes went by as I made cut after cut, cauterizing as I went to stop the bleeding and to keep the surgical site clean and clear. I'll never forget the smell of singed flesh or the sound of the bone saw as I went through the tibia. It reminded me a bit of the chain saws I'd used as a kid on the farm, but that sound had a rough, gritty quality to it, while this one was finer, more delicate, and also more gruesome. There was something surreal to me about this moment—I couldn't really believe that it was me in the surgical gown and face mask. It was so improbable that I would have ended up here.

I was painfully quiet as a teenager. Perhaps my shyness was partly because I grew up in a fundamentalist family, never feeling like I fit in anywhere. In high school, I was voted Most Shy. I always felt out of place in my homemade clothes, getting off the school bus and returning to my family's house, which felt like walking back through time. TV and radio were not allowed, and the world seemed small to me then. The adults I knew worked the farms and occasionally had blue-collar jobs. My mother worked part-time as a nurse at a Lutheran hospital in Fort Wayne, and when I turned seventeen, she suggested I apply for a job there as an orderly. I was tall and strong—used to carrying heavy bales of hay and buckets of water or grain—and so I could easily lift a grown man onto a gurney or transfer a patient into a wheelchair.

In that job, I saw the full spectrum of the human experience. I wheeled mothers out to the curb with their newborns in their arms. I lowered people onto bedpans and carried the waste out. I collected laundry; I cleaned up the blood on the floor after a difficult procedure. I watched a kid with cancer lose his hair; months later, he walked out with his fuzz growing back in, carrying a bouquet of balloons in his little fist. I helped roll patients over for the nurses, holding them in my arms as they were bathed and bandaged. I wheeled people to the morgue, a sheet pulled over their faces.

I got to know the nurses better than the doctors. They were the ones who were always around, ever present at bedsides. They coached me, taught me how to draw blood, how to attach the leads and do EKGs.

"You have a good bedside manner," the nurses told me. "You should become a doctor."

It was a startling idea, and it landed in the fertile soil of my brain like a seed. It germinated and grew. It had never occurred to me that such a future might be possible.

And now I was here, performing surgery in an OR, just like the one I'd once wheeled patients out of after the surgeons were done, tossing their masks and caps onto the floor.

With an amputation, you have to keep enough muscle below the bone edge to shape a stump that will fit nicely, and ideally painlessly, into a prosthetic leg someday. As I put in the stitches with a long, curved needle, I worked to mold a limb that would do just that, even though I doubted that this man would be getting up out of his wheelchair on a prosthesis. The surgery had gone fine, but I worried for this man. He was elderly and ill; the insulin he'd been on for most of his life was failing him, and his body was starting to shut down, limb by limb. I wondered if there was more we could have done for him, long ago, to get him on a different path.

I got into medicine because I thought I could help people. I imagined helping patients have healthier lives—better lives. But so much of what we did as physicians was too little, too late. I watched my fellow doctors working long hours, around the clock, rushing from patient to patient. It wasn't because of a lack of hard work or dedication that we so often struggled to help people get better. But we were always operating with such a narrow slice of the story, missing the bigger picture, and we were treating the symptoms of disease, rather than the root causes. Every day I was seeing people suffering from real illnesses, who needed real solutions.

Years later, I still thought about this man—my first surgical patient—who'd developed diabetes long before he'd been in my OR, the disease that had sent his health into a tailspin from which he was never able to recover. And I thought about how these unexplored cases of spontaneous remission could hold the clues we needed in order to help people like him before it was too late. So, in 2003, I bought a ticket to Brazil.

DISSECTING A "MIRACLE"

When I stepped off the plane in Brasília, the capital of Brazil, the air was smooth and warm as bathwater. It was March, late summer in the Southern Hemisphere. The sun seemed to sink right into my bones, and the chill of the Boston winter I'd left behind began to fade. *Maybe this trip wasn't such a bad idea after all,* I thought. But I still had my doubts.

When I'd made the decision to check out reports of "miraculous" recoveries at a few healing centers in Brazil, I'd had no idea what I was getting myself into. I figured I'd go down for a week, investigate, and resolve the questions that had been unsettling me about whether or not there was any legitimacy to these claims. I'm embarrassed to admit it now, but I'd pretty much made up my mind that there wasn't. I was sure that as soon as I scratched the surface, the shiny veneer of "miracle healings" would peel off, exposing the fraud underneath. A quick trip, a clear conscience, and then I'd move on with my life and career, not worrying about spontaneous healings and whether or not they represented anything real.

For the previous year, I'd been hearing reports from Brazil and elsewhere of sudden recoveries from incurable diseases. It had started with Nikki and then rapidly expanded. I began getting phone calls from all over the country from people desperate to share their stories of recovery. It turned out that, when I declined to investigate,

Nikki had asked friends she'd made in Brazil to get in touch, and word had spread quickly that I was researching the phenomenon of spontaneous healing. Some of the recoveries I heard seemed unbelievable. But people were incredibly open. They typed out their stories and emailed them to me. They attached x-rays, MRI scans, and medical records with their doctors' scribblings in the corners.

Some cases just didn't have enough evidence to substantiate the claim of spontaneous healing, or the original diagnosis seemed shaky to me. Some looked promising, but the time frame was too short—they might just be temporary remissions, a brief respite in the course of an ultimately terminal trajectory. Others were instances of people so desperate to be healed that they believed they had been, even as their disease progressed. My heart ached for these people; I understood their wanting to be better, yearning for it so much they convinced themselves it had happened. But that didn't mean it had. When people called with and emailed their stories, I listened, but that was all. The weight of my administrative, clinical, and teaching responsibilities had settled on me like a yoke. Now was not the time to go on a wild-goose chase, searching for a difficult-to-define phenomenon that would almost certainly vanish like a mirage, a modern-day Fountain of Youth.

"You have the training, you have the perspective," Nikki kept insisting, referring to my combination of medical training and a degree in theology. She felt I was uniquely positioned to investigate the phenomenon of spontaneous healing with an open mind. And the stories being reported were compelling—tumors melting like ice cubes, the paralyzed standing to walk, the terminally ill alive and thriving years after they were supposed to be gone. But they were just stories—there was no proof, at least not yet—and I worried that I'd take this leap, risking my career and reputation, and find no actual evidence to back up any of these claims.

But could I continue to turn my back on what might be an entire untapped field of groundbreaking research and inquiry? Some of the cases coming in were hard to turn away from. These people had real evidence of diagnosis and remission. Looking at their medical files, I struggled to explain them. What if something real *was* happening—something that modern medicine refused to see?

Once I realized how incorrect the data was on the frequency of spontaneous healing, I kicked my research into a higher gear. Night after night, once I finished my evening rounds, I found myself at the computer, clicking through journal articles, typing the words *spontaneous remission* into medical databases and following the trail of bread crumbs where it led. I was shocked at the volume of what I found.

Instances of spontaneous remission from incurable diseases were everywhere—it was just hard to see them. Considered "outliers," they were typically not mentioned in discussions of disease progression and treatment options. When data was collected and aggregated, cases of remarkable recoveries, looking like flukes or errors on a graph of data points, vanished into the mass of averages. Medical science is built on averages, on what *normally* happens and on what the *average* person does. But when I searched specifically for cases of spontaneous remission, they seemed to be under every rock I flipped over. This whole time, they'd been hidden in plain sight.

A long time ago, when I decided to give up my cloistered rural life and pursue higher education, I'd vowed that I would follow truth wherever it led me. Science is about going where you don't want to go sometimes, even if it's not politically comfortable. Now the time had come to start asking the questions that weren't being asked in medicine, about why these cases of spontaneous remission were happening. Even if my investigation led to debunking these claims, I had a responsibility to follow the questions. I kept thinking of my mentor at Princeton and his mantra: *The quality of your question determines the quality of your answer.* How were we ever going to arrive at any kind of answers if we never asked the questions to begin with?

The taxi ride from the airport to the first of several "spiritual" healing centers would take an hour and a half. As we slid out of the outskirts of Brasília, the landscape opened up, turning into rolling green hills. I tried to distract myself and enjoy the view, but my mind was spinning with questions and doubts. Would this all turn out to be a mistake? I had to remember to keep an open mind. I was ready to start asking questions, but I needed them to lead somewhere.

The healing centers were tucked away in little towns in rural Brazil. They showed me what a deep spirituality the people of Brazil possess. It is a markedly different culture from my own. They operate with a belief system that accepts a healer could communicate with and channel spirits, or energy, from another plane—an invisible world that is realer and more important than the visible world we can see and touch. The physical world, in their view, is a faint shadow of this deeper, truer world. In this belief system, ineffable qualities like love and the human soul are thought to be extremely powerful forces, especially in regard to illness and healing—illness begins in the soul, and when a healing occurs there, the physical body then "catches up" to this new reality.

People flocked to these centers from all over the country, sometimes selling possessions to afford the trip. The center that was the focus of my trip, however, was the Casa de dom Inácio Loyola, in Abadiânia. This place was a little different from the others because it attracted people from all over the world. More reports of remission were coming from this population, and at least a few of the ones I'd vetted before coming down looked interesting enough to pursue. And this was the place that Nikki had urged me to investigate.

Arriving, I took in the setting of the Casa, a largely open-air villa surrounded by rolling green countryside. There were spaces for meditation and prayer. Outdoor gardens full of winding pathways, with benches shadowed by rosewood trees. Certainly, coming to a place like this, which felt so far from one's normal life and all its stresses and concerns, could help the mind and body *reset,* in a sense—and perhaps find reserves for battling certain illnesses and conditions, both mental and physical. Even I was beginning to feel my worries lifting, the stress and anxiety I'd carried with me from Boston evaporating under the warm sun and gentle breeze of Abadiânia. But of course, going on vacation doesn't cure the incurable. If the reports I was hearing were true, there had to be more going on.

When I met João Teixeira de Faria, also known as John of God, the healer to whom so many visitors attributed their recoveries, he was sitting in a large chair at one end of a vast sea of meditators. He had dark thinning hair, wore glasses, and was dressed in all white. People waited in a long line to see him, passing briefly before him to receive their diagnosis and prescription in a matter of seconds, before returning to meditation. I shook his hand, aware that some people thought of him as a miracle maker, and others, a con man (later, even worse accusations would surface).

I had reason to be skeptical of Faria. I knew that he claimed to perform "spiritual surgeries," and that although the healing sessions were completely free, as was the daily lunch, his healing center made money off the sale of a proprietary blend of herbs, among other things. And any time people ascribe "miracle" healings to a specific person or a place, a red flag goes up in my mind. Hundreds of years ago, people claimed healings from the holy water at Lourdes, France, but when a panel convened to begin investigating claims, it wasn't able to tie recoveries to the water itself in any statistically significant way. Had I been able to investigate the healings at Lourdes all those years ago, I'd have turned my attention to the people experiencing the recoveries, not the spring of water. Similarly, here in Abadiânia, I was most interested in the community of people—this was a unique population, with a high concentration of reports of remissions.

Privately, I drew my line in the sand: I would deal only with cases that had indisputable medical evidence that something inexplicable had happened.[1]

One of the first people I interviewed was Juan, a vigorous older man in his eighties who went to the Casa each year with his family.

He was a soybean farmer from another part of rural Brazil, and his sun-darkened hands, worn and polished like wood, showed his years of outdoor work. Decades earlier, he'd been diagnosed by biopsy with glioblastoma multiforme, a deadly and fast-moving type of brain cancer. Glioblastoma multiforme is not the type of cancer that people survive—within five years of diagnosis, only 2 to 5 percent of patients are still alive. And that small percentage drops to zero pretty quickly after that. There is no cure for glioblastoma multiforme; treatment is palliative, with the intent to make patients comfortable and, if possible, extend their lives a bit. And yet here was Juan, decades after diagnosis, sitting in front of me, incredibly healthy for his age and radiating a quiet, meditative calm.

I asked him to what he attributed his impossible recovery. He shrugged, opened his palms. Who could know? He told me he started coming to the Casa after his diagnosis. Since then, he'd come every year to sit in the energy room and meditate. He thought of it as an annual tune-up, like an oil change.

"Did you change anything about your life after you were diagnosed?" I asked him.

He thought, then shook his head. He didn't know, he said. He didn't think so.

His wife, who'd been sitting next to him during the interview, listening in, suddenly began to cry. We all turned to her in surprise.

"*Everything* changed," she said. She began to describe how, pre-diagnosis, Juan barely spent any time with her or their children. He was either out working, off drinking, or who knew where. There was a lot of tension, a lot of strife. To her, he felt like a boat drifting farther and farther out to sea, on its own course. When he was diagnosed, and death was suddenly staring him in the face, his life and priorities were completely reordered. He seemed, almost overnight, like a different person.

"He came home to us," she said. "He's so much more connected to us now."

Over and over, from interview to interview, I heard the same thing: *everything changed.* The people who went to Abadiânia didn't just show up expecting a miracle. They had changed fundamental things about their lives, how they operated in the world, even who they were. They left jobs and marriages. They resurrected lost dreams and threw themselves into pursuing them. They completely shifted their priorities and how they spent their time. They went to the Casa hoping to find some guidance and to dig down into a deeper level of faith, where they believed that healing *was* possible. And sometimes, it was. I examined MRIs of deadly, inoperable tumors, and then follow-up MRIs as the tumors shrank and vanished. I tried to make sense of what I was witnessing. It was, of course, more complex than it looked.

Before the trip, I'd scoured all the material on the Casa that I could get my hands on. Several sources, approved by the Casa, claimed a healing rate of 90 to 95 percent. *Ninety-five percent!* If true, the statistic was staggering. Sources referenced studies done in Brazil that supposedly backed up this statistic. I searched but was unable to locate these studies, hindered in part by the language barrier, which made it even more difficult to track things down. Later, I was able to uncover one or two studies that had been done, but at the time, they were obscure, still untranslated from the original Portuguese.

From the information I gathered over my week of intensive investigation—interviewing patients, sifting through records, and plumbing medical databases for studies that might back up what was going on—it became clear to me that the healing rate wasn't anywhere near 95 percent as the place claimed. It was true that many people did feel better after visiting, and at first glance, these cases could seem like true remissions. But when I peeled back the "miracle" label, the real stories began to emerge.

As I had initially expected, some people did experience a dramatic regression of symptoms but then later relapsed. Some people recovered while pursuing other, mainstream treatments, and while they insisted that the Casa was the real catalyst for their recovery, it was impossible to tell if their time there had been the real cause.

Others got moderately better, and their quality of life did truly improve. It was great to hear how much better their lives had become since illness had loosened its grip, but I couldn't categorize these instances as definite spontaneous healings. And in the final, most heartbreaking category were the people who believed fervently that they *had* healed, while all the medical evidence pointed to the contrary. Belief had carried them a certain distance like an airplane coasting without an engine. But the problem persisted—the illness remained in the body, despite the patient's wish for it to vanish—and soon enough, the airplane would begin to crash.

It was difficult to break the news to people when I couldn't use their cases. These were human stories, full of complexity and contradiction, and they were coming from real people sitting across from me, who so deeply wanted to believe that they were better. Listening to someone describe how it felt to be in his or her body—to experience a debilitating disease wash from the body like a receding tide—was so different from reading a printout of columns showing a patient's tumor load, or holding an MRI up to the light, an impersonal black-and-white scan of a torso that could have belonged to anyone.

It was tricky at first to determine what was real and what was a mirage. I followed some promising leads that took me nowhere; in other instances, I had to circle back to cases months later that I had initially passed over, thinking them too far-fetched, once I was confronted with medical documentation that backed them up. As I scribbled notes in interview after interview and checked the stories people told against the stories their medical files revealed, certain cases began to emerge. These were irrefutable, documented diagnoses, which were then followed up—weeks, months, or sometimes years later—by documented evidence of complete remission, usually recorded by baffled and surprised physicians and technicians. Out of the murk, real cases of spontaneous healing began to reveal themselves, bright as diamonds.

Matthew, diagnosed by biopsy with an aggressive type of brain tumor, went to Brazil, stayed for weeks, then months, and fell in love. His tumor vanished, leaving only a small scar in his brain where the cancer had been—an impossible result. Jan, who'd arrived with end-stage lupus, on the brink of multiple organ failure, accompanied by a doctor who was sure she wouldn't survive the trip, now sat in front of me, healthy and radiant, with a smile that reached her eyes. Lynn, saying that she had been healed of breast cancer. Sam, describing how the tumor on his spine had vanished.

They continued to surface, improbable and even impossible recoveries. It wasn't anything close to a rate of 95 percent, but it was significantly more than could be explained by modern medicine. It was more than enough to convince me that something real was happening; people *were* making unprecedented recoveries in Brazil. And neither my medical training nor my theological studies would allow me to chalk this up to an inexplicable "miracle." A miracle, after all, is just an amazing quirk of nature that we haven't quite figured out yet. We are constantly in the process of overtaking the inexplicable, of rendering the miraculous rational and routine. As doctors, we use medicines all the time, even though we don't know how or why some of them work. Many of the technologies that we take for granted today—cell phones, radio, TV, and so on—would have been considered miracles in the past. Imagine what it would feel like as an individual living in the 1600s to look up at the sky and see a massive jumbo jet roar overhead—a million-pound hunk of metal flying through the air. *Impossible.* Yet now we know Bernoulli's principle and can create jets that fly safely and regularly. It's probably fair to say that, given the progress of history, today's miracles are tomorrow's "normal."

The week in Brazil flew by, over as soon as it had started. I threw my bag of files and notes over my shoulder and looked around one last time as I walked toward the taxi. A chicken idled across the road, looking for corn. A donkey labored to pull a cart with its wizened driver. I was leaving a world I didn't understand and returning to a world that I now realized I understood less well than I had thought just one week earlier. I had come away with more questions and fewer answers. This was a different culture, with different assumptions about the nature of health and healing and the relationship between mind and body. I was on the edge of a mystery. I felt both drawn to the mystery and afraid of what I might find.

On the plane home, I flipped through my notes, trying to sort out everything I had seen and heard. Something real was happening, I was sure of that. But I was missing too many important pieces of the puzzle to make sense of it just yet.

Nothing I unearthed in Brazil had convinced me that this was fundamentally a case about a miracle healer. In fact, just the opposite. Vague reports circulated that John of God invited women to have private sessions that resulted in sexual encounters and sometimes even assaults. While I wasn't able to substantiate the rumors at the time, they were concerning enough that I decided not to refer interested people who could potentially be vulnerable. When television and media outlets contacted me about speaking about the Casa, I turned them down, not wanting to encourage travel there. I didn't want to take even the slightest chance that individuals could end up hurt or confused.

I decided that I wouldn't turn my back on the intriguing cases I'd uncovered, the ones that showed healing had occurred—instead, I'd focus more clearly on the shifts and changes made by the individuals themselves, in the hopes of understanding the internal roots that lead to recovery. I didn't believe that unexpected healings or improbable recoveries had much to do with the healer or physician, outside of the role that they can potentially play in activating something that already exists within all of us. But as the accusations against John of God showed, people in healing traditions can also potentially play a harmful role, making it all the more urgent to uncover the actual factors associated with healing, so we can recognize and activate them for ourselves.

I don't want to disparage the impact a great healer or doctor can have on an individual; the connection between healer and patient can be profound and can become an essential piece of the healing process. But as I thought about what I'd learned from the process of sifting the real cases of spontaneous healing from the chaff, I knew that whatever was happening wasn't primarily caused by something external. It wasn't a pill, a medicine, a surgery, or a healer's miraculous hands that held the key to these people's recoveries, as tempting as it might be to believe in these simple and seemingly clear solutions. Something was happening *within* these individuals that made their recoveries possible.

A CLUE, BURIED IN HISTORY

A few months later, I was getting ready for a presentation, digging through old notes and textbooks, when I stumbled upon a story I remembered vaguely from medical school. I'd come across it a number of times back then, but it was only a brief mention—a paragraph here or there in a pathology textbook, a side comment in a professor's lecture. It was presented as a footnote of history, always skimmed over. This time, with the question of spontaneous healing on my mind, the anecdote caught my attention. I set my presentation aside and sat down to read it.

It started in the fall of 1890, when a young surgeon at New York Memorial Hospital, William Coley, saw a new patient. A young woman named Bessie Dashiell came in with an injury that wouldn't heal, a wound on her hand that had been bothering her for weeks. In the exam room, she told Coley her story: While traveling on summer vacation, she'd gotten her hand smashed between two seats on a rickety passenger train. The resulting swelling and pain didn't worry her at first, but it persisted, growing worse instead of better. Coley biopsied the site of the injury, fully expecting to find signs of infection. Instead, he discovered a very rare and aggressive type of bone tumor called a sarcoma.

At the time, the only treatment available for Bessie's type of cancer was amputation. She was put under with a low dose of sweet-smelling chloroform, and Coley removed her arm just below the elbow.

It was too late. The cancer had already spread. Bessie failed to improve, and a few weeks later, Coley found a tender, almond-sized nodule in her right breast. The next day, it had doubled in size, and two more had appeared in her left breast. Sarcomas grew rapidly throughout her body, swelling up under the skin, as big as golf balls, then grapefruits. In her abdomen, Coley palpated a tumor "the size of a child's head."[2] Just a few months after diagnosis, in January of 1891, she died at the age of eighteen.

Bessie Dashiell's story, though it features a particularly rare form of cancer, isn't unusual for the period and wouldn't normally warrant a mention in the history books of medicine. But Coley, devastated by the loss of his patient—she was so young, and her death had been painful—couldn't let it go. Instead of moving on to the next case, he began to investigate what he might have done differently. He combed through the hospital's records until he found a case almost identical to Bessie's, except for one thing: the patient survived.

What was different about the two cases? The surviving patient, a German man by the name of Stein, developed a dangerously high fever in the days following his amputation surgery. The associated infection—likely a skin infection called erysipelas—almost killed him. However, his immune system was able to beat back the erysipelas bacteria, and his fever began to drop. And bizarrely, his sarcoma tumors began to shrink. By the time he had recovered from the infection, the tumors had melted completely away. His doctors discharged him, baffled—it was a miracle.

By cross-referencing with other instances of erysipelas, Coley found more evidence of patients recovering unexpectedly from cancer after falling ill with a fever and infection after undergoing surgery to remove a cancerous tumor. He noticed that other medical pioneers such as Louis Pasteur had reported similar findings with erysipelas and began to suspect that postsurgical infections in some cases actually *helped* patients recover from cancer. Coley hypothesized that the infections triggered an immune response that not only ridded the body of the invading bacteria, as a fever is intended to do, but also stimulated the body's immune system to attack the cancer cells.

Coley immediately tested his theory on a cancer patient on whom all other treatments had failed, injecting him directly with live streptococcus bacteria. The man, who had a tumor the size of a chicken egg on his neck, could barely speak or swallow and had been given only weeks to live. After the injection, his fever flared and he grew alarmingly ill. But then, as he recovered from the infection, he and Coley watched the tumor dissolve and disappear. The man survived and went home cancer-free.

The implications were astounding—somehow, the body's natural processes of fighting infection were also breaking down cancerous tumors, liquefying and flushing them away as if they'd never been there.

Rereading the story of Dr. Coley and Bessie Dashiell, I was struck by the visionary nature of his discoveries, so long ago. Coley, now called "the father of immunotherapy," uncovered something essential about the power of the human immune system—a way to potentially turn it on to fight an incurable illness. He went on to develop a mixture of dead bacteria that he began to use as a cancer treatment, safer to use since this mixture was less likely to make sick people sicker to the point of death. But the idea of introducing "bad" bacteria into the body was difficult for people to accept.

Coley was an innovator ahead of his time. While he sought to provoke a strong immune response that spurred the body to do what it was supposed to—flush the mutating cancer cells out itself—the zeitgeist was moving in the direction of *suppressing* immune response. At the time, medicine was in the early stage of discovering the power of medications, and things rapidly tilted in the direction of the new immunosuppressants and antipyretics, drugs designed to suppress the immune system and fevers and kill off cancer cells. Radiation also eventually became part of this new tool kit. A side effect of these new treatments was that they killed off a lot of healthy cells, too. But they saved lives, and so we embraced the practice of suppressing the immune system to treat disease, rather than stimulating it. Coley's work was brushed into the dustbin of history—he had the right ideas but was trying to get them out into the world at the wrong time.

These immune-suppressing treatments are important and have proven to be a lifesaving development in medicine, but I couldn't help but wonder where we'd be today if we'd *also* kept hold of the lessons learned from Coley—that our own immune systems can become our secret weapon in rolling back incurable diseases.

RECLAIMING A LESSON FROM THE PAST

As I did my rounds at the hospital and prepared talks, I continued seeing things through the lens of spontaneous healing—where it came from and how it could be replicated. Old, passed-over lessons from medical school like that of Coley and his quest bobbed to the surface of my brain like apples; comments by current patients who were recovering unusually well snagged in my mind, echoes of what I'd heard from survivors in Brazil.

I'd expected to go to Brazil and debunk the claims of miraculous healing—cross it off my list and move on with my life. Instead, I'd found a new passion. I knew that something real was happening. I still didn't understand exactly why, but I had a feeling that it was rooted at least to some degree in what science has recently been discovering about the immune system and the various factors that affect it.

We all know that our immune systems are our greatest asset in fighting off colds and other viruses we encounter. "I've gotten run down," we tell our friends and colleagues as we blow our noses or cover a sneeze. We understand and accept that when we catch a cold, a chink in our immune systems has let in a virus that otherwise might have bounced off our armor, perhaps because we didn't get enough sleep or we've been stressed at work or home. But when it comes to cancer, heart disease, diabetes, and other chronic and incurable diseases that plague so many of us, we tend not to think about how our bodies and immune systems might be working for us—or not. We immediately turn outward, often to interventions designed to treat the worst *symptoms* of those diseases, rather than

turning inward and seeking out the underlying *cause*. And perhaps the cause is from an immune system gone awry with chronic
inflammation—an immune system that has not only ceased to be
as effective as it should be but is now creating its own problems and
diseases. While we have a medical system that is brilliant in some
ways, it very often treats patients by providing medicines that help
them tread water with their illnesses—at best. But we don't usually study health, and—to a degree that defies common sense—we
don't study those who have found ways to heal.

Coley's experiment showed that a fever could sometimes reset
the human immune system so that it could "see" and attack cancer
cells that it had previously allowed to flourish and grow, almost
like rebooting a computer to reset the hard drive. From my studies
in medical school and my years of practicing psychiatry, I've seen
how everything we put into our bodies—from foods and toxins to
thoughts and feelings—can shift immune function at a base level.
What we eat affects how our immune systems perform, in terms
of whether or not we are giving our body systems and cells the
micronutrients they need to perform at the top of their game. Our
immediate environments affect it; a recent study out of Stanford
University[3] found that the world around you, from your mother's
womb to your childhood home to where you live and work today,
shapes and determines your immune function *even more than your
genes*. In fact, 90 percent of chronic illness is driven not by the
genome, but by disease-creating factors in our environments.[4] How
we manage stress affects it; we have long known that chronic stress
suppresses immune function, and groundbreaking work in the
fields of psychoneuroimmunology and now positive health—which
plumb the intricate connection between the brain and the immune
system—are proving that positive emotions and happiness literally
make us healthier by boosting immune function.

In Brazil and elsewhere, people were occasionally healing from
incurable illnesses, either without medical intervention or else with
treatment but wildly outperforming the projected outcomes of
those treatments. Some essential, unseen shift was occurring across

a diverse cross section of individuals and diseases that was allowing their immune systems to somehow rise up and turn the tide against disease. The "how" of this was what I needed to focus on. Questions about whether or not João de Deus was really a "miracle healer" or whether every claim made by the Casa was legitimate were ultimately irrelevant. If spontaneous remission occurred at all, even occasionally, science could investigate it if I could scrape away all the surface distractions: the false stories, the dismissiveness of the medical mainstream, and my own fears about how I would be perceived.

I'd launched my investigation into spontaneous remissions in part to begin asking better questions. So my first question was about immune function and why it isn't more of a priority in medicine today. When someone comes to us with a chronic or incurable disease, why isn't immune function the *first* thing we look at?

2

Natural-Born Killers

> The important thing in science is not so much to obtain
> new facts as to discover new ways of thinking about them.
> —*Sir William Bragg*

Medicine today is like a long line of ambulances parked at the bottom of a tall cliff. High above, people walk off the cliff and fall, plummeting to the bottom. The ambulances pick up the broken bodies and whisk them off to the hospital, where the latest technology and medications will fix them up as best they can. And they do a pretty good job! But the only real way to help people is to have guardrails at the top—methods to support people in developing vital, healthy lives, from the immune system up, so they don't go over the cliff to begin with.[1]

What the people profiled in this book will show—these "ultimate achievers" in health—is that all of us can use the principles and practices they used. These transdiagnostic factors, applicable across a wide range of diseases and that keep some people at the top of the cliff via guardrail, can also serve as a ladder for those at the bottom. When used more intensely, they can perhaps be accessed by those of us at the bottom to climb part of the way back up—or even, in these "miraculous" cases of spontaneous healing, all the way to the top.

That being said, staying at the top of the cliff can be difficult until you really understand what's entailed. And getting back up there, if you're one of the many who's been failed by our lack of guardrails, can be even more challenging. But for a clue as to where to begin, let's look at the burgeoning field of immunotherapy.

In this rapidly developing arena, doctors and researchers are trying to push beyond the very edge of what we know and understand about the human body's natural defenses against disease. *Immunotherapy* means, essentially, manipulating the patient's own immune cells to combat disease, usually cancer. Jedd Wolchok, an oncologist and immunotherapy innovator at the groundbreaking cancer clinic Memorial Sloan Kettering, has said that spontaneous remissions "are either divine intervention or the immune system."[2]

What is your immune system? Usually, we only notice it when it fails us. And for something so essential to our survival, it can be hard to picture. It may seem pretty abstract—an invisible shield that we hope continues to work for us. But your immune system is quite real and tangible. Along with the nervous system, it's the most complex system in the human body. It's made up of organs, tissues, and cells that form an intricate and multipurpose web of protection throughout your entire body. It starts, in some ways, with your skin, your saliva, and the mucus membranes inside your nasal passages, which stop, trap, and neutralize many pathogens before they even enter the body. And it goes as deep as your bone marrow, where your white blood cells are born: the intelligent, specialized, rapid, and ruthless soldiers of your immune system, which hunt down and take out everything from invading pathogens to burgeoning cancer cells.

Here's how your immune system functions on a moment-to-moment basis. Every second, whether you're awake or asleep, your immune system works vigorously to defend you from foreign invaders and internal problems that arise. Like a top-of-the-line burglar alarm system, it's always humming silently in the background—

running internal diagnostics, scanning for problems, correcting bugs, and thwarting viruses. Even as you're sitting here reading this book, your immune system is hard at work. Each breath you take in is screened for invaders. At night, while you're sleeping, your immune system increases the production of certain proteins that help it to identify and flush out harmful pathogens and rogue cells. When properly fortified with the physical and emotional nutrition it needs, your immune system is ingenious at figuring out how to best protect you, developing unique solutions tailored to each individual situation. When it doesn't receive what it needs to be at its best, the cells and messaging are sluggish, prone to mistakes and miscommunication.

To maintain such constant vigilance, new white blood cells are constantly being born in your bone marrow. From there, they are sent to your thymus—a small organ that sits behind your breastbone—where they grow and mature before fanning out into your bloodstream, fully grown and ready to fight. They move through your body even faster than your blood does, which is a pretty amazing feat, given that a red blood cell completes a full circuit of your body in about one minute. The many different types of white blood cells, each with its own specific job, can develop hundreds of tiny legs, grip the blood vessel walls, and move millipede-like when they are rushing to the site of a cut, infection, or other breach in the immune system's barrier, or to the site of an internal emergency like a rogue cell that has mutated into something dangerous.[3]

Many symptoms in the body that we think of as "bad"—and that we are in the habit of medicating away—are actually an important part of your immune system's pathogen-fighting process. Take, for example, the redness and swelling that appears around a cut or a scrape. The redness is caused by your veins and capillaries dilating to allow infection-fighting immune system cells to arrive as quickly as possible to the site—like traffic opening up for an ambulance. Once at the site, the cells organize themselves into teams—some in charge of cleaning, others repair, and others generating new tissue. This causes swelling as the cells do their work. As long as they are successful in preventing infection from setting in, this type of inflammation is a normal and healthy response that is necessary for you to heal.

But the best example of an immune response we often misunderstand has to be fever.

When we get a fever, we tend to immediately try to figure out a way to get rid of it. Up until very recently, it was standard practice in medicine to recommend controlling a fever with over-the-counter medications called *antipyretics*. But theories began to emerge that fevers might actually *help* our immune systems—as long as they aren't dangerously high.

In 2011, a team of researchers at the Department of Immunology at the Roswell Park Cancer Institute in Buffalo, New York, decided to investigate a little further. They'd observed that in nature, animals who developed fevers did not try to alleviate them by cooling down. Instead, they actually tried to *preserve* their febrile state by moving to a warmer location.

Why would they do this?

When they ran an experiment on a group of mice, inducing fever in one group and not in another, they found that the group with the fever produced significantly more pathogen-fighting T cells than the control group. Plus, the higher temperature seemed to help the cells of the immune system operate more rapidly and with improved accuracy. Essentially, the T cells were already doing a pretty good job, but when something got past their sweeps and scans, *heat* was the factor that could unlock their superpower and kick them into high gear.

Fevers, uncomfortable as they are, are one of the immune system's many ingenious tools. They help your body produce extra virus-fighting cells to get rid of a cold or flu faster. This finding loops back to Coley's discovery over a hundred years ago—that a high fever somehow corresponded with the disappearance of cancerous tumors. What Coley had stumbled upon, without completely understanding it, was that when the immune system turned the heat on to kick itself into gear to fight an infection, an unexpected side effect was that it got better at fighting cancer, too. Thus, when we take medications to suppress a fever response, we may also be suppressing our immune systems' efforts to guide us toward recovery.

Of course, as brilliant as the human immune system is, it doesn't always work perfectly. Sometimes, things go wrong. Your immune system, when lacking the physical and emotional nutrition it needs, can become confused when it deploys to attack a threat; it can overreact or set its sights on the wrong target. Allergies, for example, are an instance where the immune system overreacts to something that doesn't really pose a threat to you. For some people, it's a whiff of pollen that leaves their head pounding and nose draining; for others, a speck of peanut can cause them to spiral into anaphylactic shock. The reactions are different—one an inconvenience and the other a life-threatening emergency—but the mechanism is the same. It's a glitch in the immune system, a bug in the programming that, once written into our bodies' codes, can be difficult to eradicate. In the United States alone, fifty million people suffer from allergies of some kind, and for the most part, all we do is treat the symptoms. Although some research is beginning to indicate that processed foods and chemicals may play a role, we still don't completely understand why this very common immune system glitch occurs or how to reverse it.

In the case of autoimmune disorders, our immune systems go especially haywire. With these diseases, your own body turns on you, attacking what it was sworn to protect. It flags your own cells, tissues, or organs as "foreign" and assaults them. Type 1 diabetes is an example of this: the immune system destroys the cells of the pancreas, making it impossible for the body to produce the insulin it needs to metabolize sugars and survive. Some autoimmune diseases, such as type 1 diabetes, are present from a young age, coded into the DNA of the person who suffers from it. But many other autoimmune disorders don't appear until much later in life and often don't have a strong genetic component. However, once they appear and begin to progress, most are considered "incurable," and the focus becomes how to live *with* the disease and manage it, as opposed to how to cure it. Some of the individuals I will profile in the first section of this book are those who recovered completely from autoimmune diseases thought to be incurable—diseases such as type 2 diabetes, lupus, and ankylosing spondylitis, a devastating and rapidly progressive form of arthritis that "freezes" the bones of the spine and pelvis. In all these cases, the individuals stumbled upon a way to reset their immune systems—to wipe out the bad programming that had it attacking its own cells and tissues, and reset completely to normal, healthy immune function.

DEPLOYING YOUR SECRET WEAPON

How did these individuals achieve this reset, and what triggers the onset of these autoimmune disorders to begin with? In some cases, we suspect the triggers are likely related to our environment and our diet. A few decades ago, autoimmune disorders were barely a blip on the radar, but as our routine use of chemicals in agriculture and commerce skyrockets, so do cases of autoimmune disease. In fact, autoimmune disorders are one of the leading causes of death in young and middle-aged women today.[4] There's evidence that everything from environmental toxins to a onetime infection to the long-term wear and tear of chronic stress can trigger an autoimmune disorder. Even pregnancy can do it! Running a study on women in Denmark, researchers found that women who gave birth developed autoimmune diseases of all types at a markedly higher rate than their nonparent counterparts. They already knew that during pregnancy, fetal cells mix into the mother's bloodstream and settle throughout the body—decades later, fetal cells from the children she carried can be found in a mother's brain tissue or bone marrow. They theorized that for many women, as the body attempts to unearth and attack those cells, it gets locked into a pattern of attacking itself.

There are a lot of unknowns surrounding autoimmune diseases like diabetes, rheumatoid arthritis, lupus, and many more. What triggers them varies from person to person and is highly individual, but what it boils down to is that something derailed the immune system like a rock on a train track. Whether that rock was a gene sequence you were born with, a toxin your body absorbed, or a much-wanted pregnancy, the mission afterward is the same: get that train back on track instead of spinning its wheels, doing more damage to your body.

It would be incredible if our immune systems never got off track or misdirected—if they stayed in perfect working order like a well-oiled machine. But even machines need maintenance. How can we expect our immune systems to continue to function at their peak, with healthy cells responding crisply and correctly to instructions from above, if we don't service them the way we do our cars? I know I've gone through long phases in my life where I paid less attention to my body and immune system than I did to my car, which I brought in for regular oil changes and recommended services. It's funny, because my car is ultimately replaceable, while my body is not.

So how do we keep our immune systems running at top-notch levels or, if they're currently depleted, how do we replenish them? How can we avoid the kinds of triggers that can set off one of the autoimmune disorders that are becoming all too common, or hit the Reset button on our immune systems if we are currently suffering from one?

One of the immune system's secret weapons, built into our biology from the beginning of human life on earth, is the "natural killer cell." It's one of the various types of white blood cells that are born in your bone marrow and programmed to do a very specific job. Other types include the helper cells that flag problematic cells for removal, and the memory cells that remember viruses and bacteria so that you can fight them off more effectively the next time they turn up. As for the natural killer cell, think of it as the James Bond of your immune system. It's a specially trained spy, a secret agent, a hunter of master villains. This type of cell plays an essential role in eliminating tumors and virally infected cells, tracking them down, gobbling them up, and flushing them out of the body.

Natural killer cells are among those types of white blood cells that get a superpower boost from a fever and were undoubtedly part of the team responsible for dismantling the tumors in Coley's experiments. Of course, we can't just run around trying to catch infections, inducing dangerously high fevers in our bodies in the hopes that it will spur our immune systems into action. But we can certainly learn from Coley's experiment, which proved that the immune system *could* be prodded into doing its job better.

Seventy-five years after William Coley sat next to a dying Bessie Dashiell, wondering how he could have saved her, another young surgeon picked up his scalpel and prepared to begin a routine gallbladder removal. His patient was not exactly the picture of health; the patient was an older man who had been a lifelong alcoholic, known for polishing off a few quarts of bourbon a week. And during one of their first meetings, he revealed that he'd been diagnosed with terminal gastric cancer with metastases to the liver years earlier, but that it had apparently just "gone away."[5]

Dr. Steven Rosenberg didn't believe him. *Sure,* he thought. He knew this particular form of stomach cancer was incurable. The man must be confused. But he found the original pathology report and was shocked to find the old guy had been telling the truth. At the time of diagnosis, doctors had removed the tumor to buy the man some time and make him more comfortable. But the cancer had already spread, and there were many tumors swelling in his liver. The illness was terminal; it was only a matter of time. He was expected to die in a matter of months.

That this man was lying on Dr. Rosenberg's operating table for a gallbladder removal twelve years later was impossible. Dr. Rosenberg couldn't imagine how the man was still alive, and he wasn't sure what he would find when he went in to remove the gallbladder.

He made a sideways incision just below the rib cage, following the angle of the lowest rib. To get to the gallbladder, a pear-shaped organ that dispenses bile and assists with digestion, you have to reach under the liver, which sits on top of it like a blanket. Before Dr. Rosenberg proceeded with the cholecystectomy, he paused,

curious, and palpated the liver. By now, it should have been absolutely riddled with tumors. Twelve years earlier, the patient's surgeon had recorded dense, rock-hard lumps scattered throughout
the organ like gravel. But the liver was silky smooth. *Not bad for an
alcoholic,* he thought. *What does he drink?*

Baffled, Dr. Rosenberg completed the cholecystectomy and
closed up the patient. The man lying there, seemingly ordinary in
every way, had experienced the extraordinary.

Questions whirled through the young surgeon's mind in the
days following the procedure. What an incredible discovery—that
a man expected to die within months of one of the most fatal, viru-
lent forms of cancer out there had watched his body simply flush
the cancer away like it was nothing more than the common cold.
And nobody had even known. Feeling better instead of worse, the
patient had simply never returned to the hospital after his tumor
was removed. Nobody had followed up with him when he failed
to return; they probably assumed he'd gone elsewhere for care or
simply died. To the hospital that had treated him, he became a
piece of paper in a file. Meanwhile, he'd simply walked off into his
life, happy and healthy without knowing why. The only reason his
unprecedented recovery had finally come to light was because of a
gallstone. To Dr. Rosenberg, it felt like "a mystery of ultimately
enormous dimensions,"[6] like striking crude oil while digging a
backyard well. There had to be a way to refine it into something
usable—something that could help others.

Assuming the mechanism was biological—something unique
to this patient's physiology—he tried injecting the man's blood into
another patient with gastric cancer. But there was nothing special
about the blood that he could find—nothing that could be trans-
ferred in such a way, anyway—and the other patient eventually
died. Dr. Rosenberg realized that it wasn't something magical or
miraculous about his patient's blood or body that had caused the
tumors to melt away. It was something else, some switch that had
been flipped somehow in this man's immune system that caused it
to turn itself on and eradicate the cancer cells on its own. And if

this was the case, it wasn't a onetime event—it was repeatable. It was possible to figure out how to turn those switches on in other people's immune systems, too, like flipping a switch to banish disease.

As it did for Coley with Bessie Dashiell, the case of the vanishing gastric cancer set Steven Rosenberg on a lifelong quest to better understand the human immune system and how its innate skills and powers could be harnessed and honed to fight the deadliest diseases. Today, he directs the Tumor Immunology Section at the National Cancer Institute and has pioneered a new direction in cancer treatment—that of cancer immunotherapy, which looks for ways to use the immune system to fight cancer rather than suppress the immune system. He's spent the past four decades uncovering many of the secrets of the immune system, one by one, like an archaeologist slowly uncovering a buried skeleton bone by bone, getting closer and closer to revealing the big picture.

Steven Rosenberg never did figure out what caused that case of spontaneous remission back in 1968 when he was just starting his career in medicine; the man's vanishing stomach cancer remains a mystery. As with so many cases of spontaneous remission, it happened in the dark, when nobody was looking. Investigating cases of spontaneous healing are so often a detective story—trying to piece together what might have happened when, based on an always incomplete set of clues.

Today, cases like these are "miracles." Tomorrow, we'll look back at them and see them for what they were: steps in the long, steep staircase toward knowledge. But even now, we are already unearthing new ways to gain access to our immune systems, like hacking into software to fix faulty code.

While we can't yet use immunotherapy to fight every type of cancer or incurable disease, the progress that Rosenberg and other immunologists have made has been groundbreaking. He figured out how to take certain cells out, "train" them to do their jobs better, and then release them back into the body to hunt and kill cancer cells. More recently, he and his team have been working on a new therapy called *checkpoint inhibitors,* reactivating immune system cells that have been turned off by a growing tumor—one of cancer's many tricks for slipping past the immune system's network of detection.

These are incredible advancements that have been lifesaving for people with certain types of cancer. But immunotherapy in its current state doesn't work for everyone, or for all diseases. It's still a niche therapy, available only in specific situations. So what can the rest of us learn from this?

Successes in immunotherapy today tell us that the power to overcome incurable illness may very well be locked inside each of us. Immunotherapy is a highly technical, precise way of targeting specific cells in the immune system and making them work against cancer. While you can't practice immunotherapy yourself at home, you *can* communicate with your immune system, perhaps even—like so many of those who experience spontaneous healing—to the point of changing the way it functions, turning the tide against disease.

OPENING THE LINES OF COMMUNICATION: HOW TO TALK TO YOUR IMMUNE SYSTEM

Why do our natural killer cells sometimes target and remove mutating cancer cells and other times overlook them? When do they work *for* us, hunting down pathogens and viral invaders, and when do they turn against us, attacking our own tissues and biological systems?

In the 1950s, a young seminary student made spontaneous remission history by being the first person to become ill with a serious disease and then experience a startling spontaneous healing, all while under the care and close observation of multiple doctors.[7]

Daniel began therapy in his early twenties. He was struggling. Brought up in a strict religious family, he wrestled with deep-seated guilt surrounding sex and sin. He had enormous difficulty with social interaction. His doctor described him as "rebellious, frightened, rigid and anxious." He didn't know what he wanted to do with his life, and this tortured him. He described his college years to his therapist as "a walking nightmare." After he graduated, things only got worse. He'd always thought he'd become a pastor, but he didn't feel worthy of the profession that he'd considered his calling. He refused to be ordained. He met a woman he thought he might be able to forge a relationship with, but it was rocky—he held her at a distance, was rigid and controlling. Therapy stopped helping. Utterly lost, he retreated into a virtual prison of anger, guilt, and shame.

In January of 1959, when he was twenty-six years old, Daniel noticed a hardness in his left testicle. His diagnosis: embryonal cell carcinoma of the testes. His doctors attempted to excise the cancer by operating immediately to remove the tumor. Initially, they hoped they had succeeded. But after the surgery, Daniel fell into an even deeper depression. He felt that his illness was a punishment sent by God for his sins, and he was overwhelmed with anxiety over his medical bills, which he struggled to pay. Four months after the surgery, his doctors discovered that the cancer had in fact blossomed once again, spreading into his lymphatic system and throughout his body. Tumors swelled in his axillary and neck lymph nodes, making it difficult for him to hold up his head. He had metastases scattered through his lungs and chest cavity. Node biopsy confirmed that it was the same embryonal cell carcinoma.

The prognosis was as bad as it could be: his chances of surviving one year were zero. When he asked his doctors to be honest about how much time he had left, they told him, "Weeks."

His therapist had a question for him: "What do you want to do before you die?"

He replied without a moment's hesitation, "I want to be ordained and get married."[8]

In the face of a devastating illness, his desires and dreams had lifted into sharp relief. Even with death on the horizon, Daniel experienced a sense of peace and clarity that he had never before felt. Arrangements were made immediately for him to be ordained, and his family began to throw together a wedding. Despite everything, he and Constance were happy.

A few weeks later, on July 13, they were married. Daniel was ghostlike in his wedding suit, looking as if he might not make it through the ceremony. But oddly, the tumors on his neck were significantly smaller. Daniel and his new bride took it to be a momentary reprieve—a sort of last hurrah before the cancer killed him.

Within days of the ceremony, however, the tumors that had swelled from his neck had vanished completely. A week later, on July 20, his curious doctors ordered an x-ray. Shockingly, it showed not only that the visible tumors in his lymphatic system were completely gone but also that the pulmonary metastases in his chest cavity seemed to be shrinking. They could think of no explanation; the only treatment he'd undergone since discovering the extent of the cancer had been palliative. On July 31, a follow-up x-ray showed that the metastases were gone. The dark spots on the scan had been seemingly erased.

A few days later, Daniel was ordained as a minister. And on August 8, 1959, he was informed that his cancer had fully regressed. There was absolutely no evidence of disease in his body. He was completely well.

The fact that the psychological factors of this case were known and recorded in great detail make it an incredible window into the link between the mind and the immune system. This is the only known recorded case of spontaneous remission where the patient was in therapy and under psychiatric observation before his illness and then through the onset, development, and startling regression. The ups and downs of Daniel's aggressive cancer mirrored his psychological state at every turn, raising many important questions: What was it about the specter of death that freed him to live? Given all that changed for him both medically and psychologically in the course of his recovery, was this about the death of his false self and the birth of his true self? About moving through fear to embrace life and purpose? About liberation inspired by feeling loved?

Let's look, for a moment, at the nervous system. Your nervous system is an intricate network of nerve cells that winds and sparkles through your entire body. You have literally *billions* of nerve cells, or neurons, that allow you to do everything from lifting your finger to feeling an intense emotion. Nervous system cells are unceasingly sending messages through your system, whisking through the body as fast as electricity.

We now know that the immune system and the nervous system are, in fact, intricately interwoven. They are not separate systems operating independently in different sectors of the body but overlapping networks that can swap information and "talk" to each other.

First of all, the nervous system connects directly to the thymus, one of the powerhouses of the immune system, which nurtures and deploys natural killer cells and other types of white blood cells into your body on command. But even more fascinating, researchers now know that the cells of your immune system actually have *neuroreceptors* on them. Neuroreceptors were believed to be limited to the brain and the nervous system until Candace Pert, often called "the mother of psychoneuroimmunology," discovered the presence of neurotransmitter and neuropeptide receptors on the walls of cells in both the immune system and the brain. And what are neuroreceptors, exactly? Basically, they're a way for the nervous system to communicate cell to cell. It's like having a certain radio frequency turned on so that you can talk to someone via walkie-talkie. The cells of the immune system, roaming throughout your entire body at all times, have that radio channel turned on. They are in direct communication with your nervous system, meaning whatever's going on in your mind is being broadcast directly into your immune system. Cases like Daniel's show us that it is possible for our emotions to talk to our immune systems—sometimes with dramatic and unexpected results.[9]

When I dug into the details of Daniel's case, I found that during the days of his amazing and rapid recovery, he underwent an age-regression hypnosis session with his therapist, where he relived the deep and unconditional love of his beloved great-grandmother. Daniel later attributed an important part of his healing to an ongoing, unshakable feeling of being loved by this person who'd been so important to him. Could this powerful feeling of being loved have been broadcast into his immune system, revivifying something deep within him? Whether it comes from a therapeutic session, a loving relationship, deep meditation, or focused imagery, love touches and heals something that medications can't touch.

And it's not only your immune and nervous systems that are operating on the same frequency. Ever have a *gut feeling* about something? Well, there's a reason for that.

Your gut (or the entire digestive system: esophagus, stomach, and large and small intestine) contains over one hundred million neurons—more than there are in your spinal cord. Serotonin, one of the neurochemicals that helps regulate mood, memory, social behavior, sexual desire and function, as well as appetite, digestion, and sleep (and which is one of the main targets of antidepressants),[10] basically originates in the gut; it turns out that more than 90 percent of the serotonin in our bodies is synthesized there.[11] The gut's effect on mood, emotions, and even thoughts is so significant that researchers now think of it as a "brain" in its own right. And the cells in your gut aren't working alone to produce all that serotonin; they're teaming up with the microbes in your gut, also called the *microbiome*.[12]

The microbiome is an entire microscopic ecosystem that is living and thriving inside your body. It is complex, smart, and influential, to the point that it could very well be determining your ability to heal . . . or not.

WHAT IS THE MICROBIOME?

When we talk about the microbiome, what we are essentially talking about is you—and the trillions of bacteria that reside on the outside and inside of your body. Most of them live in your gut, but they are in fact spread throughout your body, an interconnected web of life that in many ways functions like an additional organ. The vast majority of these bacteria living in every sector and on every surface of your body are actually beneficial bacteria. You give them a home, and they work for you, digesting food, producing certain vitamins and neurochemicals that your body needs, and even preventing "bad" bacteria from gaining a foothold. These beneficial microorganisms, which live in symbiosis with you, actually account for up to 3 percent of your body mass. And you're outnumbered; for every human cell in your body, there are one hundred bacteria cells.

The question, then, is where do *you* end and your bacteria begin? That's not as easy to answer as we might wish. The bacteria in our microbiomes have an enormous impact on our health and can play a big role in whether or not we get sick—and if we do, whether or not we recover.

Our individual microbiomes are as unique as a fingerprint. Your microbiome was shaped at birth, when you were colonized by the bacteria in your mother's birth canal as you moved through it. From that moment forward, your microbiome has been shaped by your environment, by the foods you ate, the places you traveled, the kinds of jobs you worked. Every new environment you're exposed to adds to your ever-shifting microbiome, ideally making it richer and more diverse. But one thing can massively set back your microbiome: antibiotics.

Antibiotics, a major leap forward for medicine and a lifesaving intervention, come with their own set of adverse effects. And one of those is that in the process of wiping out "bad" bacteria that are attacking you, they also wipe out the "good" bacteria that support healthy immune function. In fact, approximately *80 percent* of your immune system cells are in your gut, and we are finding more and more evidence that a healthy, rich, diverse microbiome can shape an immune system that is more effective against both external threats like viruses and infections, as well as internal threats like mutating cells that may turn into cancer if not caught.

So how do the "good" bacteria in your microbiome play a role in shaping a healthy immune system? The one hundred trillion bacteria that live in your body come with their own set of DNA. Collectively, the DNA of those bacteria are their "genome." We are beginning to discover that the human genome, which comes preprogrammed to resist certain diseases and can be taught to resist others through exposure to them or through vaccines, doesn't actually have enough "code" to protect us from all the disease threats that exist. It's like we've filled up our hard drive already; we just don't have the space. We rely on the genome of our microbiomes—our gut-brains—to store more information, tactics, and disease-fighting knowledge for us. Wipe that out by taking too many antibiotics, and it's like burning a library.

A single round of antibiotics can impact your gut bacteria for up to a year. Of course, antibiotics and other immunosuppressive interventions that affect the microbiome—like chemotherapy—are at times necessary, even lifesaving. The trick is knowing when to use them and using them wisely. And the problem is that instead of taking care of our lives and bodies so that we are less likely to get ill in the first place, we've created a trigger-happy culture in medicine that leaps to these sorts of late interventions instead of helping you create those guardrails and ladders we saw at the beginning of the chapter. The microbiome is essentially an extension of our immune systems. And yet, our default approach to treating major illnesses usually involves decimating the microbiome while we do so.

If we know how important the microbiome is to immune function, then why are we still treating disease, for the most part, with a scorched-earth approach that takes out the good along with the bad? How did we get here?

WHAT CREATES DISEASE—THE MICROBE OR THE SOIL?
A hundred and fifty years ago, we still believed in "spontaneous generation." This was the idea that illness was generated and born within the body, appearing out of nowhere inside human cells. We also thought disease was a moral affliction—a side effect of poverty or making poor choices. If you were sick, it was probably something you'd done wrong that had caused it—a judgment from God.

By the time Pasteur set about disproving spontaneous generation, plenty of his predecessors had already tried. One attempt in particular stands out. In the early 1800s, "childbed fever," which cropped up in women in the days after they'd given birth, killed up to a quarter of all new mothers. There were all kinds of ideas about what caused it and what cured it. The doctors who treated these women were certain it wasn't contagious and didn't worry about contracting it themselves. Spontaneous generation was the general assumption about the origins of disease at the time, so it was clear to everyone that childbed fever "spontaneously generated" in the female organs in the days after delivering a baby.

But in Austria, a surgeon named Ignaz Semmelweis questioned this assumption. Semmelweis worked at a hospital with two maternity clinics. The first clinic had rates of maternal mortality that were consistent with the average at the time—childbirth was an even more dangerous business in the nineteenth century, and labor and delivery were risky. This clinic certainly lost women to preeclampsia and other complications of labor and birth, but the rates of childbed fever were extremely low. The second clinic that Semmelweis ran was a completely different story. It had such a terrible reputation for new mothers dying from childbed fever that women, terrified to go, got on their knees and begged not to be taken there. Some even refused to go and instead stopped and gave birth right out in the street. It happened so frequently, the practice was referred to as *street births*. Semmelweis looked into the cases of street births, expecting to find poor outcomes—after all, how could squatting in the gutter be preferable to giving birth in a hospital, attended by trained doctors and top medical students? What he found shocked him: the street births had a vanishingly small rate of death by childbed fever, barely registering at all on a chart of mortality rates.

Semmelweis began to look more closely for differences between the two clinics. The clinic with the better outcomes was staffed with midwives, and the other with medical students, so perhaps, he thought, they were using different strategies? For example, the midwives had women lie on their sides, while the medical students had them lie on their backs. Semmelweis instructed his medical students to have women deliver on their sides instead, but it had no effect. He ran through a list of possible differences, changing one thing and then another, always with the same result: no effect. It was a personal tragedy that finally brought him a flash of insight.

Another surgeon, a colleague and good friend, pricked his finger with a scalpel while performing an autopsy on a woman recently deceased from childbed fever. Within days, he died of the same illness that was killing thousands of women each year in Semmelweis's maternity clinic.

Semmelweis was devastated by the loss of his friend, but it was the clue he needed; childbed fever was not spontaneously generated in the female organs but passed to the patient by a doctor who'd recently done an autopsy and not sufficiently cleaned his hands. There was a type of bacteria that doctors picked up on their skin when they performed an autopsy, and when they went straight to the bed of a laboring woman and used those unsterilized hands to deliver a baby, they passed the bacteria on to her, condemning her to the same painful death. This was the difference between the two clinics: the midwives at the first clinic did not perform autopsies, while the medical students at the second one did. They'd been killing their own patients by carrying microbes from corpse to patient.

We know now that childbed fever was actually a type of sepsis, a strain of the virile streptococcus bacteria that—once introduced into the body—causes a painful and lethal infection. The solution was to kill the bacteria before it could be passed to another victim. Semmelweis, without exactly knowing why, stumbled upon the solution: he had his medical students wash their hands in a chlorine/lime solution after performing autopsies and before delivering babies. The death rate from childbed fever immediately plummeted from a soaring high of close to 25 percent down to only 1 to 2 percent.

It was a dramatic and undeniable success. But the medical world couldn't, or wouldn't, accept the theory that diseases were spread in this way. First of all, the notion that doctors carried some kind of infectious substance on their hands was laughed off as utter nonsense—to think there were tiny, invisible creatures covering surfaces and flying through the air spreading illness seemed absurd. And second, the idea that doctors had been responsible for their patients' suffering and death all along was impossible to believe, anathema to the image of physicians as saviors. "Doctors are gentlemen," said one prominent Philadelphia physician, "and a gentleman's hands are clean."

Semmelweis was mocked and threatened and eventually run out of the medical profession entirely. He reportedly took to stopping pregnant women in the street and urging them to "make sure your doctor washes his hands." Judged insane, he was committed to a psychiatric institution, where he died—quite possibly of the very same strain of sepsis that had once killed so many of his female patients.

Meanwhile, Pasteur, a French chemist, had also long suspected that the concept of "spontaneous generation" was off the mark. He noticed mold growing on bread, fermentation in wine, and milk not only spoiling but causing potentially fatal illnesses when it went bad and people drank it. He figured that it had to be something in the air causing these changes. He'd watched three of his children die from typhoid fever, one after the other. He believed that microorganisms all around us were contaminating foods, invading the human body, and causing illnesses. He just had to prove it. And in 1862, with his swan-neck flask experiment, he did.

Using a special flask with a long, narrow, S-shaped opening, he boiled a nutrient-rich broth to kill off any microorganisms. He then let the broth sit. Nothing happened—the broth remained clear. But when he tipped the flasks, letting the liquid run into the swan-neck and collecting the microbes that had been gathering there—settling in the opening of the flask along with dust and other microparticles—the broth turned cloudy, blooming with bacteria.

With the swan-neck flask experiment, Pasteur effectively debunked "spontaneous generation" and proved germ theory—exactly the concept that Semmelweis had fought so hard for. Like "spontaneous remission," the term "spontaneous generation"—once an accepted "fact" of medicine—turned out to be a sort of false container that was hiding a wealth of lifesaving knowledge. And in the years immediately following, a cascade of advancements helped solidify it: stronger microscopes were developed that could visualize the tiny, invisible creatures that had once just seemed like a crazy, improbable theory. It couldn't be denied anymore—germs were real.

The stories of Ignaz Semmelweis, Louis Pasteur, and the development of germ theory show us not only how reluctant the medical establishment was (and so often, still is!) to shift in response to new information but also what a profound effect germ theory had on public health. The discovery that microbes were the cause of the devastating infections and epidemics that routinely swept through human populations, killing off millions, was groundbreaking. Once researchers understood that bacteria and other microorganisms spread illness, they devoted themselves to developing public health standards, medications, and sterilization processes (like pasteurization) that could kill germs. Mortality rates from typhus, typhoid, cholera, and tuberculosis plummeted. Food and waterborne illnesses began to disappear. By the time the first antibiotics were being developed in the 1930s, life had changed drastically in just a handful of decades—women could expect to live through childbirth and see their children grow up.

It seemed we had unlocked the secret to health: *kill the germ.*

But at the same time, another scientist had been working on a germ theory of his own—an opposing one. Antoine Béchamp was a colleague of Pasteur's, and they didn't get along particularly well. The two men had clashed multiple times over the course of their careers, each accusing the other of plagiarism and theft, racing to make discoveries and announcements. Their rivalry grew even more bitter as germ theory gained wider acceptance and researchers began to work to develop chemical agents that could wipe out bacteria and stop the spread of infectious diseases.

Béchamp found Pasteur's "kill the germ at all costs" approach to be a dangerous proposition. He was one of the first to discuss what we now talk about as the microbiome. He believed that most microorganisms that lived in, on, and around the human body were beneficial, even symbiotic. Instead of taking a scorched-earth, take-no-prisoners approach to microbes, Béchamp urged physicians to focus on what he called the "inner terrain" of the human body. He maintained that when tissues are healthy, and not diseased, and when cells have the nutrients they need to function optimally, germs are unable to gain traction in the body. He compared the situation to a pile of excrement sitting on the ground, attracting flies. Do you keep swatting the flies away one by one, indefinitely? Or do you remove the pile of excrement? Establishing a foundation of health and vitality, free of toxins, and fostering a strong, balanced immune system, he argued, was more important than killing pathogens.

His friend and colleague Claude Bernard agreed—the *milieu intérieur,* or inner environment, was paramount. In a speech on the topic to a group of students and physicians, Bernard declared, "The terrain is everything; the germ is nothing." He then lifted a glass of water, contaminated with deadly cholera bacteria, and drank it down.

He didn't get sick, proving that his "terrain" was as healthy as he claimed it was.[13] He made his point—germs don't cause disease. Their ability to cause disease is a symptom of breakdown in the body.[14] But this didn't stop the tide of public opinion from flowing toward Pasteur's approach to medicine and away from his and Béchamp's. Theirs was a murkier proposition: that microbes could be both bad and good and that health depends on consistent, tending to the "soil" of the body, and not on "magic bullets" that could take out disease in an instant.

The argument boiled down to: Which mattered more, the soil or the microbe? Béchamp and Bernard said soil. Pasteur said microbe, and he won. Ambulances: 1. Guardrails: 0.

FROM "SILVER BULLET" TO "SUPERBUG"

As medicine swept forward into the twentieth century, we remained fixated on one task: *destroy the microbe.* Antibiotics came along and wiped out the infections that used to kill with impunity. Insulin was developed, and suddenly, survival was possible for children with type 1 diabetes—their whole lives opened up before them. It must have seemed like a miracle to the generation of people who had watched the "destroy the microbe" approach take down many of the terrifying serial killers of their era—typhus, typhoid, gonorrhea, syphilis, tuberculosis, diphtheria, and more. No wonder we've spent the last century searching for more of these silver bullets— the medications or other interventions that can take out illness in a single shot. But as much progress as we've made, we haven't been able to heal some of the most serious diseases out there, ones that continue to defy many of our current treatment models.

There are still many deadly blind spots in medicine today, holding us back from lifesaving progress in medicine. And one major holdover blind spot is that we continue to operate on a model of pathology: we fixate on tearing down disease at all costs instead of building up flourishing health and immunity. Since Pasteur's time, we have developed a philosophy of medicine that is primarily a science of disease rather than a science of health and vitality. We've become locked into this mode where destroying the microbe is our only tool—and we all know the adage "If the only tool you have is a hammer, everything gets treated like a nail."

We have been overprescribing antibiotics to patients at an alarming rate for decades now. That rate is finally beginning to slow, but it's late in the game, and we still aren't helping people create a healthy inner terrain. Plus, the overuse has already begun to take its toll. We know now, for example, that antibiotics increase a woman's risk of developing breast cancer. Studies found a strong link between repeated use of antibiotics and breast cancer— for women who had multiple courses of antibiotics before the age of eighteen, their risk had almost *doubled*. And it's a dose-response relationship: the more they used, the higher the risk. Researchers aren't sure exactly how antibiotics contribute to breast cancer, but guess that the antibiotics weaken the immune system and affect its ability to naturally combat mutating cancer cells. It's also possible that the antibiotics wipe out the microbiome, affecting the body's ability to digest and use nutrients that would aid in fighting off cancer before it takes root. Either way, it's clear that firing off what we've thought of as silver bullets at the first sign of trouble, instead of creating healthy immune systems and microbiomes, is costing us dearly. While we once thought there were no downsides to using an antibiotic "just in case," it turns out that we were dead wrong.

This is just one of the devastating consequences of chasing silver bullets. Harmful bacteria have also become increasingly resistant to the very antibiotics that were engineered to kill them. They've adapted and become stronger. Today, the CDC estimates that twenty-three thousand people die each year from antibiotic-resistant infections, when the antibiotics they are prescribed fail to work against the bacteria that have gained a foothold in their bodies. An additional fifteen thousand die from a specific bacterial infection called *Clostridium difficile* (*C. diff*), which can actually be *caused* by heavy antibiotic use. When antibiotics decimate the microbiome, they scrape away the good bacteria that have been helping protect the body from potentially lethal bacteria like *C. diff*. With the protective armor of the microbiome scraped away, *C. diff* moves in and flourishes.

And if all this isn't ominous enough, we recently saw the emergence of the first completely antibiotic-resistant superbug. In early 2017, a Nevada woman developed an infection that failed to respond to any of the increasingly strong antibiotics used by her doctors. There are twenty-six types of antibiotics available in the United States, and her medical team tried them all. None of them worked, and she died of her infection. We've gone full circle: there are now, once again, infections that are "incurable," just as there were before antibiotics were developed. And we're going to be seeing more and more of these incurable infections as the bacteria we've been coexisting with learn to dodge our silver bullets even more effectively. Over the course of a century of watershed advancements in medicine and technology, we've gone from "silver bullet" to "superbug."

One thing we forgot about in this sweeping march of progress:

the incredible potential of the human immune system. "If I could live my life over again," wrote Rudolf Virchow, who is now known as the Father of Pathology, "I would devote it to proving that germs seek their natural habitat—diseased tissue—rather than being the cause of the diseased tissue; e.g., mosquitoes seek the stagnant water, but do not cause the pool to become stagnant."

Imagine where medicine could be today if we had kept *both* Pasteur's and Béchamp's discoveries with us, holding Pasteur's knowledge in one hand and Béchamp's in the other? If we had put as much effort into building up health and immunity as we do into tearing down disease?

The Pasteur approach spurred progress in leaps and bounds, but we have reached the end of its effectiveness. It's time to turn in a different direction: back to Béchamp.

What we want is an immune system with well-nourished cells that are fast, smart, accurate, and ready to fight for us. We want our immune systems to be fully staffed, not depleted and sluggish, sending out sloppy troops that hit the wrong targets or are ineffective. We want our immune systems to have twenty-twenty vision, able to see viruses as they enter our bodies and rogue cells that threaten to mutate into cancer. The unfortunate truth is that a lot of us are walking around with immune systems that are chronically worn down. They are sluggish, exhausted, impeded by our poorly managed relationship with stress and nutrition. We are missing key positions in our army of fighter cells, leaving it sparse and thinned out. This leaves us more vulnerable not only to routine colds and flus but, as we will continue to see, to cancer, heart disease, diabetes, and a wide range of serious autoimmune disorders.

Spontaneous remissions give us enormous insight into how we can bolster our immune systems to prevent these diseases from taking hold, or roll back their damage if they already have. As new studies into the immune system emerge, I continue to notice how the kinds of things that stimulate natural killer cell activity line up with the kinds of changes that survivors of incurable diseases make before they experience their spontaneous healings. Certain diet changes, such as increasing one's nutritional level, turn out to support natural killer cell activity, as does reducing (or more effectively managing) stress. Studies even show *forgiveness* to be linked to a spike in natural killer cells.

It's easy to look at these new findings and leap to the conclusion that simply changing your meal plan or learning to meditate can spur your natural killer cells into action and turn off your disease like hitting a switch. But what my work with remarkable recoverers has taught me is that it's not that simple. There are no silver bullets or quick fixes with spontaneous healing. In fact, there is nothing spontaneous about spontaneous remission. In many cases, the stage had been set well before the "miraculous" remission occurred.

The best way to repair a cracked and ineffective immunological wall is to build health and vitality from the ground up. The body—if you can get out of its way—is a brilliant self-correcting organism that *wants* to get better. Cases of spontaneous remission, as unique and individual as they are, offer clues on how to get out of your body's way and give it everything it needs to build and maintain a thriving, *smart* immune system.

PREPARING THE SOIL FOR SPONTANEOUS HEALING

When Claire Haser (whom we met in the introduction) walked out of her doctor's office after declining the Whipple procedure recommended by her surgeon, she knew what she needed to do. She went home and began to prepare herself to die.

For Claire, that meant a couple of things. It meant facing her fear of death. It meant accepting that her life would end. It meant reaching out to her community of family and friends, surrounding herself with supportive people, deepening her relationships. She spent time working on forgiving people in her life. She let go of grudges. She didn't want to spend the time she had left on earth hating or resenting anyone. She didn't want to waste time being stressed and anxious, so she worked on responding differently to stressful situations. You can't change the world or eliminate stresses and worries completely, but you can change the way you interact with them, and that was her goal.

Early on, when she didn't know how much time she had left, she rented a beach house on the Oregon coast with all her closest friends, people she'd known since she was a kid. They made her cards, wrote messages about how they felt about her, and stood in a circle to present them to her. It was one of the most deeply moving experiences of her life.

"But it wasn't all so serious," she says now. "We had so much fun. We decorated cupcakes—pretty erotically, as I recall. We laughed ourselves silly for three straight days."

When Claire returned home to Portland after the weekend, the love and support of her friends was like a boat she coasted on.[15]

"I cannot stress how important it was," she says now. It helped her find the strength to make all the other changes in her life that she felt she had to make to live well while she was dying. It helped her resist the tendency to fall into a hole of hate or resentment, asking why this happened to her. It helped her "stay focused on the beautiful." She did deep breathing exercises every day to keep the fear at bay and keep herself calm and centered—*four seconds in, four seconds hold, four seconds out.*

She did change her diet gradually—she shifted toward foods that made her feel better and away from ones that seemed to keep her fatigued or uncomfortable or that caused the irritable bowel syndrome (IBS) symptoms she'd always struggled with to flare up. She noticed her diet getting cleaner, more plant-heavy. She eliminated sugar. But she kept certain things that she loved—pizza, coffee—because they made her happy.

"I was just trying to live well," she says. "I wasn't trying to save my life."

For months, she continued to feel worse. More exhaustion, more pain, more weakness and abdominal discomfort. Then it seemed to plateau. And then one day she realized she'd been feeling a little better lately. She expected it to be a brief reprieve—the eye at the middle of a hurricane. But she kept feeling better, stronger. It wasn't that she'd rebounded to the way she'd been before she got sick. The disease had been a kind of fire she'd walked through, and she'd been melted down and re-formed. She felt utterly changed. She had a completely new understanding of who she was and what she was doing in the world.

She didn't go back to the doctor to find out what was going on. She figured, why bother? Was she going to march back into those windowless waiting rooms that she'd vowed never to spend another minute in and demand to know why she wasn't dead yet?

For whatever reason, she'd been granted extra time—extra time in which she felt good. Healthier and healthier. She could enjoy life. So she did. And five years later, when a scan taken for another purpose showed her pancreas clean and free of tumors, she was as shocked as the doctors.

When I first interviewed Claire about the mysterious disappearance of her pancreatic cancer, the old feud over the importance of "the soil" came flooding back. Claire didn't know to what she should attribute her remarkable remission; she just knew that at some point between walking out of her surgeon's office and returning to the hospital years later for an unrelated issue, it had vanished. The profound changes that Claire made in her life were not made with the intent to cure herself; she fully expected pancreatic cancer to take her life. The changes she made were about living fully and more authentically with the time she had left. They were about confronting fears and other obstacles that had held her back from doing the things she really wanted to do. But perhaps this combination of factors—diet changes, lifestyle changes, and deep emotional and spiritual changes—had in fact altered the terrain of her body like nutrient-rich compost added to thin, barren dirt.

With cases of spontaneous remission, something shifts that allows the immune system to once again do its job. In several healing centers in Brazil, I'd witnessed a higher-than-usual rate of spontaneous remission. There was something about these healing centers that was allowing these deep, fundamental shifts to occur in the immune system so that healing could be unlocked. Perhaps they represented a cluster of cases for a phenomenon that is happening everywhere, invisibly, swallowed up by statistics and averages. In Abadiânia, for example, people ate nutrient-dense foods. They exercised and meditated. They left behind the stresses of their everyday lives. They turned inward and faced themselves: their fears, their forgotten dreams, their beliefs about themselves and the world they had never before questioned. They reinvented themselves, often completely rearranging the bedrock of their lives. They believed that healing was possible.

Somewhere in these physical, mental, and spiritual transformations that so many visitors experienced—and which were also described by other survivors who emailed me from around the country with their startling stories of recovery—there may lie the code to spontaneous healing: the precise combination of numbers that have to be punched in *together* to unlock the door to healing. I suspected that it couldn't all be boiled down to one single trigger but instead was a serendipitous combination of all the right factors that lined up to create a rare and "miraculous" phenomenon—like an eclipse.

Everything we put into our bodies affects our terrain. The foods we eat, the toxins that filter in, the medicines we take, the types of bacteria that colonize our bodies. Even thoughts, feelings, and beliefs about ourselves and the world affect the "soil" that are our immune systems. The strength of your team of natural killer cells and other disease-fighting cells within your immune system are linked not only to what you eat, how you exercise, and other lifestyle choices but also to how you manage stress, relationships, old traumas, what you believe, and how you see and understand yourself.

According to a biography of Pasteur written by his son-in-law, even "the father of germ theory" himself recanted during his final days. Suffering from the effects of a stroke, he knew his life was drawing to a close, and looking back over his life and career, reconsidered his stance.

"Bernard was right," he said, referring to Claude Bernard, the colleague of Béchamp's who, as the tales goes, drank the glass of cholera. "The pathogen is nothing; the terrain is everything."

THE TERRAIN IS EVERYTHING

Most people at the Casa had said they believed their healing to be divine intervention—the hand of God.

I didn't dismiss the possibility that these people's deep faith in the divine as they conceived it could be playing a large part in their remarkable recoveries; we are only in the early stages of studying the impact of deep psychological and spiritual experience on the physical body. As a psychiatrist, I knew that both the conscious and subconscious minds can impact the workings of the body, right down to its very cells and how they function. But if something was happening, then it was happening *within* the individual, deep in the biological systems and cells, in its mechanisms. And if it was happening, we should be able to detect that.

Well after my trip, I continued to hear from other people who hadn't made this type of pilgrimage to a healer or spiritual center and who nevertheless experienced the same type of spontaneous healing. What did the people who experienced healings in Brazil share with people who experienced healings elsewhere? I tried to look for common threads, but it was difficult to clear away the clutter in the stories to find the core truths. A cluster of people in Abadiânia, a single individual in Iowa, many cases without adequate medical documentation to support the claims, a historical case of sudden remission documented hundreds of years ago or in a medical journal two decades ago—among this broad array, a handful of similarities would appear, along with confounding differences.

What I couldn't find were randomized, double-blind, controlled studies on spontaneous remission—because they don't exist. This kind of study, in which neither the participants nor the researchers know who's receiving the treatment, is the gold standard of medicine, and they're great for evaluating the efficacy of different kinds of treatments, but spontaneous remission cannot be boxed in and controlled in this way. In the same way we can't predict who is going to be the next Steve Jobs or Elon Musk, the next Serena Williams or Tom Brady, it's impossible at this early stage in the research to predict who will be the person to break through to health and vitality when such is thought to be impossible or highly unlikely. It's not something that we can create or control for—yet.

Spontaneous remissions currently happen when nobody is looking—often, not even the patient. They occur when a patient has been treated to the end of the doctor's capacity to help and is then sent home on palliative care. They happen when people have resigned themselves to living with a disease with as much quality of life as possible, or even when they make plans to die. They happen when someone decides to take their health into their own hands and do something, because nothing else seems to have worked and, after all, "This is *my* life and no one else's." Or people make pilgrimages to alternative healing centers, where much attention is paid to their spiritual healing, but no physician is present to witness or document the changes in their physiology.

The recoveries I'd witnessed in Brazil should not have been possible. And the reasons that people there gave for their recoveries stretched the limits of what I could believe until they snapped. I became acutely aware of the gulf between cultures. For one thing, the culture in Brazil was much more accepting of the idea that powers of the mind and heart exist that we don't yet understand. As a product of Western culture, this was a hard concept for me to accept. At the same time, pushing it away felt wrong—like the opposite of good science.

I decided to go back to several healing centers in Brazil in 2004. I arrived quietly and didn't call ahead to say I was coming. The first time I'd gone down, I'd been both the observer and the observed—I'd gone with a detective mission, to investigate, to dig through medical records and sit in on surgeries. But I was also being filmed doing these things, performing the role of "doctor." It was difficult to understand what the experience of visiting these centers was really like when I had cast myself—and been cast—as an outsider, an anthropologist, a Harvard physician. This time, I wanted to be just a person—to experience what it was like to be a part of this community for a short time. Perhaps that would provide more understanding and more room for my own interpretation.

I did a handful of interviews while there, but mostly tried to be invisible and participate in the rhythms of the place. In Abadiâna, I sat in the "current rooms," a series of rooms in a U shape where participants meditated. I felt the pulse of energy that moved through the crowd like a heartbeat. There was something about being here, in the midst of a group of people who believed in miracles. I thought about how incredibly powerful it must be for people to come here and be immersed in community like this, so full of hope, so unshakable in the belief that healing was possible. But I had resolved to start by looking at the basics: How did people live while they were here? And how was it different from their "normal" lives?

Most visitors to Abadiânia stay in *pousadas*—small hotels run out of local residents' homes, which operate like large bed-and-breakfasts, with meals included. The food served was mostly vegetarian, full of bright, fresh colors that caught my eye every time I sat down to a meal. Perhaps hearkening back to my days on the farm, I've always had a hearty appetite, and I soon came to love the endless varieties of fabulous-tasting vegetable dishes and colorful tropical fruits. The meals served were dense in nutrients, light on refined carbohydrates and refined sugar, and largely free of animal products. The emphasis was clearly on natural, whole foods with little that was processed. Instead of gathering for cocktails, people met up at the open-air juice bars and shared their stories over tall glasses of mango, papaya, passion fruit, and guava, all of which flooded their bodies with a wide range of micronutrients. I particularly enjoyed the popular açai bowls, which are considered by many to be a superfood because of the purported high level of antioxidants. This was the kind of food that was thought to be medicine for the body, and the people who arrived looking for a miracle were eating it around the clock. For even the healthiest of eaters, it likely represented a significant shift in their eating habits. It certainly did for me.

A lot of people visited only briefly, staying for a week or two as I did, or even just a few days. But some stayed longer, for weeks, months, or even years. More than a few, deeply inspired by the place and the community, relocated to Brazil and stayed long term. Real estate and rents were cheap, and the exchange rate was good.

I thought about all the shifts and changes, both large and small, that would accompany such a drastic move to a community like this one. Not only the total immersion into a close-knit, faith-based community full of hope and mutual support but the accompanying lifestyle changes, including exercise (people walked everywhere), daily intensive group meditations, and yes, diet.

This is not to reduce what has happened to people in Brazil and elsewhere to a simple menu edit. Certainly that doesn't explain what happens for people who experience a dramatic remission after only brief visits. Plus, the vast majority of those I've spoken to about their remarkable remission will tell you that their recovery was about so much more than what they ate.

At the same time, Abadiânia was unique from the other Brazilian healing centers I visited because it drew international visitors. Many who traveled to Abadiânia to stay made immediate and drastic changes to their diet—simply by virtue of immersing themselves in a new and very different food culture. Perhaps people who were experiencing spontaneous healings elsewhere were able to make similarly dramatic changes on their own. One researcher, I discovered, had analyzed two hundred cases of spontaneous remission and reported that nearly 88 percent of people studied made dramatic nutritional changes, mostly to a vegetarian diet.[16] We can't skim over the importance of the sweeping lifestyle changes that survivors of incurable diseases tend to make when they're diagnosed, and nutrition is an important place to start.

Common sense would suggest that a significant change in one's nutritional level can be associated with a significant change in one's biochemistry, creating a bodily environment that's less hospitable to disease. After years of interviews and research, I have come to believe that, depending on its nutritional value, food can be medicine or it can be poison, and that although healing ultimately comes from a higher place than food, it's still not a small issue.

One of the most immediate, most impactful ways we can change our terrain is to look at what we put into it. Hippocrates, often called "the father of modern medicine," once said, "All disease begins in the gut." Perhaps health begins there, too—just as life can begin from a seed planted in soil.

3

Eat to Heal

The person who takes medicine must recover twice.
Once from the disease and once from the medicine.
—William Osler, M.D.

Imagine your body, for a moment, as a garden. Most gardeners will tell you that you need to cultivate the soil carefully. You need to turn it, aerate it, add fertilizer and the right amount of moisture. If you really want to be successful, you need to address its pH, need for nutrients, and even beneficial microorganisms. Sometimes it's important to evaluate for toxins such as lead. And gardens vary widely, which means they often need different things. The makeup of soil changes from garden to garden. An intervention that is beneficial to one garden might not be for the one next door. Some need more nitrogen or phosphorus, some less. Some need compost, others need lime to shift the pH.

Now think of the microbiome, which we talked about in the previous chapter. The microbiome of your gut is a *literal* garden, the living microculture that can determine how you process and react to foods and nutrients, and it has immense power over your health. Just as gardens can be different from one yard to another, we each have a unique microbiome, depending on what part of the world our ancestors came from, what kinds of foods both we and our parents have tended to eat, and how well cultivated we are when it comes to our relationship with stress and emotional nutrition. As we discussed, the microbiome has long been underestimated, but it is emerging as a leading field of research with the potential to transform our approach to health and medicine. Some researchers believe that learning about and making adjustments to your microbiome may be the key to turning around the trajectory of many diseases.

I grew up tending crops on the farm. I know that a good yield for the harvest doesn't come from randomly tossing seeds and hoping for the best. Yet many of us, myself included for many years, treat our bodies with little consideration or respect as if it's a garbage pit—not paying much attention to the makeup of the soil or doing anything to care for it. We fill it with junk and just hope for the best. Sometimes we get lucky. Usually we don't, but by the time we realize this, there's a lot of work to be undone and not a lot to help us find our way back.

Imagine how much more success we might have if we cared for and fine-tuned our soil—especially that of our microbiomes—by treating our bodies with love and gratitude, making them as healthy as possible. Anything less seems like self-sabotage, really; our bodies are our vehicles, our vessels of transport, and they are deserving of our respect.

Every day, we are bombarded with conflicting messages about what we should eat. What is "proven" by one study to be healthy is then immediately proven to be unhealthy. Publishing cycles seem to run on the next diet fad, soon to be replaced by another. Patients ask me constantly what they should and shouldn't eat, saying that all the books seem to contradict one another. We flip-flop from year to year on everything from red wine to coffee to fish and red meat. The food pyramid says one thing. Nutritionists and doctors say something else. The new book you just bought says something completely different. When individual nutrients are found to have health benefits—omega 3s, for example—health writers will crow about the miraculous effects of eating walnuts. And when a famous actress or athlete publishes a book about nutrition, a doctor will often criticize some aspect of the nutritional plan but fail to understand or see the overall big picture. Yes, eating walnuts *is* good for you, but this fixation on the perceived healthiness of specific individual foods or nutrients keeps us from seeing the forest for the trees. A healing nutritional plan isn't about counting calories, eating certain proportions of the major food groups, or adding and subtracting certain nutrients. It's about gaining a big-picture, sustainable approach to food that isn't about "hot" foods or fad diets.

In his excellent 2008 book, *In Defense of Food,* Michael Pollan laid out his entire case in the opening sentences of the book: "Eat food. Not too much. Mostly plants." By "Eat food," he meant to eat the kind of food that your grandmother would've recognized as food—simple whole foods that are natural enough to decay when not fresh, unlike the processed foods that will look and taste the same a year—or a decade—from now. He admitted in the next paragraph that this was the entirety of his message, joking that reading the rest of the book wasn't strictly necessary—all the reader really needed to hear to drastically improve their health and well-being were those first seven words. The book goes on to make an impassioned plea to all of us to drastically change our eating habits and our ingrained ideas about food and health.

I remember reading that book, being struck by the simplicity and truth of that opening statement—*Eat food. Not too much. Mostly plants*—and then failing to make any real change to my own diet. At the time, I didn't have the motivation or wherewithal to make such a dramatic change and stick to it. It was just easier to remain unconscious and do what most others seemed to be doing around me. Brownies, pizza, and cookies were ubiquitous in my busy life, available at nursing stations, easy to eat between meetings or as snacks throughout the day. What's true is that what we eat, along with most of our daily habits and addictions, is deeply ingrained in us and is shaped by our families, our cultures, what's most available where we live, the logistics of our lives. Often, it takes something dramatic happening—like an illness—for us to wake up and decide to change. Perhaps what's unique about healing centers in Brazil is that when you go there to stay, changing your diet is almost effortless; it's built into the community and culture.

When I returned home from Brazil, I went back to my job with its long hours, where I barely had time to step away to grab a slice of cold pizza from the nurses' station, much less cook the nutrient-rich, medicinal meals I'd eaten in Brazil. And because I didn't eat "too much," I thought I was doing okay. In med school, we'd been taught that the developed world suffered from *overnutrition* rather than malnutrition—when in fact, so much of what we eat is empty of nutrition that the opposite is true.[1] It's difficult to make changes alone. So I continued to not think much about what I ate; it wasn't a priority. My patients were the priority, and there was a long line of them waiting to be seen. My career came first. In the medical profession, it's easy to get into this kind of pattern. You're so busy taking care of other people, you don't take care of yourself. I barely noticed at first, but my numbers were creeping up—weight, cholesterol, blood pressure. I rationalized it away, promising myself that I'd make a change soon, when I wasn't so busy.

As the months scrolled by, I noticed a pattern of people making diet changes once they were diagnosed with a disease. But those changes varied widely. When I heard from Claire for the first time, she said that changing her diet was the first thing she'd done. She'd discovered in her research that salt was especially bad for patients with pancreatic cancer. *You wouldn't believe how fast I got salt out of my diet,* she wrote. *Fear is a powerful motivator!*

But she also mentioned that while she took out most processed and salty foods, gravitating toward a whole-foods diet, she also left in some things that she really enjoyed that on a strict "anticancer diet" would not be allowed. I noticed this in others as well. A Pilates instructor in Florida with a dangerous lymphoma dramatically increased the nutritional quality in her life but retained her nightly glass of wine. Another person loved cheese and continued to enjoy it but otherwise eliminated refined carbohydrates and animal products.

One man with gastric carcinoma almost exclusively ate meat and took supplements. Over a span of fifteen years, I saw many people make improbable recoveries, but considerable variation existed in the changes they made regarding food. I saw up close how it's not "one size fits all" when it comes to food and nutrition, though certain clear trends existed.

A young man in Britain, Pablo Kelly, wrote out of the blue to tell me of the success he was having shrinking his glioblastoma multiforme. As we saw earlier, this type of brain cancer has historically been untreatable and is always fatal. The five-year survival rate—a good measure of the deadliness of any given disease—is an extremely low 2 to 5 percent. Most people die within six months. Yet Pablo's tumor was doing what is considered impossible for this particular type of cancer—shrinking instead of progressing. His doctors were baffled, and he'd been written up already in a number of British publications. He told me that he attributed his success to a ketogenic diet, which he'd been incredibly strict about—no "cheating" to leave in foods that he loved, as Claire had done. Low in carbs and high in fats, the ketogenic diet encourages the body to enter a state of ketosis where it burns its own fats.

Normally, the body converts the carbohydrates that we eat into glucose, which is used as fuel for the body and the brain. But cancer loves glucose; this is what it feeds on more than anything else. In fact, doctors routinely find cancer by injecting radiolabeled glucose into a patient's body and then putting her or him into a scanner to see if any part of the body is avidly sucking up the glucose. Pablo did a lot of research and decided that he was going to try "starving the cancer to death." And he is right that the ketogenic diet is thought by some researchers to starve cancer cells of the nutrients they need to grow. But we don't know the long-term effects of a high-fat diet yet, and there are big differences between high- and low-quality fats. It's also considered risky for a person who is already ill to undertake such a strict diet, and most doctors don't recommend it. It should only be done under medical supervision when it is done, and with a strict diet such as this, one needs to be very disciplined about obtaining certain vitamins and minerals through supplements. Pablo, however, did meticulous research and carried out his plan with dedication—and also with attention to his positive psychological health and attitude. Against all odds, he is alive and improving long after he was supposed to be dead.

I also met with Juniper Stein—whose case I'll discuss in the next chapter—a woman who recovered from a progressive and incurable form of arthritis called ankylosing spondylitis. Sitting in Central Park in New York City, with the trees rustling around us and the distant rush of traffic, the lithe, vibrant woman in front of me described how she and her husband made dramatic dietary changes years earlier following her diagnosis. Since then, they had come to recognize that those changes had created a healthier microbiome.

Mirae Bunnell, whom I interviewed by phone after reviewing the CAT scans of her metastatic melanoma—which surely should have killed her—talked both about cleaning up her diet and also about her relationship with food. She saw her terminal diagnosis as a "wake-up call" from her body.

"My body said to me, 'You've been treating me like crap for years. You've been throwing caffeine and alcohol at me, no sleep, eating like a racehorse.' My body said, 'I'm done.'"

Describing the kinds of changes she made, Mirae focused on the *process* of eating.

"I realized that I needed to really think about the food I was eating," she said. "I needed to slow it down. Focus on the nutrition that was flowing into my body." Others spoke of learning to eat with gratitude, and some said that making healthy changes from a place of fear is worthless, even destructive. The *how* and *why* of healthy eating are as important as the *what*.

The ways that people changed their diets before an improbable recovery initially seemed vastly different. When I looked at the people I'd interviewed or corresponded with as a group, it was like looking at the cookbook section at a bookstore—every fad diet under the sun seemed to be represented. Were there any common threads?

Wanting to drill down beneath the surface of fad diets and

health benefits, I reached out to colleagues in the field of medicine and nutrition to ask if they were aware of any cases of spontaneous healing that hinged mostly or completely on diet. One wrote back: *You have to talk to Tom Wood.*

A LIFE-CHANGING EMAIL

Tom Wood is a detail-oriented person. When I first reached out to him, he replied back from his work email—he runs a consulting firm on the East Coast—with extensive records documenting his multi-decade struggle with diabetes. I could see the fluctuations and overall trends for his blood sugars across a span of many years. His record keeping was impeccable.

In conversation, he is similarly thorough. He's also confident and at ease discussing his health and body—like most of the people I've spoken with over the years, he has become accustomed to thinking and talking about his health and what he believes is helpful and not so helpful from the medical system as it is currently designed. His voice when he speaks on the subject is weary but warm. As always, the story is a long one, and there is much to say. When I ask him to tell me his story, he lets out a long breath.

"How much time have you got?" he says, laughing.

He asks where he should start. I answer simply, "The beginning."

Whenever I ask people to start at "the beginning," they tend to go back to the same place: not when they were sick or back further to when they were diagnosed, or even further back to when they were healthy. They go back all the way to their childhoods. I don't have to ask them to. Something in them knows intuitively that the true roots of their stories are there. And no matter what the disease process is, it's always about the story.

Tom always thought of himself as a healthy person. It was part of his identity and had been since he was a kid growing up in Ithaca, New York, where in high school he captained the intramural soccer and tennis teams. His father was director of athletics at Ithaca College, and they were always doing something physical together as a family—hiking, biking, being outdoors.

He carried that love of activity instilled by his upbringing into his adult years. After he finished college at Cornell, he found an office job that paid well and moved downstate. He married, and not long after that, he and his wife had a son. He ended up running his own company that offered recruiting, staffing, and consulting services. He was well on his way to a happy and successful life. He set his alarm early every morning, drove to the gym in the chilly dark, the pink sunrise just seeping into the sky, to get in a racquetball game before work. He lifted weights, jogged on the treadmill. At lunchtime, he drove to the fast-food restaurant near his office to get a burger, fries, and a Coke.

He says now, a little ruefully, "I ate more Burger King than anyone alive."

The years swept by like a river—he was busy at work, his son was growing up too fast. His weight started to go up. Intermittent back pain came and went. He tried some diets, including the Atkins—he'd lose a few pounds, enough to feel slightly encouraged, then gain it back. He wasn't terribly overweight, but he was heavier than he used to be. He felt his age, and it wore on him.

Then one Friday afternoon, coming home on the train from a meeting in the city, he started to feel that something wasn't right. All day, he'd been feeling run-down and out of sorts but had assumed he was just tired. Driving home from the train station, his chest began to well up with pain. A band tightened around his rib cage, and his left arm started to tingle. Recognizing the signs of a heart attack, he turned off his route home and drove himself straight to the hospital.

"They took me right in," he says, "and stuck one of those beautiful gowns on me. Slapped on an EKG. I was on it for hours."

By 11:00 that night, the doctors had found what they thought was the source of the problem: one of the blood tests had revealed a protein that is released into the bloodstream when the heart muscle is damaged. It was high, about four or five times above what it should have been. So there it was: a cardiac event. They suspected artery blockage.

A needle catheterization was scheduled for first thing Monday morning. They threaded the catheter through the femoral artery up to his heart. He was awake, under local anesthesia, as they began the procedure. He could see on the screen as the catheter reached his heart and released a squirt of dye into the bloodstream. An x-ray image tracked the dye as it flowed through the arteries of his heart, allowing the doctors to see any areas of narrowing or blockage. Based on his test results, they anticipated significant blockage. But the catheterization results were surprising—he had less than 5 percent blockage, great for a man his age.

They wheeled him back to his room—and back to the drawing board. It was a nurse who finally walked in with the necessary clue, holding a readout, clearly a little irritated that nobody had figured this out yet.

"Excuse me!" she said. "Do you realize he's running a blood sugar of 300?"

A follow-up blood panel revealed the true culprit: type 2 diabetes.[2] Tom had insulin resistance. Insulin, a hormone that helps drive glucose from the bloodstream into cells where it can be used for energy, was having difficulty doing its job. This is called *insulin resistance,* and it is different from type 1 diabetes, where the cells in the pancreas aren't able to make enough insulin for the body's needs. In Tom's case, since the insulin was prevented from doing its job, blood sugar was building up in his system with nowhere to go, causing a number of harmful changes in the structure and function of his heart.

Type 2 diabetes, untreated, leads to heart failure, kidney damage, blindness, stroke, and amputations, among other problems. Ninety-five percent of new cases of diabetes are type 2, and it's the seventh-leading cause of death each year. The CDC reports that a staggering 20 percent of spending in health care in the United States is on diabetes alone. The day that Tom Wood drove himself to the ER with what he thought was a heart attack, he became one of the 422 million people worldwide known to be suffering from diabetes.[3] Experts estimate that eighty million Americans over the age of twenty have prediabetes and report that one in four people have diabetes but don't know it. And rates have been climbing stratospherically in recent decades, not only in the United States and developed nations but all around the world.[4]

In practical terms, type 2 diabetes is treated as an incurable illness—thought of as irreversible and progressive. If caught early enough, some doctors will encourage diet changes, exercise, and weight loss to help slow or mitigate the symptoms, but usually only as an afterthought. And misunderstandings about genuine nutrition abound, not only in patients but also in doctors and nutritionists. Our usual approach to this disease (along with most other chronic illnesses that come through our waiting room doors) is to "treat 'em and street 'em"—basically, make an accurate diagnosis, start a medication, and then discharge to home.

It seemed to Tom that the approach to diabetes hadn't changed much in the past fifty years. His mother had been diagnosed with diabetes when he was a kid, but she continued to cook the same classic 1950s foods, heavy on carbs and starches. One day, as a teenager, standing in the kitchen, he noticed her lift her shirt to give herself an insulin shot. He realized she'd been doing it for years.

"The attitude was that taking insulin was just as good as making your own insulin," he says. "It was basically the same when I was diagnosed." It's true that our ability to provide insulin to people with diabetes, starting in 1922, was a game changer for medicine. That year, a fourteen-year-old boy named Leonard Thompson was given the first ever dose of artificial insulin made for human treatment. As a type 1 diabetic in that era, he typically would have been placed on a starvation diet and would have had only months to live. He lived for another thirteen years.

The discovery of insulin has saved millions of lives and played its own role in prompting medicine's search for "magic bullets" that would eradicate disease and suffering. But as a new era opens in medicine, built on both the successes and limitations of the old, we now know more clearly that medications like insulin treat symptoms but not causes. In the case of type 2 diabetes, the insulin resistance remains, even as we treat a patient. Nothing really gets better if the causes aren't addressed; one is left treading water at best. With diabetes, disease progression often continues, and therefore one often still ends up with a painful and progressive disease course involving damage to multiple organs, physical pain, and a sharply diminished quality of life. If what Tom's mother experienced was similar to what we often see, what she called "aging" was actually the progression of the diabetes and, perhaps, other illnesses that are often associated.

True to form, Tom's diabetes progressed. He was placed first on metformin, a drug that attempts to convince your body to use insulin more effectively, but when that began to fail, he was switched to regular shots of insulin, which he took before meals, snacks, and bed. In total, he took approximately forty-five units of insulin per day for the next decade. One problem with taking insulin is that it causes weight gain, which worsens insulin resistance, which then causes even higher blood sugars, causing more insulin to be needed. And so the spiral continued; Tom's weight crept up, he stopped working out, he developed chronic back pain.

"I couldn't walk one hundred feet through a mall," he says. "I was in bad shape."

Now, we need to understand: Tom was a smart guy. He was an Ivy League grad and president of a company, had long valued exercise, and had many resources available to him. He had prided himself on not only seeing the best endocrinologists but on seeing the best endocrinologists who treated only diabetes. He said that he had seen perhaps twenty to twenty-five doctors total, including at least eight of these highly specialized diabetes experts over a period of fifteen or more years. And, disciplined and numbers-oriented by nature, he had been more rigorous than most about monitoring and treating his blood sugar as directed. Yet in spite of all this, his blood glucose readings were through the roof—the efficacy of the medication he'd been pumping into his body for fifteen years was wearing thin. He developed a cataract in one eye, and his feet went numb: diabetic neuropathy. And he was increasingly at risk for the common comorbidities—the ever-threatening complications that occur in conjunction with diabetes like heart disease, kidney problems, eye damage, even cancer.

It was the weekend after Thanksgiving 2014, when an email swooshed into Tom's in-box. Glancing at it, he immediately saw that it was spam, an advertisement promising to turn his life around. If he signed up today, the message urged, he would receive the secrets of their "special diet," lose weight, and be off his diabetes medication and showing normal biomarkers within a month! Tom hovered his mouse over the Delete button, but the money-back guarantee caught his eye. He was tired of being sick. He was tired of the continual shots every day, the chronic pain, extra weight, of feeling like each day was a struggle. He read the message again. "Change your diet, change your life! Only $39.95!" The program was four weeks long. It included a promise: if at the end of four weeks he wasn't nondiabetic and off his medications, he could have his money back.

What the hell, he thought. *What do I have to lose?*

He punched in his credit card number and downloaded the instructions. The meal plan included no meat and no dairy. The list of foods he'd be able to eat—mostly vegetables, fruits, and beans—looked long and full of options at first glance, but Tom was at a loss. A lot of them were things he'd never eaten or things he didn't know how to prepare. But he was in for forty bucks, and he figured he could do anything for a month.

Four weeks later, Tom had dropped ten pounds. He'd cut his diabetes medications in half. He felt more energetic, lighter on his feet. He wasn't completely off his insulin, though, as the program had guaranteed. Still a little suspicious of the program and its promises, he called the company. They refunded his money.

But he was impressed. In just four weeks, he had eliminated half his medications and dropped weight for the first time in decades, through nothing more than adjusting the ratio of food types he put on his plate at each meal. How could such relatively modest changes in diet and almost no increase in exercise change his body and his blood sugar so drastically?

He started researching diet and diabetes in depth. He discovered

The End of Diabetes by Dr. Joel Fuhrman. Tom and his wife both read the book. For the first time in years, he felt a tingling of energy and hope, the possibility of truly revolutionizing his health and life. He launched into the program with the support of his wife, who joined him in both the diet and the cooking. Initially, it felt like a lot to learn. But in some ways, it was much easier than the calorie counting that is recommended by many doctors and the American Diabetes Association. Dr. Fuhrman focuses simply on making sure people are eating the foods loaded with the highest percentage of vitamins, minerals, and phytochemicals, rather than counting calories or paying attention to food groups. There are lists of "unlimited" foods you can eat anytime, and food is organized into tiers, based on their nutritional density.

What is nutritional density? According to Fuhrman (and, in fact, the World Health Organization), nutritionally dense foods are loaded with vitamins, minerals, and phytochemicals, but low in calories. They are low in sugar and refined carbs, salt, starches, and unhealthy fats. Included are fruit and vegetables, fish, whole grains, nuts, legumes, seeds, and small amounts of chemical-free fish and lean meats. Dr. Fuhrman created ANDI—the Aggregate Nutritional Density Index—to help patients construct a diet that is high in nutrient-dense foods. The index can easily be found online and provides a great visual aid to use for internalizing the concept of nutritional density and begin building your diet around it. It's hard starting out, when you have to analyze each meal and each choice that you make—you might need to frequently reference the ANDI and do the creative work of learning new recipes and habits. But with use, it does become second nature.

The ANDI will probably change as the science of phytochemicals takes off,[5] but as it currently stands, it's absolutely a better tool for health and healing than the food pyramid most of us were brought up with. Zoom out, and essentially the nutrition plan boils down to this: eat mostly vegetables. Tom didn't completely eliminate foods like pasta, bread, meat, and dairy, but he drastically reduced his intake of those foods to *less than 5 percent of calories consumed.* He essentially turned his diet upside down, making fresh fruits and vegetables the base of his personal food pyramid.

It worked. As of this writing, Tom has been completely non-diabetic, without medication, for almost three years. He's remained on Dr. Fuhrman's antidiabetic nutritional plan ever since finding it after that trial promo in Thanksgiving 2014. He says he "stuffs himself" with what Dr. Fuhrman calls "nutritarian meals"—a daily menu organized around great-tasting, high-nutrient eating. It mostly consists of beans, green veggies, nuts and seeds, and berries—a lot like the meals I ate in Brazil. "I'm never hungry," Tom says. "I wouldn't go back to my old way of eating for anything."

But does he cheat, every once in a while? Does he have a piece of cake?

"Very rarely, almost never," he says. "I don't feel the compulsion to do it. The cravings for the foods I used to eat were gone after the first month."

So many of the people I've spoken with say their taste buds have come alive again upon changing their diets. They find that the nutritional lifestyle is no longer difficult once you start following it, and the benefits are so tangible and life-changing that nothing could prompt them to return to the old foods. Fruits and vegetables can be prepared in fabulous ways, though most of us start off not realizing how to do this and not realizing it doesn't need to be costly or time-consuming. In this case, ignorance is decidedly not bliss. Even eating out is fine, once one knows how to recognize what has nutritional density and what does not.

Notice how Tom uses the language of addiction above: "I don't feel the *compulsion* to do it. The *cravings* . . . were gone." This language is important, and people often use similar language when, in retrospect, they talk about the nutritional changes they have made. They say they had felt addicted to refined flours and sugars in general, and it's these habits that make the transition to food with a higher nutritional density initially difficult. It's not uncommon for people to experience headaches and other temporary symptoms as the body goes through a detox from years of accumulated toxins.

Tom is healthier now than he has ever been. Whereas before he couldn't walk a hundred feet without doubling over in pain, now he walks three miles each day with no pain at all. Now in his seventies, he is lean, flexible, and without any trace of the diabetes that ravaged his body for more than fifteen years.

Tom's doctor, an endocrinologist, has been shocked by his progress. A few years ago, she had him come in for lab tests, nervous that he might be neglecting his illness. She walked into the exam room holding his file, looking at the current lab report, then at the one from the previous year, when he was still taking forty-five units of insulin per day, shaking her head.

"I can't count how many patients I've had in my career," she said, "but in the past twenty years, I've never seen anybody do this."

Tom's story resonated with me. Like Tom, I'd always thought of my diet as generally healthy, other than the junk I ate occasionally while busy at work. But for the most part, I thought of myself as making pretty good choices around food, and I didn't pay attention to how often I simply ate what was around. And I've noticed that other people do the same. As a doctor, I ask what people eat, and often see what is on their hospital trays. The truth is, almost everyone thinks they eat healthy, even though they don't.

Growing up on a farm, with that Amish mentality, we ate all home-cooked meals. We never had takeout or packaged foods. My mother made nearly everything from scratch; she even ground the wheat we grew on the farm to make her own flour for baking bread, pancakes, and muffins. We ate meat at nearly every meal, often three times a day. We also ate a lot of heavy carbs like bread and potatoes. I replicated many of these eating patterns into adulthood, and with college added the chips, cookies, and snacks of modern life. I still held on to the traditional food pyramid, with animal products like meat and dairy occupying large structural stripes holding the pyramid up. The message was, they were essential. The pyramid would collapse without them.

Ironically, it was med school more than any other place that encouraged terrible eating habits. We ate what was convenient, fast, and filling. We ate on the go, as an afterthought—fast food, takeout, things out of packages and boxes. In medical school, you take in an immense amount of information. The schedule is relentless, and nutrition was rarely addressed in the curriculum. When it was, we failed to make the larger connections that would have emphasized how important it was to put these lines from the textbook into practice.

My fellow students and I sat together in class, memorizing chemical and neurochemical equations that required certain vitamins and minerals at key points to complete important chemical reactions in the body and brain. But then the professor would blithely say that in Western cultures people receive plenty of nutrition, and we would move on. We got up, walked out, and ate pizza and chips for dinner, in the middle of the night, in between study sessions. On tests, we checked boxes to answer questions about how the absence or presence of certain nutrients in the bloodstream could affect the brain's ability to produce neurotransmitters like serotonin, dopamine, or acetylcholine. And yet now, when someone comes into a doctor's office with an issue, most of us don't think to ask, "What are you eating?" It makes sense that if you put the wrong type of gas into your car, sooner or later, the car is going to have problems. Could our mind and bodies really be any different?

After Brazil, and after listening to story after story of those who had experienced healing, I began to realize that I also needed to make some major changes, before I found myself fighting one or more of the many illnesses I was seeing in these cases. I knew that I would have to custom-design a nutritional plan to work for me—like Tom, Claire, Juniper, and so many other people who experienced remarkable recoveries had done. Claire in particular emphasized how individual it must be. On her excellent blog, *Living with Pancreatic Cancer,* where she chronicles her journey to recovery, Claire tells a story about sharing details of her own diet changes early on in her blogging experience. Shortly after she had launched the blog in an effort to reach out to other sick people who were suffering, a woman wrote to her, asking for more detail on Claire's diet. She gave it, generously I'm sure—Claire is as generous, open, and giving a person as you can find. The woman replied to say she had gone out and bought all the items Claire listed and would follow in her footsteps exactly. Sometime later, she died.

From then on, Claire has made it a rule not to share the specific menu that she followed after her diagnosis.

"Obviously what worked for me didn't work for her," she writes. "I believe that each of us responds to and needs different things. . . . I don't believe there's any one thing, any silver bullet out there for everyone. We need to find out what works for us individually."[6]

What she is comfortable sharing is that she eliminated refined flours and sugar, as well as processed foods and additives (food coloring, preservatives, etc.). Unlike some, she left in a moderate amount of organic meat and dairy. Her overarching rule that she used as a touchstone: eat fresh and seasonally.

There were certainly some common truths emerging from the stories of remission I was collecting, but they were broad strokes, not specific rules. The repeating echoes were: eat fresh, eat plants, eat whole foods, and don't put refined sugar and flours, or anything processed or artificial, into your body. This lined up with research I was seeing that indicated that cancer cells, just like bacteria and fungi, "feed" and grow avidly on their favorite food—refined sugar in the bloodstream—and that the chemicals and additives present in processed foods can serve as disruptors that let cancer and other diseases get a toehold in your body.

A study with mice at Georgia State University[7] revealed a disturbing correlation between emulsifiers, a very common additive, and cancer. Emulsifiers like carboxymethylcellulose and polysorbate-80—just to name two—are ubiquitously present in processed foods, in everything from mayonnaise to ice cream. They are added frequently to grocery products to extend the shelf life of these foods and "improve the mouthfeel," as those in the food science industry are fond of saying. The FDA puts limits of how much of any one emulsifier can go in a product, but many companies dodge this by using different *types* of emulsifiers—each one a distinct chemical compound. This is technically allowed, but it adds more potential chemical disruptors to the foodstuffs we pull off the shelf and into our baskets. Once in our bodies, the emulsifiers—having ridden in on the processed breads and meats we eat, the salad dressing and sauces, and more—disperse through our digestive tract and unbalance the microbiome—that delicate, flourishing ecosystem in our guts.

The Georgia State study and others suggest that by disrupting the microbiome and triggering chronic inflammation, emulsifiers may contribute to weight gain, inflammatory illnesses, autoimmune disorders, and even cancer.

It can be hard to imagine how such a tiny, microscopic chemical element in a food product—a tiny portion of the overall item—could be responsible for such a wave of illnesses. But when I think about how regularly I used to consume such products—really at every meal (along with my salad, potatoes, and grilled chicken), it's not so surprising after all. It's like a tiny pebble that slips into your boot and rubs your whole heel raw. And this is just *one* of the many chemical additives that you might encounter in a typical food product that you pull off the shelf at your local grocery store.

I saw how these broad guidelines on basing my diet around fresh, green, whole foods could serve as a template for me as I developed an individual diet that satisfied me and turned food into a daily medicine for my body—while noting they ran completely contrary to the way that most of us are taught to eat. For evidence, I didn't need to look much further than the most comprehensive study of nutrition ever conducted.

LESSONS FROM A CANCER-RESISTANT COUNTRY

Around the time that Tom Wood was graduating from Cornell—about to embark on his career and unaware of how his diet might alter the function of his cells—a new professor arrived and joined the Division of Nutritional Sciences right there at the very same university. T. Colin Campbell had been teaching and researching nutrition and biochemistry at Virginia Tech for the previous ten years and was rapidly developing an interest in the link between diet and disease. This wasn't something that was being talked about at the time, but mounting evidence had Campbell convinced that it was a dangerously understudied subject. He was fresh from an experience in the Philippines, working on childhood malnutrition, and what he found had already changed the course of his career.

While there, he'd stumbled, almost accidentally, on a link between the consumption of animal protein and cancer. While working with families across the country to combat the effects of a devastating epidemic of malnutrition, he'd discovered that Filipino children were dying of liver cancer at an alarming rate. Usually, liver cancer doesn't occur until much later in adulthood, yet many Filipino children were succumbing by the age of ten. Campbell and his colleagues were initially able to trace this phenomenon to a contaminant in the nation's supply of peanut butter: aflatoxin, a highly toxic carcinogen produced by a type of fungi that grows on peanuts under certain conditions. Aflatoxin, according to Campbell, is "the most potent liver carcinogen known."[8]

This seemed to explain the problem, but there was a confounding detail. By a vast margin, the children developing liver cancer were from the wealthiest communities, while the ones from poorer areas seemed to escape it completely—even though both groups regularly consumed the contaminated peanut products.

Campbell was finally able to home in on one major lifestyle difference: the wealthier children ate diets rich in meat and dairy, similar to a Western diet. The less privileged, unable to afford such foods, did not. It suggested a link between the consumption of animal protein—meat and dairy, long the staples of the Western diet—and cancer, which Campbell wasn't quite prepared to believe. He'd been operating off a long-held belief in the scientific community that it was protein *deficiency* that opened the door to cancer and other diseases. But then Campbell happened across a new study out of India, published in an obscure medical journal. In the study, two groups of laboratory rats had been exposed to the aflatoxin that he'd found in the Filipino peanut butter to predispose them to developing liver cancer. One group was then given a diet high in casein—a naturally occurring protein in mammalian milk—while the other received very little. Every animal in the first group developed cancer or precursor lesions that would become cancer. In the second group, zero.

"It was not a trivial difference," Campbell writes of the obscure experiment that changed the course of his career, "it was 100% vs. 0%."[9]

Still, Campbell was not completely convinced. Perhaps the researchers had somehow transposed the two groups? Returning home, he carefully ran his own version of the study and obtained identical results.[10]

After that, Campbell fixed his sights on the link between diet and disease. In 1980, a senior researcher with China's centers for disease control named Dr. Junshi Chen visited him in his office at Cornell to discuss the possibility of doing a very small study on the link between the mineral selenium and cancer. But as they talked, the very small study quickly began to blossom into something much larger.

The profile of China at that time was unique, and it was ideal for research. First of all, it was an enormous country. The population would reach about 1.2 billion in that decade, representing a third of the globe's total inhabitants. Second, there was very little geographical mobility—97 percent of the populace had been born in the same county where they currently lived. From a research standpoint, this was paradise: a huge, homogenous population where nearly everyone lived where they were born. This dramatically limits confounding variables and other potential influences. And third, food production and consumption were highly localized. As opposed to a place like the United States or other Western countries, where goods were rapidly transported and meals looked pretty much alike from one coast to the other, meals in China were highly distinctive and determined by geography. This perfect storm of factors led Banoo Parpia, chief coordinator of the project, to call the China of the mid-1980s "a vast human laboratory."[11]

There was an additional factor that made China a potential

treasure trove of information about the origins of disease. About five years earlier, as the Chinese premier Zhou Enlai lay dying of cancer, he initiated a massive nationwide survey of 880 million people—98 percent of the population—to collect data on death rates for twelve different kinds of cancer. The landmark survey was called the most ambitious biomedical research project ever achieved. It resulted in a color-coded atlas revealing where certain types of cancer were prominent and also where they were nearly nonexistent. It revealed that counties with the highest rates of some cancers had rates that were more than one hundred times greater than those counties with the lowest rates. While intense politics and huge amounts of research and public interest are generated by small differences in cancer rates between different areas of the United States, this study revealed that some parts of China had cancer rates one hundred times (10,000 percent) lower than others.

The wide variations could not be explained away by genetics. China at the time was highly ethnically homogenous—87 percent of the population in the study were of the same ethnic group. This meant that the cancer triggers were not due to genes—they were due to environment. Disease was not destiny; it was within our control.

This was the landscape that T. Colin Campbell, Junshi Chen, and their team of researchers walked into in 1983. Two decades later, they had gathered irreplaceable information on disease mortality for more than four dozen different diseases, ranging from various types of cancers to heart disease and infectious diseases. They compiled data on 367 variables and compared each variable to every other. They administered blood tests and surveys on 6,500 adults, took urine samples and measured everything families ate over a three-day period, and analyzed food samples from marketplaces around the country.

When the project concluded, they'd found more than eight thousand statistically significant associations between lifestyle, diet, and disease variables. They had completed a study that was unmatched in size, quality, comprehensiveness, and uniqueness. *The New York Times* crowned it "the Grand Prix of epidemiology."

It proved without a doubt that the Western diet—which has now been exported to most corners of the globe—is a disease-creating diet, one that makes the soil ripe for the most deadly diseases in the world. Remember, this research was conducted in counties where people were genetically similar and where people across generations lived and ate in the same way every day. Comparisons of death rates were made between the dietary preferences of different counties, and the conclusion was that the people who lived in counties with a high consumption of animal products suffered considerably higher death rates from typical Western diseases like heart disease, diabetes, and a range of cancers compared to those counties who consumed more plant-based foods.

The study also proved, however, that individual nutrients matter less than the overall diet. Occasionally eating a bit of dairy or meat didn't seem to increase disease risk in the Chinese population, but they truly did eat only a very small amount. Mere ounces of pork to flavor a soup, for example, or a tablespoon of yogurt as a sauce base. On the flipside, simply adding a "good" nutrient to one's diet did not elicit any disease-preventing benefits. In other words, the researchers concluded that taking fish oil supplements or vitamins won't help you build health and prevent disease if your diet is based in refined carbohydrates, animal proteins, or processed foods, as many of ours are, through habit or necessity—the hectic churn of modern life that often leaves us opening a box instead of preparing a mélange of seasonal vegetables.

At the end of the day, we don't eat nutrients—we eat *foods*. Against the reductionist but popular view that some nutrients will prevent or heal certain diseases, Campbell and his fellow researchers concluded that the complex *interaction* of nutrients in food matters. What's essential to health and healing is the overall nutritional *pattern*, rather than eating as usual and then taking a vitamin. The whole is greater than the sum of the parts. And for most of us, this means large, radical changes in the way we eat.

Campbell himself became vegan by the conclusion of the study and remains so to this day—though he doesn't use the word to label himself. He doesn't like the ideological baggage the term comes with and wants the focus to remain simply on the life-sustaining benefits of a plant-based diet. And today, he is diametrically opposed, philosophically, to where he started his career. "I grew up on a dairy farm. I milked cows!" he told an interviewer from *The New York Times* shortly after former president Bill Clinton revealed that he'd reversed his own heart disease with Campbell's book. "The early part of my career was focused on protein, protein, protein." But he's flipped 180 degrees, and everything—his diet, his beliefs about health, his career—has been changed by the Cornell-China-Oxford Project.

He wrote a book about the project, called *The China Study*, which he published through a relatively obscure small press in Texas in 2005. Nobody expected a book preaching the revolutionary health benefits of eating plants to make much of a splash, but *The China Study* has now sold over one million copies—making it a runaway bestseller and one of the top-selling books on nutrition of all time. And yet, despite the success of the book and the lauding of the project itself in the scientific community, we have been shockingly slow to absorb this knowledge or to integrate it in any meaningful way into our health-care system. I know only a scattering of physicians and health-care providers who eat healthfully themselves or who teach others how to do the same. What is also astonishing is that this, the largest study on health and nutrition ever completed, seems to be unknown to most physicians and nurses, much less integrated into our practices.

Why are we pulled toward foods that are bad for us? Why do our appetites tug us toward all the types of foods that the China Study revealed to be harmful? We've built an entire culture of food around a way of eating that is not medicinal for us but that instead feeds diseases that can hamper our quality and enjoyment of life (at best), and end our lives early (at worst). The more I uncovered about spontaneous healing, the more signs pointed toward the inherent intelligence of the body and its innate ability to heal. But if our bodies and immune systems are so smart, why don't we gravitate toward foods that make us healthier, instead of sicker?

WHY AREN'T OUR BODIES SMARTER?

The short answer to this is: they *are* smart. But to understand the body's intelligence on nutrition and cravings, you have to go back in time. Really far back.

As humans, we're hardwired to experience cravings and to act on them. Cravings for certain foods, usually ones high in fat, sugar, or salt—those substances that were all too rare when we were just emerging as a species—are triggered by the pleasure centers in our brains. When you follow a craving and eat whatever you're yearning for, sinking your teeth into a chocolate bar or a crisp slice of bacon, that reward center in your brain goes nuts, dumping dopamine into your bloodstream like a slot machine spewing nickels. And that dopamine, often called the *pleasure pathway,* hits your bloodstream *fast.* You feel the impact immediately.

Sugar, one of the hardest food habits to kick (and, if the science of spontaneous healing has anything to say about it, the most necessary to kick), lights up the pleasure pathway the same way that other powerful pleasure stimulants do. Sex lights it up, too, as can less healthy habits like recreational drugs. We like things that release dopamine into the brain and body, whether they are good for us or not. We are driven to repeat them, to hunt them down again and again.

So if a lot of these things that flip on the pleasure switch aren't good for us, what's the benefit? Why are we wired this way?

For our early ancestors, where they found their next meal—and what it consisted of—was often the difference between life and death. From an evolutionary perspective, calorically dense foods—fatty, sugary foods, essentially—were not readily available. They were few and far between and hard fought. High-protein foods like meat helped our ancestors develop crucial muscle mass. And sugar, beyond the quick burst of energy it gives you (which burns off quickly), actually has a secondary function that was especially useful to our scrappy ancestors: it helps your body store fat. In a world of scarcity, you need to be able to burn your own body fat for fuel. Sugar, whether in the form of glucose or fructose, activates processes in the body that help you store and hang on to fat for later. Eat it, and you increase your chances for survival. In a study where kids were given a test to see whether they preferred a sweet solution or a salty one, those who preferred the sweet solution tended, upon follow-up years later, to be taller as adults. Our ancestors who sought out and fought for sugar probably had a better chance of passing down their genes . . . and becoming us.

So because high-sugar, high-fat foods were linked to survival, our bodies rewarded us for acquiring it—adding the squirt of dopamine that underlined how *great* it was to eat. These types of foods have a physical, mental, and emotional effect on us. They're soothing. Even just the slightest taste of sugar can give us an energy boost—studies have found that people who had just a taste of a sugary substance performed better on memory and acuity tests. Children are so hardwired to love it that studies found that it was a natural pain reliever—hospitals even used to give it to babies before circumcisions.

Cravings are natural and contributed enormously to our survival as a species. But when the pleasure pathway gets trampled too many times—when that dopamine rush becomes a habit and the stimulant-reward cycle goes on over and over again—a craving can rapidly become an addiction, especially when substances that used to be scarce are now bountiful. And in the span of human history, pure sugar has only been as bountiful as it is today for a very short time.[12] Technology has risen around us like a flood, bringing with it an availability of foods at our fingertips that our ancestors might have literally died for. And yet as the world has upgraded, our biological programming has not. As Dr. Peter Diamandis, cofounder of Singularity University, likes to put it, "Humans haven't had a software upgrade in 200,000 years."

Our bodies and minds aren't well suited to live in the modern world. What we call *hunger* is often *addiction* and may be akin to craving and withdrawal. Researchers have found that sugar can be more addictive than nicotine or even cocaine. It literally produces a high, not unlike a recreational drug.[13] Certainly, individuals have told me—and from personal experience, I agree—that the true hunger that one experiences after making the transition to whole, natural foods simply feels different and is less associated with craving. A body that is receiving the nutrition it needs simply doesn't crave in the same way.

We can't zap ourselves back in time to the Paleolithic era in order to eat to heal. Our needs are different now. We need to find a way to get what we need here and now, even while surrounded by all these foods that are *not* medicine for our bodies.

WRITING YOUR OWN (FOOD) PRESCRIPTION

For Pablo Kelly (whom we met at the beginning of this chapter), it started with what he thought was a stroke, incapacitating him as he strolled down a country road. What it led to was writing his own prescription for a radically different diet.

A slim, dark-haired twenty-five-year-old, Pablo had always been pretty healthy. It was an ordinary day; he'd just finished up some work in the garden, put away his gardening tools, brushed the dirt off his knees. He headed out to meet his girlfriend—they had plans. While he was walking, he experienced the strangest sensation. His left leg suddenly went deadweight heavy, dragging behind him. He tried to reach down and touch it, but his left arm wasn't responding. The entire left side of his body had gone completely numb.

At first, it was temporary. A doctor checked him out and suggested it was a severe migraine—a fluke. But it happened again at work, and then again while he was getting dressed for his sister's wedding, cinching up his tie: his jaw drooped, his hand went numb.

An MRI showed the tumor—a golf ball, lodged in his temporal lobe, an area of the brain that helps you process what you hear and see, and also plays a critical role in language, speech, and personality. It's also part of the memory cortex—essentially, a tape recorder that turns all those sensations into concrete memories and writes them down. A biopsy diagnosed a glioblastoma multiforme, stage IV. The tumor was inoperable, but they offered him chemo and radiation therapy. Not to cure him, of course—just to extend his life. With treatment, his doctors said, he could perhaps get himself a year. The specific type of glioblastoma multiforme he likely had, called *anaplastic astrocytoma,* might mean that he had only months to live.

In the radiotherapy room, they trimmed his beard with scissors, laid him down on the table, and draped a warm sheet over his face—it was light, made of mesh. As it cooled, hardening into a mask, Pablo's treatment team made preparations for his first round of radiotherapy. Radiotherapy is a form of treatment where therapists map out the tumor site and direct a beam of radiation at it to kill the cancer cells. Like all treatments, it comes with its own set of side effects that patients have to weigh against the benefits when they make decisions surrounding possible treatments.

Lying on the hard, movable bed, waiting for the radiotherapy machine to be ready, Pablo rapidly scrolled through all the thoughts and questions he'd had about this course of treatment in the weeks leading up to it. He'd been having hesitations about doing chemo and radiotherapy. If there was a chance it would save his life, he'd do it, but that's not what they were talking about. They were talking only about *extending.* And yes, of course he wanted more time. There were so many things he wanted to do, including become a father someday. He and his girlfriend had been talking about it, as something to do a little ways down the road. Now it seemed like the pavement had crumbled away, leaving only a chasm in its wake. The future, on the other side of that gulf, was now unreachable. There was no road there.

Conversations and thoughts bounced around his head like Ping-Pong balls. He'd read over the side effects of chemo and radiotherapy and had grown more concerned. *How is this going to affect me?* he'd been asking everyone on his treatment team. *Is it going to make me better, or is it going to make me worse?* Nobody seemed to have a clear answer. He'd also been researching diet and the potential impact it could have on the trajectory of different types of cancer. He'd read about Patricia Daly, who'd recovered from a type of eye cancer using the ketogenic diet, and he was curious if it could work for him. Maybe it was worth a try? Research seemed to indicate that it could starve tumor cells and bring down inflammation and swelling around the site. But when he asked about it, his doctors brushed off the idea, even advising him against it. "It has no nutritional value," they told him. "It won't help you with the chemo and radiation." But maybe he didn't want help getting through the chemo and radiation that would only tack a couple of crappy months onto his already short life.

As the mesh on his face lightly hardened against his skin, it hit him: he didn't want quantity of life. He wanted *quality*. He wanted to *have* a life for the time he had left—not come here to lie on this table six days a week for radiation and then have chemo on Sundays.

He sat bolt upright and got off the table. The therapists stopped what they were doing and looked at him in surprise.

"I'm not going to do this," he told them, peeling the mesh off. "You can keep the mask."

He launched into the ketogenic diet. Most people find the keto diet difficult to adhere to; it's extremely specific and limiting. But Pablo was determined. He thought of it like quitting smoking, which he'd done a few years before after being a smoker for ten years. Quitting was miserable and hard and almost drove him crazy, but he'd done it. And he knew he could do this.

He started off with a few days of fasting, a quick way to achieve ketosis—a metabolic state where the body, deprived of glucose (which, as we discussed earlier, cancer cells feed on) begins to break down its own fats. For those first five days, he only broke the fast with small snacks like nuts or leafy greens. Once he achieved ketosis, he switched into the standard ketogenic diet, which allows meats, leafy greens and green vegetables, high-fat dairy like butter, and nuts and seeds. He maintained ketosis for the next three years. Here's what happened in that time.

He hit the six- to nine-month mark that his treatment team had estimated he had without chemo or radiation. He did not die. He felt better, not worse. He had quarterly scans at the clinic. He was supposed to go in, get the scan, then come back a few days later to go over the results. But scan after scan showed that the tumor growth had halted completely—a very unusual turn of events for glioblastoma multiforme. He started calling up ahead of time to ask if they could just take a look at the scan and let him know if he needed to come all the way in. Every time it was the same: "It's stable," the nurse would say. "No change." To everyone's puzzlement, the golf ball remained a golf ball.

Two years passed in that way, until Pablo's surgeon approached him with some news: he wanted to try an operation. Usually, with glioblastoma, surgery has no benefit other than the temporary relief of symptoms. Glioblastoma has long tendrils that reach out into the surrounding brain, and the only way to remove all of the tumor would be to remove too much or all of the brain, which obviously isn't possible. But the unprecedented two-year stability of his tumor was changing his options.

Surgeons performed an awake craniotomy on Pablo in the spring of 2017. Pablo lay on his side on an operating table, and the anesthesiologist briefly put him under. Nerve sensors for pain don't exist in the brain, and for such surgeries, it's desirable to have the person awake so the surgeon receives as much feedback as possible when poking and cutting into the brain. When they woke him up shortly after, the surgeon had removed a one-inch piece of his skull and set it aside. Disoriented and frightened, Pablo started to cry. But his neuropsychologist, sitting right in front of him in a mask and gown, grabbed his hand.

"Make a fist," he said. "Squeeze my hand."

He began cycling Pablo through a series of questions, showing him images, asking him to name them, periodically taking his hand again and checking his ability to squeeze. Meanwhile, the surgeon sliced into the dura, the protective membrane that surrounds the brain. Using tiny scissors, he made a snip halfway along that slice, making a T-shaped cut. He used the tip of the scissors to fold back the rubbery, translucent flaps of the dura, and there was

Pablo's brain: a pale, healthy pink, mapped with bright red veins and capillaries, slick and alive. Next, he gently parted the delicate, gelatinous lobes of Pablo's brain to reveal the tumor. It was firm and whitish, irregularly shaped, and it had tendrils like octopus arms that reached deeper into the brain. The brain tissue surrounding it had turned a pale purple, the color of a bruise. The tumor obviously didn't belong.

After hours of painstaking surgery, making microscopic cuts to the membranous edges of the tumor to loosen it from the brain tissue while a nurse dripped saline solution onto the site, the neurosurgeon was able to get 90 percent of it out. They recommended chemo and radiation therapy to shrink the remaining 10 percent. Or, they told him, he could just "keep doing what you're doing." Pablo reports that nobody seemed willing to admit that his strict adherence to the ketogenic diet was the factor that had allowed him to stabilize his tumor until he had the opportunity for surgery— but at the same time, they admitted that something unusual was going on. They just kept referring to it vaguely as "whatever it is you're doing."

Pablo kept doing "whatever it was" for the next few months. And at the next scan, the remaining tumor was gone.

Since then, quarterly scans have continued to come back clean. He remains on the ketogenic diet and plans to stay on it indefinitely. When I asked if he ever planned to go back to eating the way he used to, he was adamant: no.

"This is my life now," he says. "Glioblastoma can come back with a vengeance. I'm not going to stop eating the way my body needs me to eat just because I have clear scans now."

There's been a lot of shock and awe at his remission. His acupuncturist had initially been sure he was going to kill himself. "I thought you were crazy," he said. "I just kept waiting for you to start going downhill. And then at a certain point, I started thinking, 'Damn, maybe he's onto something.'"

His girlfriend is pregnant; they're expecting their first child in a few months. He doesn't take anything for granted. He knows that illness can come back, even after an unprecedented remission like his. But he's happy now; he's living the life he once imagined.

"I don't think about dying as a problem," he says. "Everything I aimed for is coming to fruition."

What are the commonalities between Tom's, Claire's, and Pablo's radical diet changes? Though externally different, the similarities are critical: there is a major focus on nutrient-dense, non-starchy plant-based food, and the elimination of processed foods, chemicals, sugar, and refined carbs. In other ways, they are radically different—each had to "write their own prescription" based on his or her own situation and intuition. As Claire said of developing her post-diagnosis diet, there is no silver bullet. And I have found that to be true; there is no single set of nutrients or toxins I can isolate from cases of spontaneous healing that any one of us can add or subtract from our diets in order to heal. Any book or study that attempts to do so is misleading. As we see all too often, two different studies will come out on the same isolated nutrient with opposite results; and that information goes out to the public in parcels with no real connection, context, or genuine insight.

In 1917, a pediatrician named Sidney Haas discovered a miracle cure for celiac disease, which was ravaging a large number of New York City's children. He'd been struggling for years to find relief for his young patients' painful symptoms, including gastrointestinal distress, malnutrition, stunted growth, and even death. The miracle cure was *bananas*.

Haas found that when he fed his patients a diet heavy in bananas, their symptoms rapidly subsided. They gained back weight and began to flourish. He theorized that the banana was a superfood with curative properties, and he wrote a medical paper extolling the effects the banana treatment had on his young patients, including before-and-after photos that showed their growth and amazing transformation.

I'm sure their transformations *were* amazing; their health turned around so suddenly because they were eating so many bananas that they simply weren't eating bread anymore. Gluten is the toxin for individuals with celiac disease; this simple protein found in wheat flour destroys the microvilli of the intestine, making it impossible to absorb nutrients. Dr. Haas had indeed cured his patients, but he misinterpreted his results. They didn't recover because they were eating bananas, they recovered because they *weren't* eating gluten.

The China Study almost fell prey to a similar misinterpretation of findings: the research team initially found a correlation between heart disease and wheat flour in a particular region of the country and came to the conclusion that wheat flour was bad. But with a little more digging, it turned out that the spike in heart disease they noted wasn't about what people *were* eating but what they *weren't*. In this northern region, vegetables were scarce, so people subsisted mostly on grains and starches. It wasn't that eating wheat flour *caused* heart disease—it was that eating mostly vegetables *prevented* it.

When we zoom out to look at the big picture of diet, health, disease, and the possibility of spontaneous healing, what we see is that a radical change in food philosophy is required for many of us to get on the path to health. It's not about the food pyramid as it is currently constructed; it's not about calorie counting or adding or taking away a particular food. It's about *nutritional density* and understanding what this means.

Remember the ANDI Scale? That's a great starting place. But the thing to understand and internalize is that you want to be increasing your intake of the foods that carry the most vitamins, minerals, and phytochemicals and eliminating empty calories or foods that contain a high proportion of calories and relatively little of what your body genuinely needs to be at its cellular best. And what, exactly, are phytochemicals? They are natural compounds that are found in fruits, vegetables, and whole grains (*phyto* means *plant*) and give these foods their color, flavor, and aroma. Although many of them still need to be identified and better understood, what we know so far is that at least some of them are powerful antioxidants and serve to protect plants from disease, insect invasion, and pollution. And they do the same thing for us. They protect our cells from free radicals, thereby keeping our cells healthy and reducing our risk of disease.

As this book went to press, a group of thirty-seven leading experts published their conclusions and recommendations for what they dubbed a "planetary health diet" in *The Lancet* after three years of poring over the best worldwide evidence regarding nutrition and the environment.[14] Led in part by Walter Willett at Harvard's School of Public Health and less influenced by the industry groups that have shaped and limited our understanding of nutrition for decades, they drew the same conclusions that I've seen with remarkable survivors: far more fruits and vegetables, whole grains, legumes, and nuts, and far less meat, dairy, refined flours, and sugar. They call on developed countries to slash meat consumption by 80 percent, which, for the average American, suggests eating only about one cheeseburger per week.

This is a level of unparalleled leadership regarding the problems with nutrition, hunger, and obesity that are facing us around the world and presages well the issues facing us as we move into a world with unprecedented opportunities for health and vitality, not only for the privileged but for all people.

Nutrition is a large, important topic but not the main or exclusive focus of this book, and neither is it for most survivors. I'll make just four brief but important points here. First, it's important to understand that unhealthy levels of sugar and salt are hidden in most processed foods, sugar often disguised as corn syrup or under other names. Second, just because something is advertised as "healthy," as a "health food," or as containing healthy ingredients doesn't mean that it is or does. "Whole wheat bread," for example, is almost always made mostly with enriched flour, which means that it isn't made from whole wheat. Third, eating is a way of sharing love and community, and food habits are highly linked to traditions. The goal at the end of this process is *improved* quality of life rather than less. Life, relationships, and food are complex, so being practical is important. Fourth, when making nutritional changes, it's critical to focus on the nutrition you're giving your body and being grateful for that, rather than focusing on what you can't have. This shift of focus is critical for beating the mental game, for building a mind-set that works for you rather than against what you are trying to accomplish. It takes some work to educate yourself and figure out the details of this new path, but there is no substitute for true knowledge and real understanding when it comes to what you are putting into your body.

When I look back at the videos from my first trip to Brazil more than fifteen years ago, I see a completely different man in every way. I don't recognize myself physically. I don't recognize the conflict and confusion I was clearly feeling about whether spontaneous healing was worth researching. And I have a completely different body. It's nearly impossible for me to get ill any longer, no matter the degree of exposure.

When I could no longer ignore the lessons from the stories of spontaneous healing I was hearing and seeing, I began making my own gradual changes. For the most part, I dropped sugar; I didn't realize until I did how addicted I was to it, and the initial steps were difficult. I dropped processed foods, also initially difficult. Forty pounds melted off my frame, without any other lifestyle changes. Even those two simple changes had drastic and immediate effects.

Now when I'm eating, what I think about is nutritional density. Is what I'm putting into my body loaded with nutrients?

It's important to be practical when it comes to food. We all need to eat, and most of us live busy lives in the context of particular relationships and a complex, unique mix of responsibilities, financial resources, and the availability of different kinds of foods and traditions. Whatever path you choose has to work for you. You don't want to compromise your health just because you're surrounded by a context that doesn't support your best possible health.

This is how I do it. It won't work for everyone because if you're

living in some parts of the world—rural counties, for example—
you simply won't have a Whole Foods down the street. I am usually
on the go, so I know where good salad and hot bars with healthy
items are with food to go. I mostly eat vegetables, legumes, fish,
and nuts, similar to the Mediterranean diet, and have learned over
time that knowledgeable people know how to prepare great-tasting
versions of these foods. Family dinners usually consist of a great-
tasting vegetable recipe, often with a sweet potato or, less often, a
piece of fish, and I know the restaurants where healthy versions of
the same are available. More and more books are coming out containing hundreds of fabulous, genuinely healthy recipes, illustrat-
ing how you can continue eating healthy versions of the foods you
love. For example, I love pizza and ice cream and am delighted to
see that riced cauliflower and even prepared cauliflower crusts are
increasingly available as a substitute for pizza flour and that such
indulgences as avocado ice cream can be easily made and stored.

The pattern is: survivors of incurable diseases tend to fill their
diets primarily with these nutrient-dense, medicinal foods—the
kinds of foods they served in Abadiânia in 2002 and in rural China
in 1983; the kinds that Tom Wood and his wife cooked up in their
kitchen together after throwing everything in their pantry away.
Tom, now in his early seventies, says he feels younger than he did
fifteen years ago. And his numbers support that, on many counts,
he actually *is* younger.

"I only have one regret," Tom says now, "and that is that I didn't
try this sooner. If any doctor had ever suggested to me that I might
be able to cure this disease through diet, I absolutely would have
done it fifteen years ago."

A CONUNDRUM

My deep dive into diet, and the way big changes in nutrition can
roll back illness, had been incredibly illuminating. It was clear that
for a lot of people, diet changes can be the doorway into radical
healing if you can truly shift to a way of eating where food becomes
medicine. But here's the hitch: I kept seeing cases, tossed into the

ointment of spontaneous remissions like flies, where the individual made no real diet changes and still experienced a spontaneous healing. Or conversely, there were those who made all the right dietary changes and it didn't make a dent in their illnesses. I knew diet was often a huge piece, and I wished that I could offer a perfect, nutrient-dense diet that would hand all of us the keys to healing. But it was clear that this was going to be a harder puzzle to solve.

I'd read a fascinating case study that shed some light on the problem. It focused on the Rosetan people of Pennsylvania. In the 1960s, health department investigators swooped into the tiny town of Roseto to get to the bottom of why its inhabitants had such radically lower rates of heart disease than surrounding towns. A leading theory was that the tightly knit Italian community had a remarkably healthy diet, one that investigators could learn from. What they found was the exact opposite: the Rosetans smoked cigars, drank wine, fried their meat in lard and butter. Their cholesterol consumption was off the charts. They weren't eating a "healthy" diet—what they were doing was gathering together around meals, maintaining extraordinarily close family ties. They found joy and community around the sharing and experience of food.[15]

I'm not suggesting that you can fry all your food in lard, smoke cigars all day, and expect to recover from a serious illness just because you sit down to eat with your spouse or kids. A shift *away* from toxic, nutritionally empty foods was key for most who experienced remissions. But I couldn't ignore the evidence: diet wasn't the whole picture.

"I'm contacted by a lot of desperate people," Claire Haser, our pancreatic cancer survivor, once said. "Every one of them asks me, 'What did you eat? What should I eat?' We go to diet way too much. We go to what's easy. Eating different foods, buying different supplements, is so much easier than changing yourself. Eating is the quick fix; it's the pill we want to take. And I keep telling people, 'There is no pill for this.'"

Changing your diet long term, revitalizing your terrain, and setting the stage for remarkable recovery requires a whole-life overhaul, not just in what you eat but also in how you think about and experience yourself and the world. Change is about love and respect for the body. It's also about understanding your community. What you eat is a habit, a ritual, and even part of your identity. It's also a shared experience with the people you live with and love, and it can be extraordinarily difficult to figure out how you fit into those rituals when your needs are different from those around you. When making deep nutritional changes, we should aim to do so in a way that increases the amount of life and love in our lives, from a place of opportunity rather than just fear.

Later, in the chapter "Burn Your Boat," I'll talk more about where survivors found the inner reserves to make these very challenging shifts in their diets, which then tended to ripple outward through their lives. As we move forward, we'll see that for many survivors of incurable illness, making diet changes was the "gateway drug" into making the deeper, profounder changes that they believe ultimately led them toward health. Which begs the question: If diet was the first baby step toward radical transformation, what was the next one?

I knew that one of the major things that happened when people switched their diets to a nutrient-rich one was a massive reduction in systemic inflammation. Sugar, for example, can cause a damaging inflammatory reaction throughout the body. The Western diet—the diet most of us in the developed world eat— is particularly inflammatory. The link between inflammation and the immune system is clear, since inflammation *is* an immune response—outside of an acute "repair" situation, it's the immune system in overdrive, hurting what it's meant to help. Survivors of incurable diseases who made radical changes to their diet were certainly benefiting from an anti-inflammatory boost to their immune systems when they did so. So what *else* were they doing to potentially magnify that effect?

4

Shut Down the Disease Superhighway

> Before you heal someone, ask him if he's willing to give
> up the things that made him sick.
>
> —*Hippocrates*

A weekday evening. I climb in my car and drive off the manicured
campus of McLean Southeast, an inpatient and outpatient psychiatric facility of McLean Hospital, where I serve as a medical director.
Here, families send their loved ones for the best possible psychiatric
care. This is my day job. I drive north to Brockton, Massachusetts,
to my night job, on call in a busy, urban hospital where it's not unusual for violence to erupt in the emergency room, and which is the
only Level III trauma center in the area. By the time I'm parking
outside Good Samaritan Medical Center, the sun is usually setting
behind the building, a huge industrial rectangle that blocks out the
purpling sky.

As soon as I enter, I'm engulfed in the rush and cacophony of
a large emergency facility. The waiting room is packed. Through
the doors that are staff only, people rush past carrying clipboards,
wheeling carts. The beeping of machines echoes up and down the
corridors as I walk to the computer station where I'll check for that

night's assignments. I log in to my account, and the requests pop up: a list of patients for whom consults have been ordered.

Tonight, I log in and see a female patient at the top of the list. Eileen, aged sixty-four. The brief note reads, "Admitted with chest pain. Cardiac workup so far negative. Possible panic attack."

In the ER, it's very common for people to come in with chest pain, fearing a heart attack. If there *is* a serious heart issue, part of the heart may not be receiving enough oxygen because of a blocked artery; this means waiting to act can have enormous consequences. The patient's odds of surviving begin to drop precipitously as the minutes tick by. Because of this, there's a whole protocol doctors fly down, checking rapidly for markers of a cardiac event.

If they don't find an obvious issue—if the testing reveals that the blood and oxygen are moving through the heart appropriately and the heart rhythm is healthy—they begin to suspect something anxiety-based like a panic attack. People with panic attacks suffer intensely. They experience a sense of impending doom and often believe they are about to die. They feel a squeezing sensation in the chest, which can be terrifying. By the second day of Eileen's admission to the medical floor, when they hadn't found evidence that she was experiencing a cardiac event, they put her on my list.

When I went into her room, Eileen was sitting up in bed, her posture ramrod straight. Her curly, reddish hair was streaked with gray. She definitely seemed tense; her eyes snapped to the doorway and appraised me as I walked in. Her apprehension and defensiveness were palpable.

I started the conversation with her the way I start many conversations with patients I see at Good Sam.

"So," I said, sitting down at the bedside and making myself comfortable. "It sounds like you've had some stress recently."

Her eyes softened immediately. Her shoulders sagged with relief. She began to talk.

So often in medicine, we don't try to get a patient's story. We've trained ourselves to believe that we're too busy. We have patients packed into the schedule like sardines; we feel we have to rush through our encounters with people, to get to the next one. But here's a secret: it doesn't take very long to get the story from a patient. When they sense you are open to it, it can pour out just as quickly as a description of physical symptoms.

As if waiting for permission, Eileen's story came rushing out. She tried to remain calm, but panic ran through every word like an electric current, and tears flowed. She *had* been having some stress lately, she confessed. She described how her husband had abruptly announced that he was leaving her and moving to Florida with another woman. He'd packed several suitcases with the familiar clothes that she had washed and ironed for him and left the house they'd shared for almost half a century. Yes, the years had been stressful together, but she had never imagined that he might leave.

They had been together since she was fifteen years old. She loved him; she couldn't imagine life without him. She didn't even know who she was outside of their marriage. And as a more practical concern, she couldn't imagine living alone; she never had. The idea was intolerable—it filled her with terror.

"When was this?" I asked her.

"Well, it was two days ago that he left," she said.

I eyed her with concern. This trauma was only two days old! Yesterday morning, the day after her husband had left her, she'd come into the hospital with chest pain. She'd driven herself, shaking like a leaf, after spending the night alone for the first time in her life.

When I suggested to Eileen that this very recent, devastating event might have been the trigger for her chest pain, she dismissed the idea. She couldn't or wouldn't acknowledge that her emotional state might have something to do with her physical symptoms. An old-school Catholic, she hadn't been raised to think about feelings or how to deal with them. Something was wrong with her body— her heart was sick. She was sure of it.

Her tests came back clean, and Eileen was discharged. I urged her to see a therapist. I felt strongly that if she didn't deal with the intense emotional trauma she was experiencing, the situation would simply repeat itself. She nodded, but I could tell she wouldn't follow through.

A month later, she was back in the ER. She was experiencing the same symptoms as before—chest pain, shortness of breath. This time, however, she was diagnosed with new onset atrial fibrillation.

Atrial fibrillation, or AFib, is a dangerous heart arrhythmia where the upper chambers of the heart beat irregularly—muscle fibers misfiring and twitching without coordination, rather than beating with a normal heartbeat that efficiently pumps blood to the rest of the body. When this happens, blood can sit too long in a heart chamber, leaving the person at risk of developing a blood clot that can clog an artery and cause a stroke. AFib is frequently caused by an excess of thyroid hormone or an electrical wiring problem in the heart, so Eileen underwent a battery of tests and was subsequently placed on a blood thinner (coumadin) and a medicine to stabilize the heart rhythm (flecainide), both of which will reduce her risk of stroke, heart attack, and heart failure.

While these medications prescribed to Eileen are much safer than untreated AFib, they are dangerous in their own right and are associated with all manner of side effects and interactions with other medications. The coumadin leaves her at risk for life-threatening bleeds and requires regular blood draws. The first large study to look at how common intracranial bleeding is while on coumadin among older adults at risk for falls had concerning findings: nearly one-third of patients experienced more than one episode of traumatic intracranial bleeding, and many patients also still experienced strokes during the same time period—the strokes being what the coumadin was supposed to prevent.[1] And then there's the flecainide, which has its own more moderate risks of dizziness, cardiac conduction problems, and medication interactions.

Eileen will take these medications or similar ones for the rest of her life and will have to live with or manage the side effects they cause. And yet, as is typically the case, from the standpoint of standard medical care, our work was done. The system is not designed to examine or even really consider whether a deeper cause lurked behind her symptoms.

As mentioned in the previous chapter, most of the time in medicine, we "treat 'em and street 'em." In other words, if it's chest pain from which you are suffering, your chest pain is evaluated, ruled in or out for a heart problem, and then in short order you're discharged. If you are diagnosed with a heart attack, then we'll evaluate the damage and perhaps start a medicine or two (or three). But we typically don't even ask what is really going on in your life. We don't ask or help you understand (or help ourselves understand!) whether a connection exists between factors like your lifestyle, diet, or stress levels and what is now going on in your body.

In the short term, there is nothing wrong with treating symptoms. It can be the best, most instantly effective and compassionate thing to do. And it often buys time. It allows you to tread water while you take account of this new information from your body. I frequently prescribe medications to control symptoms that are causing immediate suffering. There's something deeply reassuring about simply treating the biology and letting that be what it is. But we can't tread water forever. At some point, we have to go deeper than symptoms, to the *root cause* of illness. And today, most of our top killers—heart and lung disease, diabetes, and many types of cancer—not to mention other serious illnesses like depression, arthritis, and autoimmune disorders, have the same root cause: chronic inflammation.

Did the loss of Eileen's husband and the shattering of her marriage cause her heart problem? Was she suffering from a "broken heart"? Most likely, yes. I suspect that inflammation was building quietly and invisibly for years, predisposing her to disease in some form, and then when an acute stress or precipitant occurred, she, like so many others, was left with a life-altering illness.

MAPPING A KILLER PATHWAY

Doctors typically specialize in parts, rather than the whole picture. During medical school, we choose our specializations in certain body parts, going on to become cardiologists, gastroenterologists, neurologists, psychiatrists, and so on. And the same is true for most research funding and advocacy agencies—the American Heart Association, the American Cancer Society, the American Psychiatric Association, and others—which are also built around particular disease processes or parts of the body, rather than the living person who in every moment integrates the parts into a lived whole. This is how chronic inflammation, the underlying cause of the world's most common and fatal illnesses, managed to fly under the radar for so long. But zoom out and you can finally see the map: chronic inflammation is a superhighway that runs straight to the most deadly diseases out there. Yet how often has your doctor helped you reduce inflammation in your body or even brought it up?

The so-called lifestyle illnesses—cancer, heart disease, stroke, lung disease, and diabetes—are the top causes of death and disability in the United States, and they account for 75 percent of all health-care spending. Two-thirds of all deaths in the United States are caused by these five diseases alone, and for the most part, these statistics repeat themselves across other developed countries. Worldwide, 27 percent of deaths in 2015 were caused by heart disease and stroke, and deaths from diabetes were up approximately 60 percent compared to 2000. Death due to dementia more than doubled from 2000 to 2015.[2] And then there's depression, announced by the World Health Organization (WHO) in 2017 as the leading cause of ill health and disability worldwide. More than three hundred million people in the world are now living with depression, according to WHO estimates, and this represents an increase of more than 18 percent between 2005 and 2015. People who are depressed have less robust immune systems and are vulnerable to more illness in general and to poorer recoveries.[3]

All across the globe, it's lifestyle illnesses and depression that are ruining health and vitality. They're painful, they're expensive, and their rates are increasing. Clearly, we need to be doing something differently. Outside of the handful of individuals who experience spontaneous healings, most of us who end up with one of these illnesses *don't* end up recovering. Sometimes we learn to live with them, manage them, medicate them successfully. Mostly, though, we lose function and quality of life, and far too often end up dying early.

The statistics are staggering. If this level of mortality were being caused by a type of disease we could medicate away with one of our "silver bullets," we surely would have already declared war on these illnesses and essentially wiped them out long ago, the way we did with smallpox, polio, and tuberculosis. But the tricky thing about lifestyle illnesses—why they get to stick around and become more prevalent and aggressive, killing more of us each year—is that in many cases, they stem from fundamental ways that we, as a culture and society, operate on a daily basis: what we eat, where we live, *how* we eat and live, what we think about, how we feel. They have their roots in our values systems and how we define success and happiness. This isn't something you can just medicate away.

With inflammation-based lifestyle illnesses, we've made incredible breakthroughs in surgery, medications, and technology to mitigate or treat these illnesses when their symptoms flare up in the most painful and immediately life-threatening ways. We can insert cardiac stents when the blood vessels aren't allowing enough blood through; we can bring down blood sugar when a person is in diabetic ketoacidosis and sliding into a coma. We can brilliantly manage all manner of other crises. But to truly prevent and heal illness—to place a guardrail at the top of the cliff rather than just line up the ambulances at the bottom—we need to change a whole lot more than that. Chronic inflammation comes from how we think, how we feel, how we *live*.

Inflammation itself isn't inherently evil. In fact, *acute* inflammation is an essential, lifesaving function. This intense, laser-focused process is what creates the redness and swelling when you get cut or infected. These are the visible signs of what happens when a wide variety of highly specialized cells are sent to the scene so that efficient cleanup, clotting, and repair occurs. Without acute inflammation, you'd die, overrun by harmful bacteria and invaders, unable to heal.

Acute inflammation typically resolves within hours or, at most, three days.[4] The problem occurs when an inflammatory response persists beyond the normal physiological function and results in tissue destruction.[5] This is when inflammation gets turned on and then never turned back off. When it becomes chronic, inflammation can settle in, becoming a constant state, a kind of erosion depleting the immune system and wearing down the body's systems and cells. This unceasing wear and tear creates conditions in the body that are ripe for disease to take root and grow.

Here's an example. In the previous chapter on diet, we talked about sugar, its addictive qualities, and its potential link to cancer and infection. It's also a runway to chronic inflammation. Imagine for a moment what sugar looks like when it enters your bloodstream. At the microscopic level, it's clear crystal, covered on all sides by sharp edges. When you consistently consume sugar and it filters into your bloodstream, those geometric particles flood through your veins, bouncing off the walls as they go, tearing little micro-cuts into the endothelium of your arteries and capillary walls. The endothelium is the one-cell-thick lining of the interior surface of all your blood vessels, and damage to the endothelium is the earliest discernible precursor to atherosclerosis (the buildup of substances on the artery walls) and cardiovascular disease.[6]

As we've seen, your immune system deploys repair cells that rush in to fix the cuts. So far, so good! This is exactly how your immune system *should* be functioning, right? Sure, but if your arteries are constantly undergoing damage and repair efforts, over time, they will become stiffer, thicker, and less flexible like scar tissue does on the outside of your body. Plaque is more likely to build up on those repair sites, narrowing your arteries and veins and making it more difficult for blood and all the nutrients it carries to move through the body. When your diet includes a lot of sugar or refined carbohydrates (many of which are hidden in the Western diet), the glucose load may be much less intense in the moment, but it's still causing damage over time. For most people, glucose is a slowly dripping faucet, allowed to run for decades, leading to constant damage and scarring. And it's not just sugar and refined carbohydrates—some of the chemical additives in our food create the same type of inflammation and the same damage-and-repair cycle.

But it's more than just our diets that affect inflammation; as we saw with Eileen, the way you relate to stress can also trigger chronic inflammation. Cortisol and norepinephrine, the cocktail of hormones that your brain releases into your bloodstream in response to stress, can have the same effect over long periods of time.[7] Whether it comes from a dietary cause like sugar or other toxins, or from your body's stress response, inflammation is like an unnoticed brush fire, where the low flames spread through plants and grasses—never igniting into a full blaze but smoldering along the ground, causing damage to the landscape. This is your body when chronic inflammation is present. And all it takes is one spark to turn smolders into the full-blown flames of illness.

There are a hundred ways to push the On button for chronic inflammation. What's a lot harder is figuring out how to deactivate it once it is established in the body. But cases of spontaneous remission are showing us that some remarkable individuals—whether by accident, intuition, or trial and error—are finding that Off button and pressing it, taking out illness at its source. It's similar to getting rid of weeds in your yard; you can't just keep cutting them down with a mower. You have to dig up the roots.

UNDOING A LIFE SENTENCE

In the photo, Juniper Stein is the picture of health. She's in her midthirties but could be ten years younger. Sitting on a swing set in their backyard in Rancho Santa Fe, California, she holds her toddler son on her lap, arms wrapped around the smiling boy, next to her husband and daughter. Lit from behind by the dropping sun, she seems to glow with contentment and vitality. The photographer caught her mid-laugh, and her smile is wide and genuine.

This photo, from 1989, should not exist. At least not in the way that it does, showing a strong, healthy, vibrant woman with two children. But here it is, in front of me, paper-clipped to the inside of a manila folder that contains records on Juniper's case. I unclip the photo to look closer, amazed once again at how improbable—almost impossible—this scene is.

Seven years before it was taken, Juniper was diagnosed with a devastating, progressive, and incurable autoimmune disease that should have taken everything from her: her health, her ability to move without a wheelchair, the family she'd envisioned. Before that, her life had been like a book, the pages turning neatly and evenly: grow up, be a good student, go to college, get married, have a career. She sailed through it all. But then, the page turned, and horrifyingly, the next chapter was called "Illness." Except Juniper then tore the chapter out and rewrote the narrative.

She grew up in Brooklyn and Long Island in the 1950s and '60s, in the postwar boom where all-American houses popped up in grids all over the country. Her family was stable and loving; she grew up with two parents and two brothers. In the evenings, they ate dinner together—the typical American fare of the era. Meat, starch, canned vegetable. She studied a lot, excelled academically.

"There was no trauma, no drama," she says of her childhood. "It was a very normal childhood, very traditional."

There wasn't any particular attention to health; it wasn't something they discussed or pursued. It wasn't on anybody's radar. If you got sick, you went to the doctor and walked out with a scribbled script for an antibiotic or cough syrup with codeine. And Juniper wasn't athletic; she was more the studious type. She didn't do sports and didn't have much awareness of her body. Her body wasn't something she noticed at all—unless something went wrong with it, and usually, nothing did. It was just the vehicle that got her around, the house for her mind, which was her real self. She didn't really think about it.

She went upstate for college, to Syracuse University, an urban campus plopped in the middle of a tree-filled city that curled around murky Onondaga Lake. A lot of people played sports or attended games every weekend, but more often than not, Juniper stayed in and studied. She majored in accounting, nailed her grades. She met another accounting major—a dark-haired guy named Lee with an easy smile, who was just as ambitious as she was. In quick succession, they graduated, got married, moved to Philadelphia. Lee jumped feetfirst into law school; Juniper started a job as a certified public accountant. As a CPA, she sat at a desk all day, poring over financial statements, preparing tax documents, wrangling numbers into spreadsheets. Sometimes she'd go for a walk, strolling along the leafy city blocks of their neighborhood.

Not long after that, her back started bothering her. Sitting at her desk as she always did, it started to feel tight and achy in the lower back, down by her hips. She'd shift forward in her chair, or get up to get a cup of tea, try to walk it off. Occasionally, there'd be a very sharp stab that made her gasp—like something had struck a nerve—low down in the back of her pelvis. But then it would be gone.

At first, it wasn't that bad, and it came and went. It was more irritating than debilitating, and for a long time, she ignored it. She was only twenty-four, and this sort of thing seemed like an older person's problem. She went to the doctor, unsure if anything was really wrong and feeling a little silly. But the doctors didn't have any real ideas about what it might be and didn't seem too interested in trying to find out. One insisted it was psychosomatic. Another suggested that her legs were different lengths. Eventually, she stopped asking doctors and decided to just live with it. She was young. It would go away. It was probably a passing affliction—just one of those things.

Besides, there wasn't a lot of time to think about it. Juniper's and Lee's young careers were really starting to take off. Lee had graduated from law school, and Juniper landed a new accounting job at an international holding company with investments all around the world. When the opportunity came to take a job with even more responsibility at one of their subsidiaries in California, she jumped at the chance. At twenty-four, she became tax director, responsible for half a billion dollars' worth of revenue. She was good at what she did, and they knew it. It was an enormous amount of responsibility for a person so young, but she felt ready.

She and Lee moved across the country to San Francisco, which was vibrant, gritty, and beautiful, with the fog rolling in across the bay. Mostly, they worked. Wanting to start his own business, Lee joined an office in LA, a business management company that served clients in the entertainment industry. He commuted back and forth between LA and San Francisco. Juniper put in long hours, wanting to prove herself at her new job. It was a whirlwind time, exciting but exhausting.

Juniper's career accelerated. But then so did her illness.

The pain she'd had in her back, and the sharp pinching deep in her pelvis that had come and gone back in Philadelphia, flared up again. But this time, it didn't go away. It just started to get worse and worse.

When she woke up in the morning, she was so stiff it was hard to move. She started getting up early enough that she could run a hot bath before work, ease herself into it, and lie there long enough for her joints to soften, for the ache to subside so she could get dressed, eat breakfast, and get in the car. Sitting in the car was getting harder, though—a bump in the road could send a lightning bolt of pain through her. It came from inside her pelvis, below her tailbone, and shot through her body, liquid hot and nauseating. At night, if she rolled over in her sleep, she would wake up screaming. A sneeze that caught her off guard could leave her shaking with pain.

At work, she sat at her desk from 9:00 a.m. to 6:00 p.m. and sometimes later. Mostly, she was able to hide her rapidly worsening illness from her coworkers, but it was getting more difficult.

"Whenever I got up from my desk," she says, "I had to kind of organize my body. Remember how to move to get it all going again. The first few steps were always awkward and stiff, but once I started moving it would get better."

She walked hanging on to walls and learned to arrange her body carefully in a desk chair, in just the right position to avoid breathtaking pain. Lifting herself up from her desk became ex-cruciating. What had started as an annoyance had taken over her life. Now, most of her waking hours revolved around how to get through, avoid, or manage the thought-shattering pain she lived with. She went to doctor after doctor, specialist after specialist. *Okay,* she'd say to herself. *Which type of doctor haven't I seen yet?* And then she'd move on to the next specialist, crossing them off the list.

Finally, she hit a wall. The pain was overwhelming. Her doctor began to worry that she had bone cancer. He ordered a bone scan. On the day of the scan, Juniper put on a hospital gown, and a nurse injected a minute amount of radioactive substance into her veins. She got on the exam table, the cool paper crackling, and lay very still, hoping that this time, finally, the high-tech scanning camera that the nurse was positioning above her body would yield some answers.

In a bone scan, the radioactive substance that's gone into your veins disperses through your body. It becomes attracted to areas where the body is actively repairing itself from some type of damage. In a healthy person, there may be small spots here and there where this is happening, but that's considered normal and doesn't indicate any kind of problem. But in the case of bone cancer, for example, the damage done as tumor cells grow and replicate will be much larger, along with the body's attempt to repair. The radioactive substance will rush to the repair sites, lighting up the tumors like a string of Christmas lights.

Juniper didn't have any tumors—her bones were dark and healthy, clear of repair attempts. Except for one spot.

Her sacroiliac area—the pelvis, coccyx, and lower spine—were bright under the scanner's sweep. She didn't have cancer, but Juniper's body was, for some reason, frantically attempting to repair something there. But why? Her doctor referred her to a rheumatologist, a specialist in autoimmune disorders, who would be able to look into what was going on. Something was very, very wrong.

Dr. Rodney Bluestone was based in LA and was one of the top rheumatologists in the state. Juniper and Lee flew down from San Francisco together for the appointment. Dr. Bluestone had a pretty good idea of what she had even before he had her lie on the examining table and bent and unbent her joints, before he ordered the MRI—radio imaging that would illuminate the damage already done. To him, the diagnosis was unmistakable; he'd seen it many times before. Ankylosing spondylitis (AS), a devastating form of arthritis that, as it progressed, would fuse the bones and joints of Juniper's pelvis before working its way up her spine.

Given this diagnosis, Dr. Bluestone told Juniper to expect that she would get stiffer and stiffer and lose more and more of her mobility. Her spine would calcify and curve inward. Her sacroiliac joints would turn into one solid piece of calcified bone. The nickname for ankylosing spondylitis is "bamboo spine," because that's what your spinal column looks like when the disease is finished with you. Instead of a delicately interlocking series of bones that bend and flex with your body, it becomes a single piece of bone, the spaces between the vertebrae filled in thickly, as though spackled. On x-rays, it looks exactly like a thick, smoothly knobbed stalk of bamboo.

Juniper and Lee sat across from the doctor's expansive desk, stricken, trying to understand what this meant. Dr. Bluestone recommended some medications that might slow the progress of the disease, but he warned them: this was incurable. As time passed, it would only get worse.

"If you are planning on having children," said Dr. Bluestone, "you'd better do it now."

WHEN YOUR IMMUNE SYSTEM IS YOUR OWN WORST ENEMY

As with the sugar example we saw earlier, something had triggered Juniper's body to repair damage. Except in this case, unlike the image of the sugar molecule scratching the inside of your veins, we don't yet know exactly why her body turned against itself. In most of the one hundred or so autoimmune diseases that have been identified, the exact trigger remains frustratingly out of sight. We suspect that autoimmune illnesses can be activated by everything from a genetic code you've been carrying with you all your life, to an environmental toxin, a tick bite, a pregnancy, a food allergy, or another co-occurring illness that somehow trips the switch. But doctors are rarely, if ever, able to identify the specific cause.

Whatever the cause, something had convinced Juniper's immune system that an enemy combatant was present, and in response, it sent out armies of repair cells to her sacroiliac area, where they swarmed the bones, trying to fix what did not need to be fixed. In the process, they had begun to lay out the matrix for new bone. The entire area was inflamed, full of "defend and repair" cells that were doing anything but.

By the time she was diagnosed, Juniper's body had spent years locked in a vicious cycle of inflammation fueled by desperate attempts to repair what wasn't broken. Her pelvis was already irrevocably damaged—thick striations, like scar tissue, wrapped around her pelvis where her immune cells were inadvertently creating new bone. She had AS bilaterally—on both sides of the pelvis. Once her pelvis had been ossified with bony matter, her confused immune system reaction would move up the sacroiliac joint and into the spine. Most people with AS end up with a frozen curvature of the spine and often have difficulty breathing as the ribs stiffen. There were medications available that might cool down the fire of the inflammation in her pelvic area, but they wouldn't be able to quench it or even really slow it down significantly. There is no cure for AS, only ways to buy just a little more time.

The most frustrating thing about a disease like this is that doctors could tell Juniper *what* her immune system's cells were doing—harming her by trying to help—but not *why* they were doing it. What had triggered her immune system's armies to fan out and attack what it was sworn to protect? How had such an essential, intelligent body system gotten so off track?

Autoimmune diseases and inflammation are inextricably linked. According to the American Autoimmune Related Diseases Association, there are over a hundred known autoimmune disorders,[8] and as a group, they are all categorized as "inflammatory" illnesses—causing a repeating cycle of inflammation in the body or brain. Chronic inflammation can often pave the way for an autoimmune disease, which then intensifies in the body. The illness breathes heat into the smoldering coals of inflammation, and this ground fire continues to spread through the body, preventing health from taking seed.

This happens not just with autoimmune disease. Juniper's situation repeats itself in doctors' offices every day, with almost every category of illness you can think of. Widespread inflammation in the body and brain precedes the onset of all the most deadly diseases. In multiple studies, inflammatory markers in the bloodstream increase *before* the onset of illnesses. C-reactive protein, or CRP, is a sensitive biological marker for inflammation. It's produced in the liver in response to inflammation in the body, and researchers have discovered that CRP is consistently high just before the onset of many types of diseases, from hypertension[9] and heart disease[10] to diabetes (both type 1 and type 2), autoimmune disorders, and even many types of cancer.[11] In all these cases, CRP was elevated before other markers of disease, such as blood glucose levels or blood pressure, were noted. Some studies have also shown that other inflammatory markers may be increased prior to disease onset, even when CRP isn't. In other words, inflammation appears as the original root cause across diverse illnesses.

A test for C-reactive protein that comes back high unfortunately won't tell you what's causing the inflammation—only that it's there. But it can still be an immeasurably useful tool. It's one canary in the coal mine that says, "Conditions are right for disease."

As Eileen's case from earlier in the chapter may suggest, the link between chronic stress and inflammation cannot be ignored, especially when it comes to cases of spontaneous healing. Stories like hers repeat themselves over and over in medicine, every day. Up to 80 percent of visits to primary care doctors are stress related,[12] yet most doctors are trained to focus exclusively on disease symptoms and medication management. Multiple studies have demonstrated that half of all outpatient visits, in fact, have no identifiable physiological basis. Chronic stress dramatically increases a person's risk for developing coronary heart disease (CHD) as well as a wide range of other illnesses, and there's strong evidence that a single emotional event can trigger a CHD episode.[13] Though the exact biological mechanisms are still being delineated,[14] the road that runs from stress to inflammation to disease is a well-traveled one. And people who recover from "incurable" illness seem to find an off-ramp to exit that highway, turn around, and start driving the other direction.

We're beginning to see that unmanaged chronic stress wears your immune system down over time, the same way constant, unrelenting waves wear down a rocky bluff. Anxious thoughts and feelings, the constant drip of stress hormones into your bloodstream—these internal inflammation triggers are just as powerful, if not more so, than a food you're allergic to or a dangerous toxin in your environment. In numerous studies, the majority of people (80 percent) who developed autoimmune diseases like Juniper's reported "uncommon emotional stress" just before the onset of their first symptoms.[15]

Just like inflammation itself, stress hormones are not inherently bad. In fact, they are necessary for health and survival. While your body produces a bouquet of hormones, neurotransmitters, and neuropeptides in response to stress, which work together in a complex chemical reaction, the main stress hormone is cortisol. It's a major part of the human fight-or-flight response, which rapidly recalibrates your body's many functions—blood flow, oxygen, digestion, and so on—to allow you to outfight or outrun a threat. Like acute inflammation, a rush of cortisol in our bloodstreams is meant to be a brief, occasional occurrence—our bodies are not built to be in fight or flight all the time. So when we become locked in a state of chronic fight or flight, which is for many of us the reality of living in the modern world, we expose our bodies to a chemical environment that it wasn't built to handle.

At healthy doses, cortisol is actually great for us. It helps regulate our blood sugar and even acts to *reduce* inflammation in the body. The problem comes when cortisol is rigidly flowing through our veins most hours of every day, rather than flexibly, when needed. Our tissues become acclimated to this new, constantly high level of cortisol, and its ability to regulate the inflammatory response wears off. The cells of the immune system become desensitized to cortisol's regulatory effect[16]—it's like pushing the Mute button; they can't hear the instructions anymore. They become confused, disorganized, overactive, and, as in Juniper's case, attack the body's own healthy tissues.

One particularly startling study even found that chronic stress can alter the very genes of your immune cells—the original coding that determines a cell's function and behavior. Chronic stress disrupts and rewrites that code like a malware virus wiping a hard drive and replacing it with destructive programming. Researchers evaluated the effect of stress on immune system cells first in mice and then in humans, and the effects were the same; after a prolonged exposure to stressful conditions, the stressed group had four times as many immune system cells circulating in their bloodstreams as the control group. And in that larger swarm of immune system cells, a dramatically higher proportion were "pro-inflammatory"—their gene expression had been altered by the long exposure to stress to cause inflammation.[17] Basically, what this means is that these cells had been reprogrammed to cause inflammation. And without a way to wipe that malware and reboot, they would continue to race through the body with that mission.

Your immune system is your most powerful tool in the fight against illness, but like any powerful tool, it has to function correctly so that it's making repairs, instead of doing more damage. No matter what kind of illness you're dealing with, tackling inflammation so your immune system can do its job is key to opening up more avenues to healing. But figuring out what puts out the fire of chronic inflammation in your individual situation, or for your loved one, can initially feel challenging. It may seem that everything can be fuel for this fire, another scrap of kindling tossed on—what you eat, what toxins or pollutants you're exposed to, what you think about, what you feel. So how do we stop feeding this fire, and where do we find the supply of cool water to put it out for good?

To begin, we need to start opening lines of communication with our bodies. Those who recover from incurable illness often try a lot of different things before they home in on the specific lifestyle changes that start to help them feel better. We saw this in the previous chapter with diet: while it works for some people (like Tom Wood) to launch right into a new way of eating and then stick with it, most people (like Claire Haser) needed a period of trial and error to figure out what modes of eating really worked to help them feel better, more energetic, more joyful. There is no one "anti-inflammation" prescription you can follow, though you can begin with some common tactics that help most people knock down inflammation and reclaim immune function.

It's a good idea to start with the basics: move toward a more nutrient-dense diet (nutrient-dense diets are, in general, inherently more anti-inflammatory) and get rid of processed foods and sugar, which can kick-start the inflammatory response. And start to look for your personal stress triggers. They aren't always what you think. When do you start to feel stressed or anxious? What are the major points of friction in your day when you feel overextended, worn down, overwhelmed? Sometimes these may have obvious fixes once you become aware of them—adjusting a routine, asking a partner for more support in a particular area, or even letting go of responsibilities that are simply too much for you during this era of your life. Other times, you may have to engage in a larger life overhaul to eliminate unnecessary stressors and prioritize health. Juniper, and many others who recovered from incurable illness, ended up making radical changes to how they lived their lives that may have helped reboot their immune systems into a more anti-inflammatory mode.

REFOCUSING THE IMMUNE SYSTEM

Juniper and Lee took Dr. Bluestone's advice. Fueled by the fear that they would lose their chance to ever have a family, they started trying for a baby.

By that point, it had taken more than two years from the time Juniper's back pain finally drove her to the first doctor to get an actual diagnosis. And in that time, her illness had worsened rapidly, leaving her hobbling along the halls of her workplace, gripping the walls, moving slowly and deliberately through a maze of pain. But the only time she allowed herself the use of a wheelchair was when she had to quickly move long distances through an airport. She refused to buy one for regular use. Somehow, she knew that if she got into one, she wouldn't get out; she knew that she would start to think of herself as "sick."

It wasn't that she was in denial; she understood that she *was* sick. But she refused to reconcile herself to a lifetime of illness, limitations, and pain.

"I accepted the diagnosis," she says now. "But not the prognosis."

The first thing she did after the diagnosis was fill the prescription Dr. Bluestone gave her for Naproxen, a nonsteroidal anti-inflammatory that would get her symptoms under control. She didn't want to take it for very long; she was aware of the side effects and worried that treating the symptoms of AS with medication would simply allow the disease to continue to wreak havoc on her bones under the numbing veil of medicine. But she felt that a medication like Naproxen offered urgent relief to her suffering and could buy her some time while figuring out the next steps. Only a few days after she started taking it, the pain began to recede. She realized it had been like a thick wave, engulfing her.

"The medication helped me catch my breath," she says, "and it was calming, to know that it was there as an option."

Dr. Bluestone had also given her a printout with suggestions for exercises that might help with the pain. She took one look at them and thought, *These are for an eighty-year-old woman.* She decided to try another approach.

She'd never been a very body-conscious or athletic person, but the feeling of disconnection from her body—the numb, muffled feeling of taking medication and realizing that she was missing important messages—drove her to a yoga class for the first time in her life. She knew that yoga was, in part, about stretching and flexibility. If she could push her body into those poses, perhaps she could slow down what was happening to her joints. Wouldn't it be harder for the AS to fuse the small interlocking bones of her spine, she reasoned, if she was constantly moving and stretching them?

After the first yoga class, she was in more pain than she'd ever experienced. It hurt to stand, to sit, to move—the pain was like fire licking up her back, a heat that made her dizzy and nauseous. But she decided to go back the next day. Yoga wasn't in the list of exercises the doctor had handed her; she just had a gut feeling that it was the right thing to do. She could picture the new yoga poses—which she performed clumsily, shakily—breaking up the calcifications on her bones, freeing her skeleton from their vise grip. Moving slowly and painfully into a new pose in class the next day, she visualized what she hoped would happen: the thick calcifications shattering like plaster and falling away, leaving her joints smooth, the bones sliding past one another like they were supposed to.

Juniper understood that the Naproxen she was taking wasn't going to cure her, though privately she wondered why—Naproxen was an anti-inflammatory, and AS was an inflammatory disease. Why wouldn't the medication quell the raging inflammation in her body?

The answer is that no anti-inflammatory medication that's been developed so far can make a significant dent on chronic, systemic inflammation in the body and brain. Naproxen attempts to reduce one pathway of inflammation in a body that has multiple pathways. It's like putting a Road Closed sign up when there are five other roads that run to the same location.

After about a month, Juniper felt that the medication was muffling the communication between herself and her body. She stopped taking it. But the medicine *had* given her a leg up; it had provided her a ladder out of the fog of constant pain, one that helped her remember what life was like when she felt better.

From there, Juniper threw herself into her daily yoga practice. Classes were hard, and she had to push through the same veil of pain every time. The effort was Sisyphean; it felt like climbing a mountain, and then starting over the next day back at the bottom. But slowly, gradually, she began to notice a difference. One day it felt easier—like she'd started partway up the mountain this time. The next day, she was a few more steps up the path. Progress was slow, but it was progress.

She felt her range of motion increasing, too—she began to be able to go farther into the poses. Outside of class, she walked and moved more easily. She stopped waking up screaming in pain. The electric pain that had strummed through her pelvis began to dull and fade. She started to walk through the house without hanging on to the walls.

And then, the good news: Juniper was pregnant.

As the months went by, she felt even better. For most of the pregnancy, she didn't have inflammation or pain; it temporarily faded away as the pregnancy progressed. It turns out that the hormones of pregnancy can have a positive impact on some autoimmune diseases, causing a remission of symptoms or even slowing down the progression of the illness.[18]

At twenty-eight weeks, Juniper went into premature labor and was put on bed rest, where she remained for the next month. She took a leave of absence from her busy, demanding job. She left her desk set up—picture frames propped up by the computer, cardigan draped over the back of her chair. But as it turned out, she never went back. When her pregnancy was full term, the doctors released her from the bed-rest restriction, and she started walking the hills of San Francisco, trying to urge her body into labor. She walked those hills for two weeks until her daughter, Serena, was born, a perfectly healthy baby, in February of 1982.

In the weeks after the birth, as the pregnancy hormones faded, the pain began to return. Sitting in the glider in her daughter's room, breastfeeding her new baby, she felt those excruciating electric sparks starting up again deep in her pelvis. She realized that she couldn't do it all—she couldn't work full-time, take care of an infant, and devote the kind of time to her yoga practice that her healing required. She quit her job, and in a leap of faith, she and Lee relocated to LA and started their own business management firm, Stein & Stein. It was a lot of work and stress, but at least now she controlled her schedule and could prioritize the yoga practice that she was certain was the key to treating her AS.

Encouraged by the progress she'd made so far and searching

for ways to accelerate her healing, Juniper began to look for ways to deepen her yoga practice. Like many who recover from incurable illnesses, one of the first things she began to change was what she ate. She didn't follow any particular diet or meal plan; she simply started noticing that certain foods made her feel better, stronger, lighter, and more energetic in yoga class, and others made her feel heavy and sluggish. She found herself rapidly shifting to a plant-based diet.

She pursued Rolfing—a type of bodywork that's like massage, but deeper. Its goal is to rework and reorganize the connective tissues of the body—the fascia and ligaments that bind joints together. She tried a couple of different Rolfers but didn't feel a good connection with them, and the trial sessions with them didn't seem to help much. Their technique was fine, but they didn't seem to have any real intuition about the body and what an individual might need that was different from their next client. Then she found Mark, an experienced practitioner who'd studied directly with Ida Rolf, the founder of the practice. There was something different about him. She felt a connection with him, trusted him. He had the intuition she was looking for. He told her that his approach was to visualize in his mind what he wanted to accomplish in the fascia, then use his hands, knuckles, and elbows to melt away adhesions and open up blocked stagnant areas. Juniper felt that his mental and physical energy was able to clear what she calls her "stuck spots," allowing healing to happen on multiple levels.

After Rolfing sessions with Mark, Juniper was able to go even deeper in her yoga—holding poses longer, lengthening farther into the stretches. She'd started with hot yoga, reasoning that the heat would help warm up her joints and ligaments and allow for a greater range of motion. Hot baths had always helped her loosen up her stiff and painful skeleton; it made sense that hot yoga would do the same. But the hot yoga she was practicing was limited to a repetition of twenty-six poses, and once Juniper mastered them, she began to want more. She felt that to continue to keep the aggressive autoimmune illness at bay, she needed to be progressing in her practice and not remain static.

Over the years that followed, she worked her way through various styles of yoga, adjusting her practice to suit the shifting needs of her body and to keep her healing on course. She found that the deeper she went into the Rolfing, the more effective the yoga was, and the less pain she felt—not only in sessions but anytime: lifting one of her children, sitting at her desk, going for a walk. And she discovered that microdosing with cannabis took the edge off the Rolfing sessions, which could be quite painful, and allowed Mark to get even deeper into her soft tissues and ligaments. The pain relief from the microdosing, the Rolfing, and the yoga—she was learning to use them together to transform her body and also her immune system, making it an inhospitable place for an inflammatory autoimmune disease. But there was still more to do to shut down the illness entirely.

Running Stein & Stein with Lee was better, when it came to flexible hours, than her previous position heading up the taxes of the largest trucking company in the world. Owning her own company was certainly a weight on her shoulders, but she liked having a sense of control and agency—being her own boss, in charge of her own time. Still, the job took its toll. They managed finances for a lot of Hollywood types who expected them to be available 24-7. And their business was young. "We were the new kids on the block," Juniper says. To compete with established outfits in the area, they had to work twice as hard and be twice as accommodating.

"We'd wake up at 2:00 a.m. to the phone ringing," Juniper says. "It would be a call from some rock star we represented, saying, 'I just got really mad at my wife and threw a Tiffany lamp across the room. Is it insured?'"

Eventually, she realized that to truly heal, she needed to reorganize her life. Juniper and Lee sold the business and moved to San Diego to focus more on her well-being and the kids. Lee became president of a real estate development company by the waterfront in San Diego, while Juniper committed herself to putting her healing first, even in the midst of raising—by that point—three children. She wasn't immune to the kind of guilt most mothers feel, putting themselves before their children, but she carved out the hours, every single day, for yoga. She told her kids, "I need to go to class so I can be a good mommy."

Looking back now, she isn't exactly sure when the pain stopped completely. She started having more good days than bad. Then, the bad days got fewer and further between. One day, it dawned on her that she felt good, that she had no pain, that it had been a long time since she'd noticed it.

She didn't need a new diagnosis from Dr. Bluestone to know that she was better; she could feel it. But she wanted confirmation. Back in the very same office where she'd received a diagnosis that should have been a life sentence, she lay on the exam table while Dr. Bluestone lifted one of her legs to test her flexibility. He began to gently press it backward toward her body, checking her face every couple of inches, expecting her to wince in pain. "Are you okay?" he asked, pressing her leg back farther. Juniper nodded. "Are you okay now? How about now?" Juniper's leg folded smoothly back toward her torso, and the look on Dr. Bluestone's began to shift to one of shock and amazement.

Juniper describes finding the path into what was right for her body as a long process of trial and error. "Looking back and talking it through, it might seem like a straight line," she says. "But there were a lot of wrong turns." Some of the tactics she tried, she says now, turned out to be dead ends. But when she hit on something that made her feel better, she steered toward it. She course-corrected over and over as she received information from her body. She changed how she ate, exercised, worked, and structured her days. She fundamentally changed her life to change her body and health.

Nobody told her to do any of it. The yoga, the Rolfing, the microdosing, the sweeping diet changes, the reorganization of her life to relieve stress and prioritize her health. She came to it all on her own, through trial and error, intuition, and developing a deeper connection with and awareness of her own body. Juniper integrated an array of healing tactics that now, more than thirty years later, are largely backed up by the latest science. Cannabis, for example, has not only gained widespread recognition as an effective and safe form of pain relief but also as an anti-inflammatory. Some researchers now suspect that imbalances in the microbiome may actually be at the root of autoimmune diseases like rheumatoid arthritis[19]— and that restoring a thriving, balanced microbiome in the gut and body can roll back inflammation-based diseases. There may even be a link between the health of the microbiome and cancer—a connection we'll explore in more depth later. And yoga—along with its closely related cousins, meditation and mindfulness—has emerged as an undeniably beneficial tool in fighting chronic illness, even when exceptional performers like Juniper, who go very deeply into their practice, are washed out in the means and averages of the typical double-blind study.

For Juniper, yoga was the north star that kept her on course, but that doesn't mean it has to be yoga for everyone. Yoga, for Juniper, was not only a way to keep her ligaments soft and limber but perhaps, more important, a way to achieve inner equilibrium—to transition into an anti-inflammatory lifestyle and turn off the constant *drip, drip, drip* of the stress hormone cortisol that damages her body's ability to regulate inflammation.

An anti-inflammatory lifestyle is ultimately based on changing your relationship with your body. That means being very intentional about what you're putting into it and how you're exercising it. It means, to the extent you can, moving your body every day. Depending on what level of health challenge you're facing, that might mean just going for a walk or doing some gentle stretches if you can. Studies found that even just twenty minutes of moderate exercise is enough to bring down inflammation in the body.[20] And if, like Juniper, you find something that your body and health really responds to, *lean into it.* Make room in your daily routine for it. Rearrange things to the extent you can to prioritize your body and your health.

And a big part of changing your relationship with your body is going to be revisiting the stress piece. In the next chapter, we'll look more closely at the human stress response, its potential role in disease, and the power of shifting out of a state of chronic stress and inflammation and into healing mode.

Juniper keeps a letter from Dr. Bluestone in her medical files now, a landmark of impossible recovery. He confirms both his original diagnosis and his assessment that her AS is in indefinite remission. And not only that, he observes that she has not only halted the progress of the disease but rolled back many of its damaging effects. Her joints have more range of motion than they did at her diagnosis; her white blood cell count (an indicator of autoimmune disease) has gone back to normal. In attempting to describe what happened to her, he finally concludes that she has achieved "a unique form of remission."

Thirty years later, Juniper laughs just thinking about it. "I guess I'm still in 'a unique form of remission,'" she says.

Now sixty-four, Juniper has been disease-free for three decades. There is no trace of AS left in her system. However, her pelvic bones still bear the mark of the disease. A scan will still show the old scars—a reminder etched into her bones that an incurable illness existed, which is now gone.

5

Activate Healing Mode

> We can either change the complexities of life—an unlikely
> event, for they are likely to increase—or develop ways that
> enable us to cope more effectively.
>
> —*Herbert Benson*

The year is 1897. Walter Cannon, a young physiologist, newly hired at Harvard, notices something strange about the mice in the lab that are being used in a number of different studies. For the most part, everything's been going according to plan: the studies are run, the results noted. The mice either respond the way researchers suspect they will, or they don't. But the studies are typically extremely stressful for the animals. And Cannon starts to see a pattern: when the mice are frightened, stressed, or disturbed, the peristaltic waves in their stomachs—the muscular pulses that facilitate digestion—suddenly stop completely.[1] Intrigued, he looks closer and finds that the hormone adrenaline, when released from the adrenal glands, has an immediate effect on digestion—and possibly other physiological processes.

Set off by the clue in his stressed mice, Cannon dives deeper into the physiology of emotion. He's at the vanguard of this research—nobody else has yet pushed into this territory—and the pieces don't fall together particularly fast. As he runs study after study, he notes that fright or stress causes various physiological changes in his test animals, affecting blood flow and clotting, heart rate, breathing, and more. But he doesn't know what to make of it. Later, looking back on the struggle to make sense of what he was observing, Cannon will write:

"These changes—the more rapid pulse, the deeper breathing, the increase of sugar in the blood, the secretion from the adrenal glands—were very diverse and seemed unrelated. Then, one wakeful night, after a considerable collection of these changes had been disclosed, the idea flashed through my mind that they could be nicely integrated if conceived as bodily preparations for supreme effort in flight or in fighting."[2]

In that moment, Cannon coins a phrase that will change the course of medicine (and which you're probably pretty familiar with at this point): *fight or flight*.

Cannon didn't invent fight or flight, of course—it's been around as long as animals have walked the earth. But he did identify it and name it, and in doing so, he opened the door onto a whole new world of knowledge about the mind, the body, and the effects of chronic stress.

Half a century later, in the very same lab at Harvard, a young research cardiologist named Herbert Benson picked up Cannon's baton and kept running. Thanks to Cannon, Benson was now working with a clear understanding of what happened to the body under stress, and why. I like to think about these two giants of mind-body medicine working in the very same room at Harvard, sixty years apart. As young men starting their careers, they even looked alike: dark hair parted far to one side, glasses, a heavy lab coat.

As a cardiologist, Benson's job was to look for new and innovative ways to treat the most common ailments of the heart. One of these ailments was high blood pressure, or hypertension, a precursor to serious heart disease, and the more he researched and observed patients, the more he became interested in the role of stress and emotion. This was a sticky subject among his colleagues; it was widely accepted that high blood pressure was the direct result of issues in the kidneys, and there was a lot of discomfort and suspicion about Benson mucking around with emotion. It was considered too "out there" to be real science.

But Benson, suspecting that stress was the silent, invisible culprit behind most types of heart disease, persisted. He designed a study to investigate the roots of hypertension and the possible link to stress. Three squirrel monkeys were trained to press a button over and over again until a light went on. If they didn't press the button fast enough, they'd receive a shock. Obviously, this was a pretty stressful situation, and their bodies responded—as they pressed the button, trying to avoid the shock, their blood pressures went up. Then Benson changed the scenario slightly. The button was taken away. The only thing that could turn off the shock was if the monkeys' blood pressures went up, just as it had before. And it did; even without the button, the monkeys' bodies responded to the conditioning, and their blood pressures shot up.[3] Essentially, they were "rewarded" for changing their blood pressures. The study suggested that high blood pressure was *not* exclusively caused by kidney disease or anything else physiological—the real cause was stress, and the takeaway was that behavioral changes *can* change blood pressure. This was a completely new way of thinking about things.

When the study was published, it sent shock waves through the field of cardiology. Western medicine hadn't remotely accepted the idea that physical problems could be rooted in mental or emotional activity, or that stress could create physiological problems in the body. Doctors and researchers were forced to reconsider their positions on the topic of stress and heart disease. If primates could be trained to raise their own blood pressures, resulting in hypertension—a major risk factor for coronary heart disease and stroke—

then they could presumably be trained to lower them as well, heading off one of the deadliest and most expensive diseases before it took root.

Benson designed a new version of the blood pressure study for people: using human volunteers in a lab setting, he essentially trained them to lower their own blood pressure using an associative system of stimuli and flashing lights. He wanted to see if humans, as well as primates, could regulate their blood pressures by brainpower alone. And it worked! Six out of seven test subjects were able to successfully regulate their blood pressures in response to specific stimuli after conditioning, with *no medication* or any other medical intervention. This was big, but it still required a long period of training, with stimuli *outside* of the individual, to achieve the result.

That was when a group of transcendental meditators came knocking—literally—at Benson's office door, offering themselves to science. *Study us,* they said. They claimed that what the monkeys could do, they could do—except better.

Transcendental meditation is a specific type of meditation that asks practitioners to focus their practice around a chant or a mantra. The group of meditation students believed they could adjust their physiology through this practice, even to the point of raising or lowering their blood pressures, but they had no proof. A study run by a Harvard physician could legitimize what they had long believed to be true.

It seemed like serendipity—a group of willing human guinea pigs, wrapping themselves up with a bow and dropping themselves right in his lap. But Benson refused. At that time, meditation was considered, at best, a dubious, fringe interest in the field of medicine, and at worst, total quackery, a dangerous example of wishful thinking. He worried that by appearing to legitimize it with a study, he would risk jeopardizing all his work, erasing all the hard-fought progress he'd made so far. Having found myself in Benson's shoes years later, I can say that it's a torturous crossroads: knowing that what you most need to investigate to make progress is the very thing that may erode your credibility and career. A classic catch-22.

But the group of student meditators didn't take no for an answer. They were persistent, and eventually, Benson couldn't resist any longer. So he took some precautions. He scheduled the study sessions to begin late in the evening, when the lab had emptied out. And he had them come in the back door, where they wouldn't be spotted.[4]

This time: no flashing lights, no conditioning, no stimulus-reward system. Benson hooked the participants up to sphygmomanometers and monitored their blood pressures as they entered and sustained a meditative state. He found the meditators' blood pressures did sink lower as they had believed it would. But not only that. Their heart rates fell. Their breathing became slower and deeper; their metabolisms slowed and stabilized. Essentially, they were able to engage the part of their nervous systems that allows the body to rest and relax. In this state, the body enters ideal conditions not only for the biological functions that were essential for our ancestors to survive and thrive on the savanna—like digestion and procreation—but also those that are becoming essential for surviving and thriving in the modern era: turning off the flow of stress hormones, entering homeostasis, and allowing the body to recalibrate and heal.

Critics of the study clung to the data showing that the drop in blood pressure was small—it fell by only a few points at most during meditative sessions. But Benson pointed out that these were people who meditated daily, practicing and "toning" their meditative abilities the way you would tone a muscle through exercise. They were highly trained, highly skilled, highly practiced test subjects. Their resting blood pressures were already extremely low—much lower than the average person's. In fact, their unusually low blood pressures were a direct result of their diligent daily practice of the relaxation response. And the evidence that the positive physiological effects went well beyond blood pressure told Benson that there was much more to investigate. These people, simply through meditation, could produce a wave of positive physiological changes in the body. What might that mean for their health long term?

And could a method like this open up a new road to health for others?

A memory flashed into my mind, bright as a slide in a carousel projector, of one of the first patient interviews I'd done down in Brazil. This one was etched vividly in my memory. It was the one that had forced me to begin to shift from skeptical to open-minded.

I found the tapes in a box in storage. Remembering that Jan's was the very first videotaped interview, I located the right one, blew the dust off, and slid it into the VCR. I saw myself settling into one of the chairs with a notepad and pen, and then Jan appears. Slender, tan, and smiling, she looks healthy and radiant. She shakes my hand and sits, raking her fingers through her golden-brown hair. It's difficult to see my face on the video, but I remember being shocked when I saw her. All I'd known about her before that meeting was what Nikki had told me. Before I left for Brazil, I'd asked Nikki— the nurse who'd first recommended I visit—if there was anyone in particular I should track down. I told her I wanted to talk to people who had hard evidence: accurate and indisputable diagnoses with clear evidence of remission. People who had proof: they'd been sick, and now they weren't, even though according to medical statistics they should be. Nikki was an oncology nurse with decades of experience. I knew she'd know what to look for.

She answered without hesitation: *Jan Shaw.* She told me what she knew: that Jan had arrived in Brazil on the verge of death, in multiple organ failure. Her kidneys were shutting down; her heart was badly damaged. She had a severe form of end-stage lupus that had spread through her organs, including her brain.

I knew enough about lupus to know that you don't come back from it once it's spread into the organs. I could believe that a person with that advanced form of the disease could perhaps prolong their life if they managed things very carefully, but to come back from it and recover completely? No.

So when a happy and healthy Jan Shaw shook my hand and introduced herself that sunny morning in Brazil, I was speechless. *Wow,* I remember thinking, *this stuff really does happen.*

"YOU HAVE TO LET GO"

From the beginning, Jan came across as vital, energetic, and open-hearted. She had just come from meditating in the current room, and she radiated a sense of peace and contentedness. It was hard to believe she'd ever been sick. When I expressed as much, she fished her wallet out of her bag, pulled out a photo, and handed it to me.

"This is me," she said. "It was taken two years ago, before I came down here for the first time."

The woman in the photograph was overweight and obviously ill. And even beyond that, it looked absolutely nothing like her. I thought, *If these two women were standing next to each other, I wouldn't believe they were the same person.*

It turned out that Jan and Nikki had met on Nikki's first day in Brazil. They were staying in the same *pousada,* in adjacent rooms.

"Nicki showed up *just* as things were starting to turn around for me," Jan says. "I had just started to be able to walk again."

Her comment hinted at the story to come and the long road to recovery that she had traversed.

Jan started getting sick as a teenager. At first, it was just that she was tired—*so* tired. She fell asleep on top of her homework. She couldn't stay up late enough to go out on a date. And even during the day, she had low energy. It seemed like everyone around her was running on some kind of supercharge, while her battery was just about out of juice.

In her twenties, it started to get stranger and scarier. At twenty-five, she ruptured a disc in her back, necessitating a surgery. At twenty-seven, the muscles in her back separated—another surgery. At twenty-eight, she was diagnosed with a radiculopathy, or damage to the nerve roots where they exit the spine, which had been causing her intense pain. They performed yet another back surgery to repair it, but it left her in a wheelchair for five years. It was one thing after another.

At first, all the issues seemed disconnected—the intense fatigue, the repeated spinal calamities, the unusual infection—but they began to form a web of illness, undiagnosed, though with a weak and crumbling immune system at its core. Something was very wrong, but nobody knew what.

Meanwhile, Jan tried to live. She got married, had a child. Adopted two more. She worked off and on; she tried to be a good wife and mother. She figured this was just the way it was. While everyone else was being swept down the river of life on rafts, she was struggling along in the water, her face just above the surface. She would have to try to do everything they were doing, but also while trying to survive—to make it to the next breath. This was "normal" for her. And as time progressed, things didn't get any easier. Motherhood became more difficult; her relationship with her husband started to disintegrate.

Finally, there was a break in the case. Jan had a jaw implant surgery that should have been fairly routine, but when she woke up from the fog of anesthesia, the surgeon seemed alarmed. He told her that she'd bled much more than she should have. And after the surgery, she came down with a dangerous brain infection—her body was rejecting the implant, suggesting something going haywire with her immune system. That surgeon was the first one to suggest the diagnosis: systemic lupus.

"It's easy to miss," Jan says now of the disease that almost pulled her under. "You have all these different things happening, so you go to a back doc, a joint doc, a jaw doc, and on and on and on. Nobody sees the whole picture."

Misdiagnosed for decades, the disease had run rampant in her body, doing irreversible damage to her heart muscle and spreading through her organs. For some people, lupus can be mild—presenting mainly in a "butterfly" rash on the nose and cheekbones and successfully managed through diet, lifestyle, and medications, so they are able to lead relatively normal and healthy lives. This wasn't the case for Jan. By the time doctors figured it out, her condition was already very serious. The disease was in her heart, lungs, bladder, and kidneys.

Years of treatment followed; nothing really worked. She was on prednisone, but it only dampened the effects of the disease—even while taking 100 mg of prednisone every day, an extremely high dosage. And using prednisone to decrease inflammation and suppress the immune system is a big trade-off. The side effects can be lifelong and debilitating; prednisone can erode joints, especially in the hip sockets, and can leave you with debilitating hip fractures.

This was the early 1990s, and we had yet to develop some of the more effective medications that are now available for treating lupus. But even today, there is no way to cure lupus. While some patients develop a milder form that responds to meds and management, others still progress in the way Jan did. No matter what, it's still an incurable disease.

Jan would be on prednisone for years. And while at times it would be able to suppress the raging illness in her body, in the end, the lupus would prove to be too much for the drug. She was left with lasting damage to her bones and joints. At one point, in 1992, her heart swelled to twice its normal size. Her medical team biopsied the heart muscle to see if the lupus was causing the swelling (it was) and put her on cytotoxin in an effort to protect her heart tissue. She was placed on a waiting list for a heart transplant but was never approved for one; the lupus diagnosis made her ineligible.

The lupus flare subsided, but in 1998, as she was going through the beginning phases of a very difficult divorce, it came back. With her heart once again affected and her health hanging in the balance, her medical team did another heart biopsy. This one left a permanent hole in her heart.

Jan was in and out of the hospital constantly. As time went on, she was in more than out. Her marriage had crumbled under the weight of illness and other issues and had become a major source of stress. Her children, now teenagers, were struggling with behavioral problems and drugs. Their heartbreaking cycle of drug addiction, recovery, and relapse had fractured her relationship with them, and they held her responsible for the dissolution of her marriage to their father. They weren't speaking to her at that time, and Jan described it as feeling like your heart was outside your body, lost somewhere in the world—aching and in pain, and you couldn't get it back. When Jan thinks back to being hospitalized for her increasingly severe symptoms during this time, what she remembers is that she felt alone.

"Nobody came, nobody brought me flowers," she says. "No one called."

Then the lupus progressed to her brain.

Once in the central nervous system, systemic lupus can cause a host of terrifying and debilitating symptoms, everything from memory loss and seizures to dangerous spinal inflammation. Many people have a type of migraine often called "lupus headaches," and even when they're not experiencing acute pain, they describe intense brain fog—an inability to cognitively process information. For Jan, it was a cruel twist to a disease that had seemed to be systematically breaking down her body—now it was coming after her ability to think, express herself, *be* herself.

In the early summer of 2002, she started having pain in her upper-middle back on the right side. Doctors quickly discovered the probable cause: her gallbladder was scarred from the multiple infections she'd endured. When they performed surgery to remove it, she contracted sepsis, a dangerous and life-threatening systemic infection. And then the lupus spread to her kidneys, putting her at risk for renal failure.

Renal failure is one of the leading causes of death for patients with systemic lupus. As the immune system attacks the essential organs, the kidneys, which are responsible for filtering toxins out of the body, become inflamed. This leads to *lupus nephritis,* which renders the kidneys unable to remove toxins or regulate the amount of fluid in the body. As the kidneys begin to fail, toxins build up in the body. In the doctor's office that day, Jan learned that it wasn't just her kidneys—all her major organs were involved. She was entering multiple organ failure.

And then, a friend called out of the blue to ask if she'd ever heard of spiritual healing. She mentioned a center in Brazil that she'd visited herself.

"I pooh-poohed it," she says. "It sounded crazy!"

But when the third and then fourth person brought it up, she decided to look into it. She read support for the program and the criticisms of it. She weighed it all and decided to go. But she was as weak as she had ever been. She had cerebral edema—swelling in the brain—and needed help to bathe and eat. She couldn't sit up in a chair without falling over. Jan's doctors were very concerned about her ability to survive the trip to Brazil. As her kidneys struggled to keep up, fluid was building up in her body. At any point, there was the possibility of going into septic shock. All her doctors said the same thing: "Don't get on the plane. You're going to die if you do."

Her response was, "I'm going to die if I don't."

As the bus rattled up the long road to the healing center, past green fields dotted with black cattle and windbreaks of eucalyptus trees, Jan's life was sustained by over fifteen different medications. She was on the verge of widespread organ shutdown, with massive fluid buildup, on the edge of septic shock. But she didn't die.

Initially, she felt that she was hovering at the edge of death—that life was a thin thread that could snap at any moment with the slightest pressure. But something about the rhythms of life in Brazil felt deeply restorative. She quickly fell into the routines of the town and healing center—the long hours meditating in the current rooms, the healthy meals and the juice bars, connecting with others who were going through the same thing. For the first time in decades, she didn't feel alone in her journey through illness.

Every day, she brought her bag of medicines, including everything she was taking to control her lupus—prednisone, heart medications, and chemo drugs, which are a common lupus treatment—to the current room with her to meditate. One day, the resident healer approached her, looked her right in the eyes, and said, "They don't belong to you."

She touched the woven purse at her side, assuming he was talking about the bag of meds.

"Yes, they do," she said. "They have my name on them!"

"No," he said. "Your children. They don't belong to you. They belong to God."

Jan walked out of the current room and began to sob. She couldn't stop. She cried for days.

Jan had had something reflected back to her that she already knew, deep inside—she needed to let go of her children, but she hadn't been able to acknowledge it. In hearing these words, she finally had permission to let go of the toxic aspects of her relationship with her kids, of her role as caretaker, and of assuming the responsibility for all the trauma that had happened within her family. They would be okay, she realized, without her mind and body constantly engaged in the panic and anxiety of holding them first and foremost in her thoughts and worries. They were on their own journeys and would have to navigate their own paths. At that point, in her mind, she cut them free—three little rowboats into the current. She felt immense grief, along with a release into a deep, limitless freedom.

She flushed the chemo drugs down the toilet. She began to wean herself off the prednisone—incredibly quickly. When she told me that she dropped 10 mg per day, my jaw fell open. That sort of pace is extremely dangerous. Most people need to be slowly weaned off such a high, chronic dose of prednisone in a way that their bodies can handle. The adrenals need time to adjust and react, to shift back into gear and pick up the slack created by the receding prednisone.

"You're lucky that didn't kill you," I told her. "That could have sent you into adrenal collapse."

"Well," she said with a shrug, "I felt better."

Jan was recovering faster and faster. Within ten days, she was completely off the drug she'd been taking for decades. And she felt good. Within a week or so, she was walking on her own. By the time Nikki arrived, months later, Jan was not only walking but hiking—happy, healthy, and medication-free.

How?

BEYOND RELAXATION

With his meditation studies, Herb Benson proved that the relaxation response had immediate physiological effects in terms of turning off fight or flight and allowing the body to recover. By dealing with the stresses of the present moment, we could drain stress from our bodies for a short time, achieve a window of homeostasis, and turn on the healing mode in the body. But if long-held stresses and traumas from the past were still present, lurking under the surface, could we *really* enter healing mode and stay there for any meaningful length of time?

After the success of his meditation studies, Herb Benson wrote and published a book called *The Relaxation Response*. The book, which became an instant bestseller, essentially repackaged transcendental meditation into a quick and simple exercise that anyone could use, rephrased in language that was more accessible to Western readers. His theory was that brief but daily bouts of meditation could have significant health benefits for the average person and that the process was deceptively easy.

Here are the basics of Benson's relaxation response: sit quietly, in a comfortable position. Close your eyes. Relax all your muscles. Breathe through your nose, slowly and evenly, in and out, while focusing on a word, phrase, or sound in your mind—a mantra that can help keep unwanted thoughts at bay and get us out of the "monkey mind," or our repetitive thoughts and fears. For the mantra, one could use words that are personally soothing and meaningful, or associated with one's own particular spiritual or religious practice. In his many presentations on the topic, Benson is quick to reassure audiences that unwanted thoughts will come—this doesn't mean failure. The important thing is to refocus and continue. He recommends keeping the session going for ten to twenty minutes. And that's it.

It seems so simple. And yet, the health effects were measurable. Carving out a few minutes each day to sit in a chair and follow Benson's handful of steps improved not only blood pressure but also had a noticeable positive impact on chronic headaches, cardiac rhythm irregularities, premenstrual syndrome, and even anxiety and depression. If such basic relaxation strategies could elicit these improvements, what sorts of "miraculous" effects could arise from an even deeper, more comprehensive practice?

Here's what I observed about the experiences that Jan and others had in Brazil: people spent many hours a day in deep, guided meditation. The sense of community was strong, and many people experienced genuine, deep connections in a few short days that seemed to run deeper and wider than anything they had at home. In the meditation room, there was a current of energy that ran from person to person, so electric that even I, an outsider unpracticed at meditation, could feel it.

We know now that meditation can literally change the shape of the brain. Sara Lazar and other colleagues at Harvard ran an eight-week mindfulness-based stress reduction (MBSR) program and found that it measurably increased cortical thickness in the hippocampus, the part of the brain in charge of memory, feelings, and regulation of emotions.[5] Not only that, it actually *shrank* the amygdala, the part of the brain that signals the hypothalamus, which then releases hormones associated with the fight-or-flight response. It seemed that the entire structure of life in the healing centers was anathema to the chronic stress and anxiety that so many visitors probably lived with in their day-to-day lives.

Jan stayed in Brazil for thirteen months. It wasn't easy; she wasn't wealthy, she was initially too sick to work, and things at home were complicated. But she ended up having help—a parent helped with her mortgage back home, and a new and loving partner had come into her life, who supported her in her decision to stay in Brazil and continue to get better. At the end of a year, when she returned home with the new love of her life who would become her life partner, they created a new life together, one devoted to connection, service, and compassion. Jan was a completely different person, and it showed—physically, emotionally, and spiritually.

At the end of the interview, I remember glancing down at my notepad and seeing the photo of Jan still lying in my lap. I was struck once again by how different the woman sitting in front of me was from the woman in the photo. This was a woman who'd been ill her entire life, who'd come off fifteen medications, stood up from the brink of death, and completely transformed herself. Now she was joyful, vibrant, brilliantly alive. The difference was astonishing. I leaned over to hand the photo back to her and tell her as much.

She laughed, nodded. "At home, I'll walk past someone on the street whom I've known my whole life," she said, "and they don't even recognize me."

People have a lot of interpretations about what happens when they travel to "spiritual" healing centers like the one Jan visited. As a doctor, I'm a skeptic, but I'm also humble enough to know that there are some things we just don't understand yet. And one thing that was becoming very clear as I researched spontaneous healing was how essential it was to really *listen.* We aren't usually trained to listen in this way, in either medical school or residency. Even in psychiatry, a discipline that is supposed to be about listening, we are often laser-focused on the disease or diagnosis, rather than dedicated to getting a big-picture sense of the person and all the factors that might be contributing to disease or health. I knew now that I was going to need to both expand and deepen my ideas about what it meant to really listen to a patient. The first step in untangling the many threads of spontaneous healing was to *see* all those threads, individually, and how they wove together. I'd have to look at the entire tapestry of a person's story.

Looking at the entire tapestry of Jan's story, it was clear that by profoundly changing her life, Jan was able to profoundly change her health. I knew that stress was a big piece of this, but there's only so much of our stress response that we can consciously control. To understand more about what might be going on with Jan and other survivors, I needed to look closely at the autonomic nervous system and how it operates.

THE NERVOUS SYSTEM: THE BODY'S GEARSHIFT

Your nervous system is the electrical wiring that connects every part of your body back to the brain. The *somatic* nervous system, also called the *voluntary nervous system,* is responsible for carrying sensory and motor information to and from the central nervous system. Approximately eighty-six billion neurons spark together to pass messages from the tips of your fingers and toes up to the command center in your brain, which decides whether to pull your hand away from something hot or to continue petting that soft cat. These messages shoot lightning-fast through your body, so that information about what you're touching arrives in your brain at the moment your skin makes contact. We have conscious control over parts of the somatic nervous system. You decide to stand up, and an intricate series of electrical and chemical reactions occur along forty-three pairs of nerves, a superspeed domino effect that starts in the brain and runs down the spine and out from the central nervous system to the peripheral nervous system, and then, with approximately eight billion nerve endings firing, you rise from your chair.

But when it comes to spontaneous healing, our focus is mainly on the *autonomic* nervous system—the branch that runs from the brain to all your essential organs, full of billions of neurons and nerve fibers. This aspect of your nervous system runs silently, not really under your conscious control. Unlike, say, deciding to lift your hand and then lifting it, the organs, blood vessels, glands, and other systems controlled by the autonomic nervous system are run by the subconscious mind.

Picture your autonomic nervous system as a car engine. Just like a car, it has different "gears" that it can shift into, depending on the situation. As anyone who's ever driven a stick shift knows, it's essential to pick the right gear for each speed. Most of us probably don't drive manual transmissions anymore, but I still remember learning to drive on one—and it was on a tractor, to boot! There's a correct gear for slow, stop-and-go driving, another for the highway, and several more in between. If you tried to drive in a low gear in the passing lane, or in a high gear in your driveway, you'd run into trouble—a whining, smoking engine, or stalling, or burning out your clutch.

These days, most of the cars on the market have automatic

transmission, meaning the computers in the cars' engines do all the shifting for you. It's easier, but sometimes I miss those old manual transmissions. There was something I deeply enjoyed about really feeling the inner workings of the engine. I was more in touch with the car's processes; I understood a little better how it worked and why. Now I drive an automatic, and I've gotten used to not thinking about it. The gears shift up and down automatically, and usually everything works fine. But when something does go wrong, I'm a little in the dark, and I don't know how to fix it.

I think that's where a lot of us have gotten with our bodies. They should be upshifting and downshifting appropriately on their own, but they're not. Something's gone wrong with the computer, and most of us don't even realize it.

Your autonomic nervous system has two basic modes: sympathetic and parasympathetic. The sympathetic nervous system, or *fight or flight,* is the gear you shift into when you're in danger or under stress. The parasympathetic, sometimes called *rest and digest,* is the gear you're *supposed* to downshift back into the rest of the time, when you don't need to be tensed and alert to deal with a threat or a problem.

You absolutely need your sympathetic nervous system—your body's natural alarm system—to engage rapidly as soon as you perceive a threat. In that instance, it should happen immediately— like a car engine turning over when you turn the key. It should roar to life. Stumble upon a tiger? Your amygdala, the twin, almond-shaped lobes that form the emotional control center of your brain, triggers a falling domino effect of responses in your body, releasing a cascade of stress hormones and neurochemicals into your bloodstream. Your blood vessels rapidly constrict, trapping blood in your limbs so you can swing, punch, run, or react as necessary. Your digestion winds down, your heart rate rises, your breathing becomes shallow and rapid. Your hearing may even grow muffled and your vision tunneled—the body's efforts to shut out distractions and focus attention on the threat.

The fight-or-flight response (often called *fight-flight-freeze,* for the additional tendency to freeze when threatened), actually turns off certain parts of your brain—the more nuanced, critical-thinking, decision-making parts. Your body doesn't want you mulling over decisions in a fight-or-flight scenario. This is not the time to think about the whole picture, consider how the tiger is feeling, or weigh the pros and cons of running versus fighting versus freezing. You should already be making tracks in the opposite direction before you even have the chance to process the word *tiger*.

The more primitive human that you once were, long ago, was able to turn fight or flight *off* after the threat was gone; the sympathetic nervous system would slowly wind down as the parasympathetic, or rest-and-digest system, booted up and took over. In this mode, the brain deploys acetylcholine, an organic chemical that hits your bloodstream like a drug. The vessels, capillaries, and arteries all through your body immediately begin to relax and dilate, letting blood rush back to your core. Your heartbeat slows. Digestion kicks back on, more efficiently processing the energy and nutrients essential to your immune system. Blood, oxygen, and immune resources immediately become available for arguably their most essential function: healing.

This is the parasympathetic system. And by design, you're supposed to be in it most of the time. But for the vast majority of us, it's the other way around—we're caught in sympathetic mode.

It's natural to wonder why we have such difficulty balancing our sympathetic and parasympathetic nervous systems if that balance is so crucial to our health and survival. Shouldn't this be instinctual? Why are we getting trapped in fight or flight when our bodies are designed to be able to flip back out of it?

GETTING YOUR GEARSHIFT STUCK

Here's the thing—I'm pretty sure you don't have a tiger in your face anymore. These days, most of us rarely have an actual need for the fight-or-flight response. Yet our bodies are wired with ancient programming, coding that needs to be consciously updated for modern life.

The fight-or-flight response is brilliant, complex, and breath-takingly fast. Your body goes from zero to sixty in the blink of an eye. And everyday stresses—any of a million ghostly tigers lurking in your world or in your mind—can flip that switch. With a barrage of other stressors coming right behind, you never manage to turn it back off. News stations report ten times the amount of bad news than good news every day. *"If it bleeds, it leads,"* is the guiding principle. Traffic is at a crawl during rush hour, the kids have the flu, and there's a deadline at work. Both as individuals and collectively, as a culture, it's just easier to focus on the bad stuff, the crises, the need to put out fires. It's the way we're programmed. In fact, social scientists call this the *negativity bias,* a phenomenon that causes us to pay more attention to potential negative aspects of our environment rather than what's positive. This was adaptive on the occasions that threats appeared on the savannas of Africa—but not now.

Unfortunately, many of us now spend a majority of our time in a low-level, chronic fight-or-flight state, and we enter the parasympathetic far too rarely and incompletely. In today's world, your sympathetic nervous system is too often stuck in the On position. Your engine revs all day, all night, all week, all year, tearing through fuel, wearing down gears, and sending you to the mechanic to diagnose problem after problem, when the real, underlying problem is the way you're driving the car.

Ideally, as was Mother Nature's intention, we should be able to toggle back and forth between systems, efficiently shifting from survival mode to healing mode, maintaining homeostasis—that healthy hormonal balance—in the body. But instead, we've run into a situation where our evolutionary biology and the modern world are at odds. The pace of civilization and technology has moved faster than our physiological ability to keep up with it.

Humans evolved for a specific set of circumstances that, for the vast majority of us on this planet, are no longer our reality. At every turn, our biology clashes with the new world we've built for ourselves. Inside every tech-savvy millennial, sitting in front of her paper-thin laptop with an iPhone next to her accumulating bright red email notifications, there's an ancestral version of her, locked in the dark of the amygdala, believing that she is scrapping for survival on the open plains or in the jungle.[6] It can seem like we are biologically doomed to find reasons to be stressed, afraid, and anxious. Surrounded by perceived stressors much of the time, and by the similar mind-sets of those around us and within our culture, it's just easier to believe the bad stuff. Long ago, it's what kept us alive. Now, it's killing us.

There's nothing new or revolutionary about the idea that chronic stress isn't great for our bodies. Herb Benson was pushing it into the mainstream back in the 1970s, and although it hasn't yet impacted medical practice anywhere *near* as much as is needed, more and more books and other media are bringing awareness to this issue. Research studies in this area now number in the thousands, and the research is showing us that it's worse than we'd thought; chronic stress has the capacity to affect our health not just today but tomorrow and for the rest of our lives. It's also showing, however, that we have the capacity to change course.

Benson's relaxation response works to improve health and stave off disease because, as it turns out, while you're sitting in a chair doing meditative breathing exercises, you're not only switching over from fight or flight to rest and digest, you're also protecting and healing your actual *cells*—the foundational building blocks of your body, which carry the detailed operating instructions for every one of the biological functions that keep you alive—from the damage wrought by chronic stress. Healing demands that you learn to recognize when you're shifting into fight or flight and do everything you can to grab that gearshift and recover back to homeostasis.

How do we do this? One way to start is by trying out the relaxation response and noticing how your body feels when you practice it. How do your muscles feel, your breathing, your heartbeat? Notice where you hold stress in your body; notice what it feels like when you let it drain out. Ask yourself: What *else* in your life helps you feel this way? For some people, it's being outside in nature, or being with certain people. For others, it's an activity like cooking or painting or even driving with the windows down and the music turned up. Sometimes the things that really relax us are the first to get bumped out of the day's schedule when things get busy, seemingly disposable, when they might actually be the most important thing you do that day. You can't spend your life sitting in a chair, practicing the relaxation response. What you *can* do is identify what else in your life helps you achieve that same feeling, that dropping out of fight or flight, and lean into it, make space for it as though it were medicine—because it is. In fact, it may be a much more powerful medicine than any of us realized.

WHAT POND SCUM CAN TEACH US ABOUT IMMORTALITY

Innovation tends to come from unexpected angles. Medicine is full of stories of discovery that start with a mistake, a miscalculation, a wrong turn that turns out not to be a wrong turn at all but the surprise answer to a long-unsolved riddle. Think back to this famous story, which you might have heard in high school science class: a bacteriologist, not known for being particularly organized or clean in the lab, finally gets around to cleaning up a pile of petri dishes that he'd recently used to culture *staphylococcus aureus,* one of the most common disease-causing bacteria. His experiment over, he'd simply dumped the petri dishes in the sink. Finally cleaning them up, he uncaps each one before sanitizing it. One of the samples makes him hesitate, and his hand pauses before tossing the dish into the cleaning solution. He looks closer. The dish has been contaminated by some type of mold. Nothing too unusual about that—in his busy, often messy lab, this can happen. What's odd is that the mold seems to have killed the bacteria surrounding it.

Instead of dropping the petri dish into the sink and carrying on with his day, Alexander Fleming, whose name is now forever etched in medical history, walks across the lab, cranks the base of his microscope in position, and discovers *penicillium notatum,* the organic basis for the first antibiotic, penicillin. And it was a complete accident. Much later, Fleming reflected back on that critical moment that he might have missed had he not been paying such close attention. "When I woke up just after dawn on September 28, 1928, I certainly didn't plan to revolutionize all medicine by discovering the world's first antibiotic, or bacteria killer," he said. "But I suppose that was exactly what I did."[7]

It's impossible to pinpoint exactly how many lives have been saved by penicillin since it was developed into a medicine, but researchers estimate the number to be somewhere around two hundred million and counting. I can't help but wonder sometimes how much longer it would have taken us to figure out how to treat deadly infectious diseases, and how many lives would have been lost in the meantime, if Fleming hadn't hesitated before dropping that petri dish in the sink. Jan Shaw's recovery from end-stage lupus—and every other case of spontaneous healing—is like that petri dish. The lesson carries over; we need to *look closer*, not toss these "accidents" of biology away.

For Elizabeth Blackburn, the molecular biologist who was awarded the Nobel Prize for her work, the aha moment came from a pretty unexpected source: pond scum.

Blackburn wanted to study *telomeres,* the protective caps at the ends of chromosomes. Often compared to the plastic tips at the ends of shoelaces keeping them from becoming frayed or damaged, telomeres protect our chromosomes in exactly this way. She chose to study *tetrahymena*—a single-celled protozoan commonly referred to as *pond scum*—simply because it happened to have a lot of telomeres. Unlike Fleming, Blackburn had hoped to discover *something* when she picked up this particular petri dish. She just didn't expect to find what she ended up uncovering: a previously completely unknown biological compound that may hold the key to health and aging.

Chromosomes, as you might remember from high school, are essentially the filing cabinets of your DNA, storing all the essential info your cells need in order to know how to function. They contain the "operating instructions" for each cell—the manual that tells the heart cell how to be a heart cell, the T cell how to be a T cell, and so on. So, pretty important! With a few very rare exceptions, your cells don't live as long as you do. To keep you going, they have to regenerate. And that means making a fresh copy of themselves to carry on the work they've been doing. Ever heard someone repeat the popular statistic that the human body regenerates every seven years? It's a common claim that's close enough to the truth that it gets passed around quite a lot—seven years pass, your cells all regenerate, and boom! You're a new person.

Well, not exactly. Depending on their jobs, different cells have different life spans, ranging from a few days (skin cells, colon cells, sperm cells) to a few years. Some types of cells (muscle and nerve cells) regenerate rarely; only a very select handful (brain cells) hang around for your entire life. What the myth does gets right, though, is that you are constantly generating new cells. Your body is made up of literally trillions of cells—37.2 trillion, according to the most recent estimates—and every moment you're alive, they are copying themselves to keep you breathing, your heart pumping, your nerve endings lighting up with electrical impulses. Every time a cell makes a copy of itself, that instruction manual (the chromosomes) has to be copied exactly. And your telomeres are what keep those instructions intact.

That is, until the telomeres wear out. And just like those plastic tips on your shoelaces, eventually they do. Each time a cell divides and copies its DNA, a little tiny bit of each telomere doesn't make it over to the new copy. It gets shorter. And eventually, when it wears all the way down and the chromosome is exposed, the cell either becomes pro-inflammatory, causing issues in the body, or it dies. This time, it is not replaced.

The faster our telomeres wear down, the faster we age. And the faster we age, the more susceptible our bodies are to the diseases of aging. As your cells die off, there are visible and measurable impacts: as skin cells die, fine lines and wrinkles begin to appear on your face. As your hair cells die off, you get gray or white streaks. And as your immune system cells die off, you are left more vulnerable to inflammation and illness—not only communicable illnesses like colds and flus but other more serious ones: cardiovascular diseases, Alzheimer's, diabetes, and some forms of cancer.

A gradual telomere shortening and eventual cell death is inevitable for all of us, right? Well, sort of. Blackburn had noticed that some people's telomeres seemed to wear away faster, while others were more resilient to the relentless copy-and-refresh cycles of cell regeneration in the human body. Some of us literally age faster than others. Why?

The clue was in tetrahymena. Blackburn and her research partner, Carol Greider, chose to study tetrahymena because it was absolutely packed with chromosomes. And the chromosomes in tetrahymena did something extraordinary: their telomeres did not shorten over time as they were copied and replaced. In some cases, they even got longer.

Blackburn and Greider discovered that tetrahymena had an unusually high level of an enzyme that nobody had ever noticed before—a nameless, mysterious protein that seemed to keep tetrahymena's chromosomes "immortal." Blackburn and Greider named it *telomerase* and figured out that it exists in humans as well—we just don't have as much of it.

So clearly, the answer is just to douse ourselves in telomerase, right? Alas, no. As it turns out, telomerase behaves differently in humans than it does in single-celled organisms. In our bodies, high levels of telomerase are strongly associated with serious cancers. In a "too much of a good thing," twist, telomerase—which for a fleeting moment seemed like the miracle antidote to aging and death—is lethal if you have too much of it. The key is to maintain a balance—not too much, and not too little. The moral of the story is that we can't artificially increase telomerase without increasing our risk of developing dangerous diseases—but at the same time, we need to fiercely protect the natural telomerase our bodies *do* make. And what Blackburn and Greider found is that outside of genetics, the single most impactful factor that throws your telomerase out of whack, leaving your telomeres vulnerable to premature shortening, is stress.

Cortisol, the stress hormone, is healthy for you in small doses, but just like telomerase, it is terrible for you in large or constant doses. Constant cortisol secretion melts away telomerase, and as your cells divide and copy, your telomeres shorten much more rapidly. Two people who are chronologically the same age can be many years apart in biological age, depending on how much telomerase or cortisol they have flowing through their systems, so how rapidly you age and how quickly you advance into the disease span has a lot to do with your stress levels. This finding proved definitively what Benson and other pioneers had been trying to push into the mainstream for years: that chronic stress was a precursor to aging and disease and that being able to shift into the parasympathetic was a matter of life and death.

"I did not invent penicillin," said Alexander Fleming. "Nature did that. I only discovered it by accident." What unfolded in Blackburn's lab wasn't an accident like the discovery of penicillin, but she *did* find something she wasn't looking for: telomerase, a previously invisible enzyme, and perhaps the key to shutting down disease at the cellular level. It's a brilliant creation of nature, and yet we've been inadvertently flushing this health-giving elixir out of our systems instead of nurturing it. If we can fold the lessons gleaned from her discovery into the way we practice medicine, we may be able to eventually save as many lives as penicillin has.

It's not about becoming immortal or even drastically extending our life spans. It's about, as Blackburn calls it, extending your "health span." She breaks down a life into two eras: the health span—the time in your life when you are thriving, vital, and energetic—and the disease span—the time when you are sick, depleted, and dying. Blackburn suggests that by reducing chronic stress and maintaining a healthy balance of telomerase in our systems by lowering our dosage of cortisol, we can dramatically extend our health spans and be biologically younger and more resistant to disease.

At this point, you may be worried that you've already done

irrevocable damage to your health span—that after years of living chronically in a sympathetic, fight-or-flight pattern, you are doomed to short, frayed telomeres and damaged, misfiring chromosomes. In fact, relatively simple changes to your routine and lifestyle can put the brakes on that damage and begin repair. Working alongside Dr. Elissa Epel, Blackburn and Epel found that simply engaging in short but routine acts of mindfulness and meditation could interrupt the cycle of chronic fight or flight and begin slowing down cellular aging almost *immediately.* Telomerase begins to regenerate. Cells get healthier; *you* get healthier.

All those years ago, when Benson was pulling concepts from transcendental meditation to repackage into his relaxation response, he knew that mitigating the stress response had a major impact on health. Now we know precisely why that is. In their research on telomeres, Blackburn and Epel found that within *weeks* of making even small changes—such as incorporating the relaxation response, regular movement or exercise, or other activities that reduce your stress—your telomeres begin to improve.[8] And this is doing the bare minimum! When we look at cases of spontaneous healing, perhaps we are seeing what can be achieved when people go above and beyond.

I see a continuing pattern of spontaneous healers making significant changes in their lives that have the side effect of radically reducing stress, usually after their diagnosis and before their unexpected remissions. Take Claire, whose choice *not* to pursue invasive treatment for her terminal cancer was partially based around how stressful and draining it would be to sit in sterile waiting rooms with other dying patients instead of spending the short time she had left with those she loved. Take Juniper, who switched careers when she realized that her job, with its inflexible nine-to-five schedule, was exacerbating her autoimmune disease. She ended up pursuing a new line of work that was still challenging and ambitious, but that allowed her the ability to organize her own schedule around the activities that healed her: yoga practice, Rolfing, and being with her children. And Jan, who removed herself from a situation that was causing an enormous amount of stress and anxiety (her toxic marriage and the immense heartache around her grown children). That these life-altering decisions occurred in the time leading up to these individuals' spontaneous remissions is, I believe, no coincidence.

The seemingly obvious solution, of course, is to eliminate stressors. But plenty of aspects of our lives that are stressful are impossible to eliminate—they are simply part of life. We all have bills to pay, commutes to navigate, life logistics to handle—there is, unfortunately, no magical world where that all goes away. And other aspects—like career paths that are difficult but rewarding, or our young children who fray our nerves, or the elderly parents we're caring for out of deep love and devotion—we of course don't want to walk away from. So what do you do when something you love and value is a major stressor in your life? And how do you identify the *right* kind of stress?

THE STRESS CONUNDRUM

Stress is inevitable. And stress hormones, which get a really bad rap, are actually necessary for your body to have healthy function. In listening to discussions of stress and human health, it's easy to start picturing the cocktail of neurochemicals that dumps into your bloodstream in response to stress—cortisol, epinephrine, certain endorphins—as inherently toxic. But stress hormones are essential to human function. They play an irreplaceable role in the body; you quite literally cannot live without them.

Cortisol, adrenaline, and norepinephrine are the three stress hormones produced by the adrenal glands, which sit on top of your kidneys. If for some reason your stress hormone production swings wildly low, you enter a state called *adrenal fatigue*. With this condition, you have no energy to get up in the morning and may experience debilitating fatigue, dizziness, weight loss, and even heart palpitations. Adrenal fatigue is usually caused by other conditions—for example, John F. Kennedy lived with Addison's disease, which meant that his adrenal glands didn't work properly.

He suffered from chronic fatigue, abdominal pain, muscle weakness, and headaches. He took steroids to control these symptoms and was always at risk for more serious complications like blackouts or seizures from the too-low dose of cortisol in his bloodstream.

What all this means is that stress hormones are essential to keeping us alive and functioning. They are not inherently bad or evil, but as with everything, *dosage* is key. There's nothing wrong with intermittent stress. Stress is a normal, natural, and inevitable part of life on this planet. And it makes sense to be aware of places where the stressors in your life are perhaps *not* normal or natural—a constantly stressful job that's a bad fit, for example, or a romantic relationship that has become toxic or abusive—and make a major change. But what we really need to do is change the way we *perceive* and *react* to stress, to learn how to downshift out of fight or flight when we find ourselves stuck in that gear.

If the healthy, ideal approach to stress is like normal driving—shifting up when necessary, but then shifting back down to a lower gear as soon as possible—then the chronic fight-or-flight state that most of us are stuck in is like trying to drive while riding the brakes. It's harder to accomplish your tasks, and at the same time, you're wearing out both the engine and the brakes. We've got to learn how to downshift.

We can't—nor do we want to—turn off the flow of stress hormones into our bodies. Stress is necessary and is often a force for good. Up to a certain point, it can be a catalyst for change, can increase our capacity to learn or achieve, or can be a sign that something in our lives needs to change on a fundamental level.

A patient of mine who is a competitive bicyclist described the physical stress on the muscles in the body that comes from intensive exercise in training. He put it this way: "Intense exercise is basically a form of stress on the body. It puts stress on your muscles to the point that it causes lots of tiny, microscopic rips and tears. And then, later on, when you're resting, your body does the real work—capillaries grow farther into the muscle because of those rips and tears, the muscle is able to expand and get stronger and more flexible. It even happens with your heart—when you exercise, you put stress on that muscle and basically break it down. Then while you're sleeping, it builds itself back up again, stronger." We need both the stress of exercise and the ability to fall back into good, solid rest, repair, and reconnect cycles. It's for this reason that top-flight athletes use tools like heart-rate variability to know when their bodies need more of the parasympathetic.

The key here is that the stress this bicyclist puts on his body while training ends up becoming good stress *because* he allows his body to rest. That's where the growth comes from. That's how we learn from stress and get stronger—by turning *off* the stress and moving into healing modes, where our minds and bodies can process stress and use it as a tool for growth and healing.

What cases of spontaneous remission show us is that it's not always about removing the stress. Some stress will always be there. Sure, sometimes removing yourself from an extremely stressful situation—as Jan did when ending a toxic, abusive relationship—is absolutely necessary. But for many of us, we need to figure out how to change our *relationship* to stress.

As a young adult, I led wilderness trips for college students designed for leadership development. As instructors, we were trained to use stress to create opportunities for growth. Whether we were scaling a cliff, or bushwhacking all day and night on a thirty-six-hour mission, the point was to find the knife-edge of stress for each individual in the group—that edge where the opportunity for growth and learning was maximal but didn't tip over into toxic stress, which is not only harmful but also results in less learning. Individuals perceive and experience situations differently; what stresses one person can be a joy for another. But finding those lines helped participants begin fundamentally changing their relationship with stress so that what was originally stressful became less so. That was the growth we were looking for on the trips, and it created better leaders.

In 1967, Michael Marmot, professor of epidemiology and public health and head of the International Centre for Health and Society at University College in London, began a ten-year study that would upend ideas about stress and health. The Whitehall study's mission was to untangle the overlapping relationships between income, work hierarchy, behavior, and disease rates. One particular idea that held strong going into the study was that CEOs and other executives in the British Civil Service, those who held the most responsibility, suffered the most stress due to their jobs and therefore higher rates of heart disease.

The study, which followed eighteen thousand men between the ages of twenty and sixty-four for ten years, yielded some surprising results. Marmot expected that the lower classes of workers would experience higher rates of morbidity and mortality; that's because such lifestyle factors as diet, smoking, less exercise, less opportunity for leisure time, and so on impacted the health of those farther down the social ladder. But what was unexpected was that those factors only accounted for 40 percent of the differences between the upper echelons of workers and the lower. After controlling for those risk factors, the lower civil servants still had more than *twice* the rate of cardiovascular disease than the upper. Why? It turned out that those higher in the hierarchy experienced the inherent stress of their jobs as less toxic. Even small differences in the civil service hierarchy revealed identifiable differences in rates of heart disease. In other words, *perception* of stress, which in part had to do with where they perceived their rank relative to their peers, was huge. The Whitehall study ultimately showed that it's not the objective amount of stress you're under that leads to chronic fight or flight. It's how you *perceive* that stress.

We tend to interpret the findings of the Whitehall study as having to do with autonomy —those in charge had more autonomy and therefore perceived their jobs as less stressful, leading to less flooding of the body with stress hormones, less inflammation, less wear and tear on the heart, and less heart disease. But a similar Finnish study found that the health boost enjoyed by those higher up on the organizational chain had more to do with self-perception or self-esteem. Perhaps another interpretation of the Whitehall study is that if you perceive yourself as "less than," your stress levels go up. But whether it's ultimately about perceived autonomy and control over what's coming or self-esteem, the point is that our relationship to the stressors out there in the world is complex and shifting—and can be changed or managed. There are plenty of things worth doing that will add stress to our lives, but one key to staying in the parasympathetic is to make sure you experience that stress as positive or motivating instead of as toxic. Perception is everything.

While doing her groundbreaking research on stress and telomeres, Elizabeth Blackburn ran a study on women who were caregivers for chronically ill or disabled children. She thought this population would offer a particularly clear window into the effect of long-term, high levels of stress on human DNA. She was surprised, however, when she found a much wider margin than she'd expected within that group in terms of telomere length. Objectively, the women in the test group had similar levels of stress for similar lengths of time; their telomere lengths should therefore also have been pretty similar. But this wasn't the case. Why? What made the difference?

What Blackburn eventually discovered was that the women were perceiving, and therefore biologically processing, the stress differently. While one group saw the stress as a challenge to be overcome, the other saw it as a threat to their well-being. Women who viewed the stress of caretaking as "threat stress" had significant telomere shortening, while the women who viewed it as "challenge stress" preserved much more length.[9] It wasn't the objective amount of stress that determined telomerase activity—it was the women's *perception* of the stress.

The science is clear: the human body processes threat stress differently from challenge stress. What's harder is answering the next question: If you're experiencing threat stress, how do you transform it into challenge stress?

Changing your lens on stress often comes down to changing

your lens on yourself. When stress feels like a threat, the basis of that is often that you feel outmatched. At the heart of feeling threatened is the ancient sensation of being *prey*—smaller, weaker, vulnerable. When your body responds to a stressful situation biologically by going into fight or flight, that's telling you that the situation or problem seems insurmountable and likely to "devour" you.

One way that I coach patients to combat this feeling is to remind themselves of the resources they possess. We all have skills, resources, and deep wells of knowledge and experience that we often forget we have because we start taking them for granted or devaluing them. Remind yourself of what your specific assets are. Are you a quick thinker, adaptable, upbeat? Are you empathetic and thorough? If you need to, make a list, in writing, of all the ways you are already prepared to navigate this situation. And if there are ways that you aren't, who can you ask for help? We often don't know how to ask for support until we've figured out what specifically we need. And most of us hate asking for help, so much so that we fail to recognize that even small gestures or "lifts" from people around us can help tremendously in feeling supported and prepared to take on obstacles.

And finally, don't avoid the stress. Avoidance makes things bigger in our imaginations. Visualize yourself confronting the situation head-on and then walking out the other side. And then do it. Once you walk toward a problem, it may turn out to be not the tiger you thought it was but a shadow on the wall that looked like one. The more stressful situations you navigate your way through, the more possible it will be to look ahead at the upcoming rapids of life and think of them as a challenge. *I got this. I can do this.* I often take a moment, in the face of stress, to be grateful for the opportunity to learn—it seems to make me larger than the stress, lessen the stress that I feel, and focus my efforts on gaining something of value from the experience.

This isn't to suggest that traumatic and stressful events won't have an impact on you—it would be naïve to think so. But it does show us that we have much more control than we might yet understand over how events beyond our control affect our cellular biology, our current health, and our future health. We can't rewrite that ancient coding for fight or flight; it is written into our biological programming—the original "software." But what we *can* do is learn to develop new software and upgrade our operating systems so that we are more adapted to the modern era. We're walking around with out-of-date software running in our brains—it's time to listen to those red flags telling us that it's time to update the program. When you use these tactics to shift your lens on stress from *threat* to *challenge,* that's essentially what you're doing.

You may also need to recognize that stress and anxiety can be a gift, letting you know that something urgently needs to be addressed. Instead of trying to turn off stress or medicate away anxiety, we sometimes need to move through it, see it as an opportunity to learn, and listen to it so we can grow, change, and live an authentic life. Take the hermit crab. Hermit crabs feel pain and discomfort as they begin to outgrow their shells. For them, that pain is the sign that it's time to shed that shell and find a new one in order to grow. So often, in medicine and psychiatry, we prescribe medications or treatments that simply help people deal with the discomfort of being in a too-small shell. But we need to recognize when stress, and its related physical symptoms, is actually a sign that we, too, need to shed our shells.

Jan Shaw is a perfect example of someone who responded to the pressure and pain of constant stress by shedding her shell. She left a life that wasn't working for her, one that was destroying her physical health, and created a new one where she could grow and thrive. I called her up recently to see how she's doing these days. She now goes by Janet Rose—a new name for a new life. She lives in Idaho now, up in the mountains near Coeur d'Alene. It's been fifteen years since I last saw her. While we're chatting, she stops trying to describe where she lives and just emails me a photo; it shows the house she shares with her husband, a honey-gold wood cabin dripping with icicles, surrounded on all sides by soft, cloudy drifts of snow. It looks like a cold and sunny heaven.

She's sixty-four now and in good health. She doesn't suffer from lupus anymore, but she does have to be careful. Back in 2012, she had a string of fainting episodes. It turned out to be her heart. Before she chased the lupus out of her system, it did irreversible damage to her heart, which is permanently weakened. She has occasional flare-ups of inflammation that may be the lupus trying to reignite—she can feel it happening. It's her heart that tells her, with arrhythmias and palpitations. But she can usually roll it back simply with stress management, by cuing in to those points of pressure in her life and making a shift.

She sees a cardiologist to monitor it and make sure everything's okay. There hasn't been anything major, but she likes seeing him anyway; she looks forward to visits, even when there's nothing going on with her health-wise. They have long discussions about philosophy and medicine. He always schedules her for the last appointment of the day so that they have time to talk as long as they want.

She's crystal clear about why her health has turned around so dramatically. "I'm a different person now," she says plainly.

She changed everything: her relationship, her job, the way she perceives the world and herself, even her name. For Jan, that's what it took to get out of chronic fight or flight and into healing mode. Some people might try to chalk Jan's healing entirely up to eliminating toxic stress and therefore changing the chemistry of her body; others might give credit to the deep spiritual healing she experienced. But why try to separate the two? In Jan's case, they are inextricably linked.

She now has a good relationship with one of her children; the others, for now, remain out of reach. But she's found peace on that front. "They're on their own journey," she says. "And I'm on mine."

For Jan, her heart is the constant reminder of the illness that almost killed her. At the same time, it's become the main line of communication between herself and her body—a very effective one, since she is such a good listener. And after everything, it still beats.

Across cases of spontaneous healing, those who have recovered responded to the uncomfortable pressure of stress by eliminating disposable stressors, changing their lenses on valuable stressors (threat to challenge), or completely "shedding their shells." But making radical changes to restructure your life is easier said than done. In upcoming chapters, we'll look more specifically at what it means to "shed your shell," how survivors of incurable diseases did just that, and how it helped them advance from just visiting healing mode to *living* in it.

6

The Healing Heart

The body is the instrument of the mind . . . the mind is
an instrument of the heart.

—*Hazrat Inayat Khan*

In astronomy, physicists talk about uncharted planets that could
potentially sustain life as being "Goldilocks planets"—not too hot,
not too cold, but just right. Conditions are in that narrow, fleetingly
perfect range that allows life to take root, grow, and blossom. The
parasympathetic is our Goldilocks planet. In this mental and physical state, conditions are absolutely perfect for health and healing.

Any astronomer will tell you how rare this phenomenon is—
out of the billions of planets in the universe, only about a dozen so
far have turned out to be Goldilocks planets. Sometimes it seems
like the odds of living in the parasympathetic, in today's world, are
just as slim. And yet, some exceptional performers in health are
figuring out how to do it and showing us the way forward. They are
our forerunners.

As we discussed in the previous chapter, strategies like the relaxation response can wobble the needle of your nervous system into the
parasympathetic for a little while, and it *does* make a difference.

But most of us can't manage to stay in the parasympathetic for any real amount of time with just this strategy alone, which gives the body very little chance for true healing. And we need to find strategies that work for all kinds of people, ones that don't feel like another task on your to-do list. For example, not everyone is a meditator, and my experience is that even meditators don't always sit down and make sure it happens regularly. I certainly don't! The relaxation response is a great first step if it appeals. But spontaneous healing shows us that healing is about more than just relaxation.

As part of our autonomic nervous system—the part we can't consciously control—the sympathetic and parasympathetic work involuntarily; we can't just think our way into the parasympathetic. So how do we gain access to the gearshift so we can shift into, and stay in, healing mode?

RELEARNING HOW TO DRIVE

You can teach yourself to shift into parasympathetic mode by managing stress, eliminating stress, or changing your lens on stress. But once you've shifted into it, the parasympathetic needs fuel in order to run. If the tank is empty, you could drop back out of healing mode soon after standing up from your relaxation response exercise. And what fuels the parasympathetic is basically this: love and connection.

Does that sound crazy? I thought so, at first. It seemed too simple. And in some ways, it *is* simple. For years, research has been accumulating showing that love—both for others and for yourself—and connecting with other people keeps you healthier, while an absence of those relationships and connections can spell trouble for your immune system. And I'm not talking exclusively about *deep* connections; you don't have to run around falling in love with everyone you meet. Even moments of "micro-connection" can deliver hits of the potent love cocktail, spool up the parasympathetic, and keep it fueled up and running.

A few months after my first visit to Brazil, a young American man arrived there with a backpack of clothes, an angry scar from a failed radiosurgery that was healing under a prickle of shaved hair on his head, very little money, and three months to live. In 2003, Matt Ireland was in his early twenties and had recently graduated from college. He'd landed his dream job in Telluride, Colorado, at an adventure sports company perched in the Rocky Mountains. In the winter, he led ski tours; in the summer, it was mountain biking. When there were no guests, he worked long days clearing trails miles and miles up on the mountain. It was a beautiful place, and he was happy—at least at first. But at a certain point, his mood shifted and darkened. He started to feel really alone, even though he was surrounded by coworkers whom he liked. He sank into a strange and surprising depression.

"I'd never felt that way before," he says now. "People usually give me shit because I'm so happy."

In retrospect, his mood changes were the first in a cascade of symptoms indicating a serious problem in the brain. He started getting headaches. They always came at the same time: ten o'clock in the morning, just as he and his colleagues were getting ready to head up to the trail for a day's work slicing through downed trees with chain saws. The first few days, he tried to ignore it. It wasn't a bad headache, but it was an odd headache. It didn't throb through his skull like a normal headache or go away when he washed down an ibuprofen with a tall glass of water. It seemed deep inside his head in a place where he'd never before felt any kind of sensation. It lodged there like a bullet, radiating more and more pain as the days went by. Soon, he couldn't go up on the mountain to work anymore. He was dizzy, nauseated, and weak. The headaches came every twenty-four hours, and they got worse every time. He vomited; he was incapacitated by the pain. His coworkers urged him to go to the doctor, and finally, scared, he went.

It didn't take long for them to make a diagnosis. The MRI showed, unmistakably, a large tumor pressing on his optic nerve. They didn't know what it was, but they told him they had to get it out immediately or it was going to kill him.

They shaved his head, prepped him for surgery. He was

whisked into the OR. *Count backward from one hundred,* said the muffled voice of the anesthesiologist, hovering over him with her blue face mask. The last thing he remembers thinking is, *I am going to die.*

When he woke up, surprised to find himself still alive, there was a shunt in his skull, draining cranial fluid. He was in a nauseous fog of anesthesia, his head aching with pressure. The surgeon told him it had all gone well—they'd removed a large amount of the tumor, which they had sent off for biopsy. In the meantime, the headaches should stop. The surgeon seemed optimistic. His initial diagnosis was brain cancer, but not the worst kind; he estimated that Matt had stage I or II and that it would be treatable.

Within days, though, Matt took a turn for the worse. Even while he was recuperating from surgery, the tumor had started to grow again. They did another biopsy, took samples of cranial fluid. Within two weeks, they had revised their initial diagnosis. This time there was no optimism, no cheerful "we can fix it" attitude. The new diagnosis was a death sentence: glioblastoma multiforme, stage IV.

There was no treatment that would work against this type of cancer—not one that would actually cure it. The long tentacles of cancer reach deep into the brain tissue, making complete removal impossible. The average survival time is twelve to eighteen months; only 2 to 5 percent of those diagnosed are still alive five years later. It is an illness that is taught as ultimately having no survivors. Matt's doctor recommended a course of chemo, but only to slow down the progression of the disease. Laser therapy as a palliative measure was also suggested, to perhaps buy him some time. *Time.* It had seemed to stretch into infinity when he was standing at the tree line in the thin air of the Rockies, looking out to the horizon miles away. Now, he had very little of it.

As a seasonal worker, he didn't have health insurance. The surgery had wiped out his tiny savings and then some. His friends had fund-raised some cash for him, but once he paid off the staggering medical bills, he only had a little bit left over. He moved home, back to Vermont, to live with his mother. He knew that any form of treatment he undertook would only give him a few extra weeks or months and could come with debilitating side effects, but he wanted to buy all the time that was for sale. Matt launched into both radiotherapy and chemo, and when a new, experimental gamma ray radiosurgery option was offered at a world-class clinic at Dartmouth, he took it.

But the chemo felt like poison in his body, and he began to think of it that way. It made him sick, numbed his senses. He rapidly lost weight. No matter what he ate, it tasted the same kind of awful. "A spoonful of sugar and a spoonful of salt tasted exactly the same," he says. "Like ash."

Matt first turned to diet, as Pablo Kelly had. He read *Beating Cancer with Nutrition* and learned that one in five cancer patients who die don't actually die from the cancer—they die from malnutrition. Cachexia, a severe wasting of the muscles, seriously limits the body's ability to fight cancer and heal, and the National Cancer Institute estimates that it kills 20 percent of cancer patients. It's possible that these patients might have eventually succumbed to their disease anyway, but when malnutrition is wiping so many out before that point, there's no way to know. Like so many other recoverers, Matt decided that he needed to focus on eating the most nutrient-dense foods he could if he was going to give himself the best shot at recovery, or even just lengthening his very short time on earth.

After two weeks, Matt decided the chemo wasn't going to work for him. "It was ruining what was left of my life," he said. He flushed the pills down the toilet.

He had higher hopes for the radiosurgery, which the doctors at Dartmouth thought might represent a new, exciting way to treat glioblastomas. But the experimental new surgery, which used a special kind of laser to more precisely target the rapidly growing tumor, was not much more helpful than other standard interventions like radiation therapy.

One day, out of the blue, a neighbor called him at his mother's house. She'd heard about his struggle from some friends in town and wanted to help. She'd had cancer, too, she said, but got better—after she'd traveled to a healing center in Brazil. She described the community there, the people who arrived, the feeling of being loved and accepted, the transformative experience of truly believing you could get better. The neighbor invited him over, poured him some tea. She showed him the scars from her surgeries. She'd had a terminal diagnosis, just like he had.

Matt was intrigued but told her traveling to Brazil was out of the question. He couldn't afford it.

"Stop," she said. "Clear your mind. If your heart tells you that you need to go, I'll buy you a ticket."

A clock ticked quietly over the sink as he considered her words; he felt a swelling sense of possibility. So many people had told him what to do, what special treatments or tactics to try. But without a cushion of money or health insurance, everything had seemed so out of reach.

"Okay," he said. "Yes, I want to go. I need to go."

He ended the experimental radiosurgery at Dartmouth. They did an MRI to check the tumor's progression and found that the growth rate had slowed slightly. They told him they'd bought him a couple of extra months—a victory, in the landscape of glioblastoma multiforme—and to wait for his scar to heal before he traveled.

Did he have doubts about going to Brazil, on what could have been a wild-goose chase? Of course, he told me.

"But I had to do something," he says now. "I couldn't just sit at home and die."

In Brazil, he rented a cheap *pousada* at the edge of town, listened to the birds screech through the wooden shutters. The first night there, he had a strange and vivid dream, which he still remembers in perfect detail. He remembers it well because he thought he was awake—everything was so clear and real. Or maybe it wasn't a dream but a vision. He isn't sure. He woke up in the middle of the night—or dreamed he did. He sat up in bed and noticed that the bathroom light was on. *Oh, shoot,* he thought, *I have to turn that off.* But before he could move, the light shifted and flickered as if someone was walking around in there. And then a figure emerged, a woman, so shrouded in light that he could barely make her out. She approached him and placed her hands on his head. In that moment, he felt the most powerful physical sensation that melted from the crown of his head, over his shoulders and down his body, all the way to his toes.

"It was a feeling of pure love, perfection, light, God, whatever you want to call it," he says. "It was like when you get the chills, only multiplied by fifty thousand."

The figure lifted her hand, stepped away, and vanished. He woke up sitting on the edge of his bed in the dark.

"I don't know what it was. I've never had a vision like that in my life, either before or since," he reports. "Or maybe it was just a dream—you decide."

Matt felt echoes of that same sensation throughout his time in Brazil. He felt those reverberations—of light, love, and acceptance—everywhere in the community.

Once back in Vermont, he did not restart any kind of treatment. He went into the clinic in Dartmouth for checkups, but he didn't want to get a brain scan. If the tumor was still growing, as it almost surely was, he didn't want to know. He didn't want the fear, the constant panicked thoughts of illness and death intruding when he was trying so hard to stay peaceful and calm. They pressed for an MRI, but he declined. So, instead, they checked his healing scar, took his vitals. He seemed healthy enough—besides the fact that he was dying, which they all knew.

Months ticked by, and he passed the "expiration date" given to him at his diagnosis. He didn't feel the disease progressing. He felt good—better than he probably deserved to feel, given his prognosis. But he also felt wobbly, on edge, like he was perched on a thin ledge, about to topple to one side or the other. But would it be into life or into death?

He tried to spend as much time with friends and family as

possible—just connecting. He felt instinctively that it helped. Friends helped out where they could, paying for acupuncture sessions and craniosacral work. It was hard at times to keep the negative voices at bay. He felt negative energy from some of the people around him—it wasn't an immersive, hopeful community as there had been in Brazil. One of his mother's friends kept telling her to force him to go back on chemo, to go to the hospital. He was too tired to explain to her that he had tried all kinds of treatments and that they hadn't really gotten him anywhere. *There's nothing more we can do for you,* the doctors had said at the end of his radiosurgery.

Finally, he felt he had to know. He asked his mother to take him to Dartmouth to get an MRI.

His doctors were shocked—the tumor had shrunk. It was not an outcome that was considered possible with glioblastoma multiforme. They tried not to give him too much hope. Perhaps it was only a fluke, a temporary remission. They didn't want him to start thinking he would be cured; there was no cure for GM.

Then one day, another friend of his mother's made a comment that changed his course. Having heard his long story, she didn't respond negatively. "Seems like it's working," she said. "He should go back to Brazil."

Reinvigorated, he scraped the money together and booked his flight.

Returning to Brazil and the close, loving community felt like slipping into a warm bath. He relaxed into the arms of the community as soon as he arrived, rejoining the rhythms of the little town. And then one night, walking into the internet café to write an email to his mother, he met a young woman whose presence, energy, and direct gaze stopped him short. They exchanged names. She was there because she was depressed, she told him. Her life had lost meaning. She'd just lost her brother to Lou Gehrig's disease and her father to cancer—the very same cancer that Matt had. They snapped together like magnets, each realizing—in one of those rare encounters—that they were made for each other.

They were together from the night they first met. Matt didn't go back to Vermont. He stayed, worked odd jobs. They got married. They rented a house in town, and his wife went to work at the local pharmacy. As before, Matt initially avoided diagnostic imaging. But finally, two years after his initial diagnosis, he agreed to an MRI. It was a very different image from the one the doctors had hung on the light board in the hospital in Denver, which had shown a huge white mass where there should have been clean, gray brain matter. In this one, there was barely anything visible—just a tiny little knot of white, like a pinkie fingerprint on the film. They weren't sure what it was—a last remnant of the shrunken tumor or perhaps just scar tissue. Either way, the impossible had happened—his cancer had turned around; the tumor had melted away.

Matt still lives in Brazil with his wife, the love of his life. After undergoing radiation therapy, he wasn't supposed to be able to have children. The doctors had warned him before he accepted treatment. He'd always wanted kids, but he went through with the treatment anyway. He had so badly wanted to live. He had some sperm frozen at the time, but after years of paying for storage, it became too expensive. He had to let the dream of biological children go.

His sons are now three and five. As it turned out, he *was* able to have children—to watch his wife carry a new life, bring a baby into the world that was part him and part her, twice. Talking to him on the phone, a fuzzy international line, I could hear the high joyous shrieks of little kids off in the distance. "It's pretty busy around here," Matt said, laughing.

It's been fifteen years now since Matt was diagnosed with glioblastoma multiforme, the most aggressive form of brain cancer, and given four months to live without treatment. Something turned his disease around in a unique way, a way that medicine today considers impossible to replicate. What was it? There are, of course, many swirling factors that could be at play here, including many of those that we've already discussed in previous chapters: major diet changes, massive reduction in stress, a changed outlook on life and the challenges ahead. But Matt has his own theory about what changed things for him.

"It was love that healed me," he says with conviction. "To me, that's what God is, that's what life is. That's what getting better is, it's love."

LOVE MEDICINE

When we experience feelings of love and connection, our brains release a cocktail of hormones and chemicals. How exactly that cocktail is mixed (i.e., *which* hormones specifically are dumped into your bloodstream) depends on what type of experience you're having. Attraction, romantic love, platonic love, and social connection all have their own specific mixture, but most involve some combination of dopamine, testosterone, estrogen, vasopressin, and most importantly, *oxytocin.* Oxytocin, first isolated in new mothers nursing their babies, is often called "the love drug" because it's both activated by, and helps to *create,* connection, attraction, love, and bonding. And beyond helping to make and deepen relationships, it has health benefits. Oxytocin is known to be a kind of anti-stress tonic, counteracting the effects of fight or flight and stress hormones. It is also both anti-inflammatory and parasympathetic in its effects.

So what controls the release of this "love medicine" into your body? The vagus nerve. *Vagus* is Latin for *wandering,* and in line with its poetic name, the vagus wanders everywhere through your body. It exits the brain stem at the base of your skull, deep in your neck. It actually runs quite close to the carotid artery. Press your fingers to the pulse point on your neck and you are as close as you can get to your vagus nerve. From that spot under your fingers, it shoots down to your heart and beyond, where it regulates heartbeat and dozens of other vital functions. If you have any doubts about how deep and rapid the connection is between the mind and the body, the vagus is that literal link between the two—a thick, humming power line that runs from your brain to your gut.

The vagus nerve, in the way that it passes information both upstream and down, works a lot like the nutrition system in a tree. Picture your body as the tree, and the vagus nerve as the xylem and phloem, the transport tissues deep inside the tree's structure that pull water up to the leaves and then pass nutrients back down through the trunk. Your vagus nerve functions the same way, but with information. Remember those old pneumatic tube systems that banks used to have—you'd put your deposit envelope in the little canister, and it would whoosh away? Imagine that happening in the vagus nerve, up and down, passing messages between mind and body millions of times over the course of a day.

Eighty percent of the vagus pulls information up into the brain. The other 20 percent sends information down into the body. This means that a great deal of sensory information is being collected for your brain and that decisions are then made in the brain and sent out all over the body. It's a rapid, constantly flowing system that allows your heartbeat, breathing, digestion, endocrine system (the network of glands that releases hormones through your body), and immune system to constantly adjust and respond to all the collected information.

Think of how often you've used the phrases *gut feeling* or *broken heart* or told someone you had *butterflies in your stomach.* You feel different emotions in different parts of your body for a good reason: these areas are hotbeds of neuroreceptors. Recent research is showing that we actually have three "brains"—the head brain, heart brain, and gut brain—and our health and development depend on keeping them in balance and alignment. With the vagus as the connecting cord, emotions flood through our systems in the form of neural messages and hormones. Some signals begin in the gut, or the heart, and flow upstream to the head brain, while others cascade from above. In this way, our thoughts and emotions have both instant and long-lasting effects on all our biological systems: nervous, endocrine, immune.

In the previous chapter, we talked about the relaxation response and why it works. What we didn't talk about was the role of the vagus in that physiological response. When you do the deep, abdominal breathing that Benson recommends, you stimulate your vagus nerve. Even a deep sigh can activate it briefly—think of brushing your fingers over guitar strings, eliciting a rich, vibrating chord that reverberates for a couple of seconds. When you experience feelings of love and connection, it's like playing a whole song for your vagus nerve. The level of cortisol in your system begins to drop, and your telomerase is allowed to build back up to a healthy, balanced level. If you can keep on strumming those strings and keep your parasympathetic activated, a host of amazing health benefits will follow.

We know that inflammation is the common pathway underlying many diverse illnesses. But renowned neurosurgeon, immunologist, and inventor Kevin Tracey made an important discovery after the death by sepsis of a young woman under his care: the vagus nerve appears to be an "inflammatory reflex" that works in the opposite direction of chronic inflammation, to offset or reverse its deleterious effects.[1] When activated, the vagus senses inflammation in the body and relays this information to the brain and central nervous system, which then reflexively powers up the immune system, inhibiting inflammation and preventing organ damage. Studies are under way to explore the extent to which stimulation of the vagus can prevent or reverse many inflammatory diseases, including arthritis, colitis, epilepsy, congestive heart failure, sepsis, Crohn's disease, headaches, tinnitus, depression, diabetes, and possibly other autoimmune diseases. But the question then becomes: How do you activate or stimulate your vagus nerve?

The vagus is a nerve, but in one important way, it's more like a muscle—the more you use it, the stronger it becomes. Using the vagus—stimulating it through everything from deep breathing to connecting with a friend or partner—is like flexing your biceps as you lift weights; it increases its strength, flexibility, and elasticity. And just like with physical exercise, the more you use it, the better you get at using it, and the more health benefits you reap.

Remember when I said that you don't have to go falling in love with every person you meet to reap the health benefits of microconnections? Well, an expert in the burgeoning field of "positive psychology" and its biological impact on the body disagrees—sort of.

Barbara Fredrickson, a lead researcher at the University of

North Carolina–Chapel Hill, has immersed herself in research on this topic for over two decades. She's run study after study[2] showing that what truly tones the vagus nerve is small moments of connection—a sort of "falling in love," if you will—with the people who surround you on a day-to-day basis, everyone from your husband or wife, to children, to the barista you're getting to know at your corner coffee shop. It could even be a total stranger you meet on the street.

Fredrickson's research was fresh in my mind one morning as I was walking to a meeting along the streets of Cambridge. I zoomed by person after person who didn't meet my gaze as we passed on the redbrick sidewalk. They were lost in thought or wrapped up in the music I could hear coming from their headphones, faint and tinny. But as I crossed over the Charles River on a busy bridge, I fell in step next to an older woman pushing a baby in a stroller. I smiled at the baby, who turned out to be her grandson, and she smiled at me; when she broke the ice by asking where a particular building was on campus (the baby's mother, a student, was waiting there to breastfeed him), we fell into an animated discussion of children, families, and life with babies. I found myself remembering the years when my kids were infants and the difficulties and joys of that time. We ended up laughing together over the baby's unselfconscious facial expressions.

Fredrickson believes that culturally, we underestimate these fleeting moments of connection. They're more important than we realize. While I was talking with this grandmother, whose name I never even caught, I was wrapped up in our conversation, laughing, making eye contact, and when we arrived at the building, it seemed like the long cold walk had flown by. I held the door for her as she struggled inside with the stroller; she waved goodbye and disappeared down a hallway. I realized that in that fleeting conversation, I'd experienced a real moment of connection with someone, and "exercised" my vagus nerve in the same way I work out my leg and heart muscles when I go for a run.

And just as exercise tones muscles, stimulating the vagus tones

it in the same way. *Vagal tone* refers to your ability to rapidly activate the parasympathetic. The higher vagal tone you have, the more
rapidly you can recover from stress and relax into healing mode.
Whereas doing reps with a hand weight will tone your biceps, positive
emotions like love actually tone your vagus.

What is love? In very important ways, it may not be what we
think it is. It's not a continuous, never-ending state that we exist
in when we're "in love" with a romantic partner. Or at least, it's not
that *exclusively*. According to Fredrickson, love is a series of "micro
moments of positivity resonance"[3] that we experience, over and over
again, as we go through life. We may have just one of these micro-
moments with a stranger at a bus stop; or a million of them over
the course of a lifetime with the person we marry. We think of the
love we share with a spouse as being the most "important" love
out there, and in certain aspects—socially, culturally—it is. What
we don't realize is that when it comes to our health and biological systems, each moment of micro-connection—whether it's with
your spouse, with a friend, or with an Uber driver you just met—is
equally as important as the next and carries the same weight.

Think of each of these moments of connection over the course
of your typical day as stars, appearing in the sky as the sun goes
down. Each one is its own individual, bright moment, and as the
stars emerge, they begin to fill the sky with points of light. There
might be a hundred stars that represent micro-moments with your
partner or child, forming constellations that represent those important relationships, and one solitary star representing the laugh you
shared with a coworker on a thirty-second elevator ride. But each
one did essential work, quietly, inside your body—it lit up your
vagus nerve.

Our narrow concept of love could be making us sick. In her
book on the topic, *Love 2.0: Finding Happiness and Health in Moments
of Connection,* Fredrickson makes the bold claim that our fixation
on the idea of love as something that can only be shared in long-
term, intimate romantic relationships shows "a worldwide collapse
of imagination." She writes: "Thinking of love purely as romance or

commitment that you share with one special person—as it appears most on earth do—surely limits the health and happiness you derive from micro-moments of positivity resonance. Put differently, your beliefs about what love is become self-fulfilling prophecies."

Essentially, Fredrickson is telling us that to feel better, we need to expand our definition of love. We need to see all moments of micro-connection as meaningful—because when we do, we are more open to connection and more open to feeling the positive emotions of love, compassion, and empathy. In this way, our vagus nerve gets stimulated again and again and again, and the positive effects begin to build on one another, growing stronger. This leads to what Fredrickson calls an "upward spiral of the heart." It turns out that vagal tone, and the ability to experience moments of love, compassion, and connection, *increase* in relationship to each other, exponentially. That means that the higher your vagal tone, the abler you are to easily engage and connect with people, and the more you engage and connect with people, the higher your vagal tone.

That might sound like a catch-22 where, if you're not very good at forging social connections, you're screwed. Luckily, that's not the case! It *is* a self-perpetuating cycle, where the better you get at it, the more health benefits you reap, and the easier it gets. Fredrickson calls it a "use it or lose it" situation. If you're rusty, you have to get back on the bike and teach yourself to ride again. It'll feel awkward and hard at first, but it doesn't take very long until it becomes second nature and you gain momentum.

To test the idea of the reciprocal loop, Fredrickson ran a study[4] where participants signed up to practice a certain type of meditation called *loving-kindness meditation,* or LKM. People were randomly selected from a pool of volunteers to take a six-week course in LKM, which focuses on training participants to cultivate feelings of love, compassion, and goodwill toward themselves and others. The study wasn't especially demanding in terms of immersion; participants were simply asked to practice the meditation tactics they'd learned at home, whenever they wanted, for however long they wanted. It was up to them. They gave the researchers daily reports on both their meditative activity and their social interactions on that day.

Fredrickson and her research partner, Bethany Kok of the Max Planck Institute for Human Cognitive and Brain Sciences, tested their subjects' vagal tone (we'll get into how that's measured a bit later) before the study and then after. They found that as study participants' positive emotions increased through LKM, so did their social interactions, and as the number of social interactions went up, so did vagal tone. And the higher your vagal tone was when you started, the more it increased over the course of the study. There it was: the upward spiral.

The good news is that there's no certain level that you need to achieve on this spiral before you can begin accessing the parasympathetic for longer stretches. It's not like Chutes and Ladders, where you have to land *exactly* on the right square to climb the ladder toward healing and health. Fredrickson emphasizes that there are "multiple points of entry" to the spiral. And the higher you get, the faster you progress. Love is a spiral that lifts you higher and faster the more you allow yourself to feel it.

To return to the idea of the guitar, the more you practice, the better at it you'll get, and the more beautiful the music you make. Strumming the strings of your vagus nerve works the same way. Make sure you're playing music, and keeping that instrument warmed up and in use. But just as with Benson's relaxation response, a little bit goes a long way. And this begs the question: What could be achieved, health- and healing-wise, if you devoted yourself even more deeply to these practices?

We talked in the previous chapter about how our bodies are, from an evolutionary perspective, preprogrammed to drop into fight or flight at the slightest provocation. Indeed, it's the reason we're here—those of us who are alive today exist because our ancestors had a very highly developed, sharply honed fight-or-flight response that allowed them to live long enough to reproduce. We discussed the idea of learning how to override this programming now that we live in the modern world, where our fight-or-flight response is turned on too much of the time. But the deeper, more complicated truth is that we also have ancient programming that runs concurrent to that—programming that actually wants us to be in the parasympathetic. In fact, we are descended from the early humans who not only were adept at dropping *into* the sympathetic but adept at shifting back *out* of it, too.

SURVIVAL OF THE FITTEST, OR SURVIVAL OF THE KINDEST?

When you're running from a tiger, social connection is not the first thing on your mind. But as soon as the threat is out of the picture, it had better be—and fast. Your life could depend on it.

In fight or flight, you're ready to hit, punch, run, or hide—you're not ready to connect. Your ability to do so is literally shut down by your body's physiological and hormonal response, for your own protection. But once you can turn off fight or flight and shift into rest and digest, your body allows you to have these moments of connection, to feel compassion, to bond with others and experience love. As we've seen when looking at the vagus nerve, this can have long-term benefits for your physical health. But there are other reasons why we developed this biological response and why that programming is there—just as strong as our fight-or-flight instinct, and just as necessary for survival.

Let's zoom out and look at all this from a biological perspective. For your ancestor on the savanna, shifting into the parasympathetic was a very evolved defense mechanism. If you can connect emotionally with someone who's a potential threat, you can perhaps defuse the situation before it escalates. Basically, love and connection can be understood in part as a highly evolved, proactive defense mechanism.

When the parasympathetic is engaged, the vagus activates a face-heart connection. At a metaphorical level, it opens your heart to others, and on a literal level, it both relaxes and constricts different facial muscles that help you to smile, focus, and express warmth and interest so that you can connect with the person you're speaking with. When you're in chronic fight-or-flight mode, you have—

without even realizing it—a flatter or forced affect. Fight or flight stiffens your body, inhibits the warmth of your gaze, limits the genuineness of your smile, and overall inhibits your ability to make connections, letting those opportunities for micro-moments of love slip by. Others can sense—if only subconsciously—if your vagus is activated or not; they can feel your genuine positive emotion and connection with them, or the lack of it. A person in fight or flight will have more difficulty, therefore, in connecting with others.

Neuroception is the brain process in which you determine whether a person or situation is safe or dangerous. It's the reason, for example, why a baby will smile at a familiar face and cry at an unfamiliar one. Stephen Porges, a psychologist at Indiana University and UNC–Chapel Hill and an expert on vagal function, has researched what happens when people lose the capacity to make social connections. Trauma victims, for example, will have a nervous system that is extremely focused on detecting a predator but totally compromised at being social. Trauma, anxiety, chronic stress—all of this can put us into the "freeze" mode of fight-flight-freeze, shutting down our ability to experience micro-connections of positivity with the people we encounter throughout our days and even with those we love over the long term. And we're seeing more and more how the long-term effects of this disrupt healing and usher us more quickly into, as Elizabeth Blackburn puts it, the "disease span."

A recent review of twenty-eight studies, involving over 180,000 adult subjects, showed in stark relief how deadly it can be if you're cut off from social connection. After examining the data, the review panel found that loneliness, social isolation, or both are associated with a 29 percent increased risk of heart attack and a 32 percent greater risk of stroke[5]—a huge increase. People who reported fewer social connections also showed disrupted sleep patterns, altered immune systems, higher inflammation, and greatly increased levels of stress hormones. And consider the sociological landscape here—in the United States, one-third of those over age sixty-five live alone, as do more than *half* of the 1.6 million people who live in Manhat-

tan. In the UK, sociologists saw a marked increase in the number
of people living alone over the course of a decade; between 2001
and 2011, it went up by 600,000 people, a 10 percent rise.

Now, there are important distinctions to make between living
alone, feeling lonely, or being socially isolated, but similar numbers
repeat across other developed countries, leading sociologists and researchers to describe this, in multiple studies and reports, as "an
epidemic of loneliness." Loneliness, if you look at the numbers,[6] is
as important a risk factor for your health as poor nutrition, lack of
exercise, obesity, or even smoking[7]—but we don't see a lot of bus
stop posters warning us about this fact. You might have seen this
with a loved one in your own life—that when they experience the
death of a spouse and are suddenly alone, their health can decline
dramatically.

Fredrickson found that moments of micro-connection—those
little power boosts that fuel the love engine—have to happen *in
person*. While positive feelings like happiness and contentment can
certainly slow down the flow of those stress hormones and tip you
over into parasympathetic mode, it turns out that in-person interactions are the most potent fuel for the vagus—the higher octane
that really makes your parasympathetic hum. This means that calling your mother to talk on the phone is good, but even though
she's emotionally closer to you, she's going to get the best health
boost from chatting with her mailman as he drops off a package or
from sitting down with her neighbor for coffee.

When a person feels alone or is without social connection most
of the time, and the vagus begins to go dark, inflammation can
flare up, the immune system is suppressed, and pathways for disease that were previously closed begin to open up. We are now
beginning to understand the science behind this: how lack of warm
social interaction boots us out of that upward spiral that we need
to be in to thrive. In fact, feeling lonely long term, or becoming
socially isolated, can suck you into a *downward spiral,* where feelings of loneliness lead to more intense feelings of loneliness as time
goes on—compounding exponentially just like Fredrickson's upward

spiral. John Cacioppo, a social psychologist working out of the University of Chicago, researched the effects of loneliness on health and found that lonely or isolated individuals had an increased risk not only of heart disease and stroke but cancer. The reason for this comes down—no surprise—to the immune system.

Cacioppo and his research partner, Steve Cole of UCLA, found that in lonely individuals, their immune system cells were altered—right down to their gene expression. In other words, there was a notable change in the way the cells of the immune system behaved in lonely individuals versus those who had more opportunity for genuine social connection. In lonely individuals who tended to view the world more as a threat (remember the differences between threat stress versus challenge stress), the cells of the immune system became more inflammatory; that means more cells were constantly cycling through the body looking for something to fight like an army unit always on patrol with no break. Because of this, they tended to fixate on the body's own tissues, as happens in many of the autoimmune illnesses we've seen in this book.

The immune system has a fixed fighting capacity. When too many of the battalions are directed toward constant inflammation, it doesn't have the bandwidth to take care of other problems like viruses, infections, and even mutating cells. In the earlier chapter "Natural-Born Killers," we talked about how important it is to keep the immune system healthy and honed so that it can efficiently find, tag, and remove mutating cells before they become full-blown cancer. Well, it turns out that one of the best ways to do that is to genuinely fall in love—over and over again, every day, with your spouse, your kids, your friends, your neighbors, your coworkers. And if you don't have those people in your life, then find a way to socially engage in a manner that feels enjoyable and life-giving to you, whether it's a book club or an exercise class at the local YMCA. It could save your life as surely as picking up a lifesaving medication at the pharmacy.

Cacioppo laid out his research in an interview[8] with *The Guardian:* loneliness is contagious (it can spread from another lonely person you interact with as they cease to make eye contact and interact) and heritable (the changes in gene expression can be passed down to your offspring), and it affects one in four people—an epidemic indeed. It increases your risk of an early death by 20 percent. As Cacioppo puts it, if we were to build a zoo for the human animal, we would include the instructions "Do not house in isolation."

Social connections turn out to be an essential nutrient like any other; you can't heal without micro-connections to light up your vagus just as you can't heal without nutrient-rich food to fuel your body. Love and connection are clearly among the most potent medicines. We should be writing prescriptions for people to spend restorative time—those micro-moments of positivity—with friends, family, and new acquaintances, just as we write prescriptions for pharmaceutical medications. We should be asking, *How is the emotional nutrition in your life?*

When you think about it, social connection is a more evolved coping strategy than fight or flight. Fight or flight, after all, came first—the amygdala, buried deep in the brain, was one of the first areas of the brain to develop after we crawled out of the proverbial soup, which is why it's often referred to as the *lizard brain.* It's been there for thousands of years. But the parasympathetic response originates from more evolved parts of the brain. As we evolved, it was only when these more advanced, complex strategies for survival— forging connections, friendships, and alliances—failed that our ancestors fell back on more primitive modes of survival. It holds true today; when we lose the ability to connect, our lizard brains kick in, and we regress to more primitive forms of coping.

The fight-or-flight response is strong and acute, and for that reason, it can seem like an insurmountable instinctual curse—we can't overcome it, because it's coded into our genes. But love and connection —the spark and fire of the parasympathetic—is coded in there, too. We are *biologically built* for positive love and connection; it's the leading edge of how we are evolving, and as a species, we now seem to be working on how to take this to the next level and drop the chronic fight or flight from being our most frequent go-to strategy.

Think of the human baby. Holding my first child, looking down at his sweet, sleeping face, his tiny body wrapped in one of those blue-and-pink-striped blankets, I was temporarily flattened by how helpless he was, how dependent on me. Growing up on a farm, I saw newborn calves clamber to their feet and wobble along next to their mothers within minutes of being born. But long ago, when we evolved from primates and began walking upright, our hips narrowed, and our brains became more complex. To give birth to a baby that would be able to function at the level of other mammals, the human mother would have to gestate her baby for up to two years—which is too taxing for the female body. In order to evolve into the upright, highly intelligent animals we are today, we needed to give birth before our babies were really ready.

So evolution, ever ingenious, worked in such a way that the benefit for another (a baby) is interlocked with ours. Love for our young, the helpless little creatures in our arms, rapidly became the most important survival tactic. The compassion, connection, and caregiving we practice with our young stimulates the vagus and improves *our* health, as well as sustaining theirs. It's a symbiotic relationship, a win-win. It might not feel that way to exhausted new parents, but even over the most sleepless nights, a breastfeeding mother's body is awash in oxytocin, and her vagus nerve is humming.

Dacher Keltner, a professor of psychology at the University of California–Berkeley, has devoted his career to investigating and understanding the link between human compassion, survival, and health. Our capacity for compassion, he says, is what helped us survive and evolve as a species, and it could be the "medicine" we need today for making radical progress in health and healing. "We became the super caregiving species, to the point where acts of care improve our physical health and lengthen our lives," he writes. "We are born to be good to each other."

Charles Darwin is famous for his "survival of the fittest" theory of natural selection. I always assumed it was the gospel truth—I'd heard it repeated so many times, even in medical school. And then it was pointed out to me that in Darwin's seminal text, *On the Origin of*

Species, the "survival of the fittest" was a flattening of his more complex ideas about who survived to evolve and why. Scholars looking with a fresh eye at Darwin's groundbreaking work are now telling us that his message was more along the lines of "survival of the kindest."

On the Origin of Species is Darwin's most famous work, where he lays out the foundations of evolutionary biology in animal populations. But his lesser-known follow-up, *The Descent of Man,* focused all its eight-hundred-plus pages on *human* evolution. In these pages, he looks at the edge we gained as a species from taking care of each other and connecting in friendship instead of fighting. In *The Descent of Man,* he spoke only twice of "survival of the fittest." Love, however, is mentioned ninety-five times.

New research is coming together to show how love, compassion, and connection are even more than a survival tactic as Darwin perceived it. These same actions that lift us up as a species or society—caring for one another, helping, having empathy, and so on—are also causing an internal shift inside our bodies. They're letting us climb into that upward spiral toward health and vitality.

What we know: stimulating the vagus nerve reduces inflammation and boosts the immune system. Recovery from injury or illness is faster in those with higher vagal tone, and Fredrickson's work tells us that vagal tone is an incredibly accurate indicator of overall health. So if that's all true, how can we tell if our vagal tone is good? We can't just look in the mirror and flex it like rolling up a sleeve to check out our biceps.

Turns out, there is a fast and simple way to check vagal tone, and by extension, your capacity for health and healing—and just like love, it has to do with your heart.

THE WISDOM OF THE HEART

There is a window into vagal function, and it's a biometric called *heart rate variability.* Heart rate variability, or HRV, is different from blood pressure or simple heart rate, which only looks at the number of beats per minute. HRV refers to the changing time interval between your heartbeats and captures a snapshot of the heart's ability to flexibly respond to situations or stimuli. Your heart is not meant to beat at the same speed at all times; it needs to be able to change depending on your level of activity, emotions, and environment. *High* heart rate variability is good; it means your body can adapt your heart rate to your circumstances. It usually indicates a high level of ability to deal with and recover from stress. *Low* heart rate variability is concerning; it means there's rigidity in the system, that it has become less responsive, perhaps due to chronic overdoses of stress hormones, hardening of the cardiovascular arteries due to inflammation, or other causes. Low HRV has been associated not only with anxiety and depression but also with an increased risk of cardiovascular disease and early death.

And most important, HRV is an excellent indicator of vagal tone. The higher your HRV, the more engaged the vagus nerve, and the more the parasympathetic is active in your system. What this boils down to is that HRV is a major, underutilized index of general health, and of vagal health specifically.

Can we use HRV in our everyday lives to help us understand our bodies better? Until recently, finding out your HRV wasn't the easiest thing to do. You'd have to go to a doctor, have them hook you up to a heart monitor, and then study the readout from the software that analyzed the electrocardiogram. But lately, there's been a proliferation of ever-more affordable devices combined with free downloadable apps that can give you a snapshot of your HRV. The technology is still developing, and some may be more effective than others, but at the rate things are going, it seems that it will only get easier to figure out your HRV and use it as a tool to navigate toward health and healing. And in the meantime, if heart rate monitors and apps aren't for you, just be aware that any of the tactics we've discussed here for getting in touch with your body, bringing down inflammation, and shifting into the parasympathetic will also positively affect HRV. Practicing the relaxation response or meditation, getting to know your stress triggers, and learning about your body's responses to stress and connection so you can more flexibly move into healing mode—all of these can only help improve HRV, and with it, vagal tone.

The heart is an important messenger, and there's a reason that it has become such a powerful metaphor in our culture—the physiological changes that happen in the body in response to emotions and stress can make it seem as if those feelings are originating from the heart. No wonder the poets have long focused on the heart as the symbol for love and loss. In medicine, however, the heart is simply a pump; its job is to keep us alive by circulating blood and oxygen. But what if the whole truth somehow includes both poles—both the literal muscle and the metaphorical symbol?

Heartbreak is something we talk about metaphorically; we don't actually believe our hearts can break like a dropped vase. But there is a rare, deadly heart complication called *takotsubo cardiomyopathy,* or more colloquially, stress cardiomyopathy. Doctors call it *broken heart syndrome* because it's essentially a situation where acute emotional pain causes potentially fatal heart complications. Until very recently, there was a lot of debate over whether broken heart syndrome was real, with doctors and surgeons choosing sides. Then, in 2016, a woman was airlifted to a Houston hospital with a clear-cut case of broken heart syndrome that was impossible to deny.

Joanie Simpson arrived by helicopter at Memorial Hermann with intense chest pain, exhibiting the classic signs of a heart attack. Doctors immediately threaded a catheter into her heart, expecting to find blocked arteries that they would have to prop open with stents. Instead, they were startled to discover that her arteries were "crystal clear."[9]

A study published a decade before in *The New England Journal of Medicine* (*NEJM*), a journal that's a standard-bearer in medicine, had confirmed that in some cases, an intense flood of stress hormones could essentially stun the heart and produce, essentially, a heart attack. Switching gears, doctors quizzed Simpson about whether she'd had any unusual stress in her life recently—and she had. She cited a number of recent family and financial stressors and then came to the most devastating: the day before, she'd watched her dog, a pet that she'd loved and treated like a child, die a painful death. She took it hard. So hard, in fact, that it interfered with the function of her heart muscle and could have damaged her heart or even killed her.

Simpson's case was written up for *The NEJM*,[10] settling the debate over whether or not broken heart syndrome was real. In an interview with *The Washington Post*, who followed up on the remarkable case, Joanie was quoted as saying that she "takes things more to heart" than other people. We think of phrases like this as being simply metaphors, a playful use of language, but they can be much more. In this case, Joanie Simpson used the well-worn phrase to offer a window into both her emotional and physical truth: she *literally* "takes things to heart."

Consider the difference between Joanie and Eileen, the woman who arrived in the ER with AFib after her husband left her. In the case of Joanie Simpson, the link between emotional upheaval and the biology of the body was quickly homed in on and explored, instead of ignored or dismissed. The vagus runs right through the heart—the nerve endings from both are intricately interwoven and constantly exchanging information. And the heart has over *forty thousand* neurons, more than any other location in the body after the brain and the gut. This means that the heart is another little brain—the heart brain—its own locus of emotion, sensation, and knowledge. And it provides a unique window into our mind-body connection and how that is helping us heal—or stopping us from doing so.

If there's one thing I've learned from caring for thousands of patients, it's that the heart is more than a pump. It is not just an organ that distributes blood throughout our bodies; it is also representative of our deepest longings, greatest joys, and most profound sorrows. Sometimes the heart reflects—like a metaphor—something going on in another, deeper part of us, something missing that we don't easily acknowledge or know how to put into words. If we listen, we might be able to find our way toward the life we truly want and deserve—a life of authenticity and fulfillment—and perhaps also toward healing.

LIVING IN HEALING MODE

A lot of us have been locked out of healing mode for a long time. Our vagus nerves haven't been lit up consistently and may need some electrical repairs. Perhaps, like Jan before she visited Brazil, stress, anxiety, or trauma have worsened our health. Perhaps constant and elevated doses of cortisol have washed away too much of our telomerase, and we have invisible telomere shortening in our cells, those all-important building blocks of life. Or it may seem that we are simply fated to become ill—that something was coded into our DNA like a computer virus, just waiting to start running its malware programming.

When you have a serious illness, it can start to seem hopeless—like your health future is already written. But it's never too late to shift gears. That Goldilocks planet, with conditions just right for health and healing, is open to all. Researchers have found that a childhood full of adversity or a life with constant stress shortens your telomeres and your health span, but they have also found that those effects could be dramatically mitigated and even rolled back. When we look back at Jan's case, we see a perfect storm of overlapping conditions that came together to allow her to heal. She completely changed her life, leaving a toxic marriage and finding a loving, supportive one. She let go of the overwhelming responsibility she felt for her children's lives. She started living a more authentic life where she understood her value.

We know now that the vagus nerve is activated by compassion for others, compassion for the self, and positive feelings in general. We know that what *really* lights up that circuit is not only the relaxation response but also love—micro-moments of positive connection with those you are intimate with and even those you barely know. Fight or flight, with its hair-trigger rush of stress chemicals, is powerful. But if you can rearrange your life to allow yourself to *more frequently* experience those higher states of love and other positive emotions, you can "inoculate" yourself against chronic fight-or-flight response as surely as you can get vaccinated against tuberculosis or the flu.

The precise lineup of conditions that make the parasympathetic possible in today's world might seem as rare as an eclipse. But unlike an eclipse, which is the product of celestial bodies drifting through space and far beyond our reach, setting the conditions for radical healing *is* within our control. From what you eat, to how you think about stress, to how you interact with others, you can change the biology of your body right down to those telomeres inside your cells.

Back when Benson was running his first studies over thirty years ago, the idea that our emotions or mental state might have any impact on blood pressure or the rhythms of the heart was considered ludicrous—so much so that it deterred researchers from investigating that area of rich potential. Today, the same biases continue to hold us back from taking the next step in finding pathways to healing. There's been a modicum of progress—a grudging acceptance that, yes, the mind *can* impact the body, and vice versa. But while this understanding has trickled into the popular culture, it has yet to be integrated in any real way into mainstream medicine; it's grabbing hold in popular culture more than in the day-to-day practice of medicine.

Fundamentally, in medicine and psychiatry, we are still operating with an understanding of the mind and body developed by the philosopher and mathematician René Descartes back in the seventeenth century: that the mind and body are separate entities, existing in completely different realms. Descartes conceived of two separate "worlds," one which contained the body, or matter, while the other contained the mind, or consciousness. The belief was that events in the physical world had no impact on the mental world and vice versa.

Where did this idea come from? Well, in many ways, Descartes developed the concept of mind-body dualism as a backlash against the prevailing ideas of his *own* time, which, back then, were effectively holding medicine back from necessary progress. In the seventeenth century, religion and medicine were braided tightly together. Humans were seen as spiritual beings—the body and soul were one entity. Very little distinction was made between mind, body, soul, or consciousness, to the point that when a person died, their body had to be preserved perfectly intact to preserve the soul. Medical dissections were not allowed; if the body was taken apart, the soul would be similarly dismembered and would never be able to ascend to heaven. And illness and disease were often blamed on wrongdoing, either by the individual or by the community as a whole, or as a judgment from God.[11] If a woman fell ill with mysterious symptoms—a growing lump in her abdomen, rapidly losing weight, sallow skin, vomiting and unable to eat—it might have been suspected that she had committed a sin. Her soul was being punished, and therefore, her body as well. If an illness swept through the town, killing children and babies with dehydration and diarrhea, the community would take the blame upon themselves. They had not been pious enough; they hadn't worked as hard as they should; there were disbelievers in their midst.

"Treatment" in these cases would be prayer, confession, a purging of the soul. The woman's body would never be dissected to reveal the cancerous tumor that was the real cause of her death. Attention would never be turned to the town's wells, contaminated with a dangerous strain of bacteria. The origins of health and illness were shrouded in superstition and fear and a firm belief that maladies of the body were punishments handed down by an omniscient god.

When Descartes peeled apart the mind and body, he assigned the "soul" to the realm of the mind, freeing up the body to be examined, dissected, experimented upon. While it might seem like only a philosophical shift, it had the groundbreaking effect of making the human body available to science. Suddenly, the anatomy of the body was allowed to be revealed. Doctors and scientists were finally free to explore the biological mechanisms of the human body, and with that, the mechanisms of disease.

The major medical advancements of the last three hundred years have essentially toppled from the separation of the mind and body like a line of dominos. But we've reached the end of that line of dominos. The last one has fallen; we are now in a lull. I believe that we've made as much progress as we could within the constraints of mind-body dualism and that we need to reach back, to reclaim what was actually right about that old idea that the body and soul were one.

Perhaps progress is more of an upward spiral than a line: we keep circling back to old ideas, but with new knowledge and technology, so that as we arrive back at the old point, we do so on a new plane, full of new possibilities. That begs the question: What will we now do with the burgeoning understanding that the mind and body are in fact deeply interconnected and that healing the soul, in many cases, can heal the body?

I'd come so far in my research after Brazil, where I'd had access to a pool of promising cases to evaluate and pull from. Though not all of them had panned out under rigorous inspection, Brazil had certainly represented a hot spot of spontaneous remissions, one that had been illuminating for my research. Looking at those cases as a group, I had to wonder: Was spontaneous healing really so "spontaneous"? While some cases of remission did seem very sudden—a tumor that was present one day disappearing the next, for example—the accumulating evidence suggested that many recoveries were weeks, months, even *years* in the making. A reversal of disease that may seem spontaneous to doctors, who are only seeing a small slice of a patient's life, or even to the patient themselves, might in fact be the result of something that's been developing for a while—like seeds planted long ago that "suddenly" burst out of the soil and bloom.

I felt close to gaining the big picture on spontaneous healing, but it reminded me of scaling a mountain peak on the wilderness trips I'd led in college—knowing you were close to the peak, even though it was obscured by clouds—only to crest the hill to see the peak still farther ahead. I needed another Brazil.

PART TWO

THE MIRACULOUS MIND

7

Faith Healing and Healing Faith

> It is better to believe than to disbelieve; in so doing you
> bring everything to the realm of possibility.
>
> —*Albert Einstein*

CLEVELAND, OHIO: 2012

I arrived in Ohio in the dead of winter. It was early March, the month that should mean a suggestion of spring, but the world was locked in ice. A recent storm had piled a layer of new snow onto old snow, the layers visible where the snowplow cut through. Cars whooshed through the icy slush as I hunched against the cold, mentally running through my interview questions. My mind flickered back to where this all started almost a decade earlier—I recalled stepping off the plane into the heat and humidity of Brazil with no idea what I was walking into. My thoughts about what I was doing there were as hazy and blurred as the steamy air. Today, though, all these years later, my plan was crystal clear. I wasn't there to debunk or prove anything this time; I was far beyond that. I was there to dig deeper into the mystery of belief and how it overlaps with healing.

My feet crunched salt crystals and ice as I walked up the stairs to a nondescript office building belonging to Dr. Issam Nemeh, a trained physician who has also been called a "faith healer." The snowy concrete streets of Cleveland were about as far as you could get from the warm dirt roads of rural Brazil. Inside, Dr. Nemeh's office was like any other American doctor's office—beige carpeting, potted plants, a big window overlooking a parking lot. On paper, this couldn't have been more different from the warm plazas full of goats and chickens, but both places seemed to be like magnets for cases of spontaneous healing. So what did they have in common? That was the burning question.

I'd first met Dr. Nemeh when we both appeared on *The Dr. Oz Show* in 2011. I'd hesitated about going on the show. With TV and radio discussions of "miraculous" healings, so often the questions don't go beyond a surface level, staying firmly in the territory of asking, *Is this real?* without going into the implications and lessons—the part that might actually help people. At the same time, I knew we had to start getting these stories of spontaneous remission out of the shadows, and these cases might offer a desperately needed antidote to the epidemic of hopelessness I was seeing in medicine.

But was *hope* really something that could change the course of an illness? Or was it, as so many in the medical profession believed, just an illusion—a mirage that led people to walk interminably through the desert, with no relief? Wary of offering "false hope," doctors shy away from expressing to patients the full spectrum of possibilities. We stay firmly, safely, within the averages, the most likely outcomes. We are conservative, careful. But are we so afraid of offering so-called false hope that we fail to offer any hope at all? And how does this impact health outcomes? So when *The Dr. Oz Show* called and wondered if I could serve as the medical expert in their investigation into a so-called faith healer from mid-Ohio, I was intrigued.

I didn't know what to expect from Issam Nemeh, a healer with a devoted following. The only thing I knew was from the short briefing the show producers had sent: Nemeh was a credentialed

M.D. with a background in anesthesiology and surgery. That didn't really jibe with my idea of a faith healer.

And when I shook Nemeh's hand for the first time in the green room backstage, neither did he. Dressed in a collared shirt and brown checked sweater, he seemed like your stereotypical family doc. And yet, I would quickly discover that Dr. Nemeh is a study in contradictions. Born in Syria, he is now a midwestern Catholic who raised a large family in the suburbs of Cleveland. Vigorous in his early sixties, he smokes cigarettes, eats what he wants. He takes few breaks, working most days of the week, often until the early hours of the morning. There is a long waiting list of people desperate to see him, either for the high-tech, electronic acupuncture he practices at his medical offices or for the healings of a different kind he performs on occasional weekends around the country. He believes the divine works through him, guides his hands. But he rejects the label *faith healer*. I quickly discovered that while others frequently refer to him using this term, he himself has never used it to describe what he does. His calling, he says, is to bridge the gap between science and spirituality. And the people who've had their eyesight mysteriously restored, bones knitted together, and tumors melted, among other startling recoveries, believe he can do just that.

Dr. Nemeh has his detractors, people who believe he is a false prophet, peddling a fantasy. But when you witness the sheer number of people who flock to be treated by him and listen to their stories of hope and recovery, you begin to wonder if there's something to it. There's a down-to-earth practicality about him that, as a doctor myself, I find refreshing; though he believes fervently in the power of prayer, he also advises those who come to him to continue seeking mainstream medical treatment. And he'll be the first to admit that his style of healing doesn't work for everybody.

From the first few moments of conversation with Nemeh, it was obvious to me that he had a tremendous capacity to connect with people one-on-one, creating a quick and genuine intimacy with his patients.

Onstage for the taping, Dr. Oz grilled him about his methods and the seemingly impossible recoveries that occurred under his care. Nemeh was modest, eschewing responsibility for the healings. It wasn't him, he said—it was God, working through him. He was only a conduit.

Dr. Oz asked for a volunteer willing to have Nemeh treat her onstage. A woman raised her hand and was ushered next to him. Her complaint was debilitating back pain. He placed his hand on her back and prayed, and the room immediately became hushed and quiet. People leaned forward in their seats to catch what he was saying, but his voice was a murmur. Even I couldn't catch it despite standing right next to them. He wasn't performative; he just did his work. He didn't seem to care about the audience at all. It was as though he and the woman were alone together.

I scanned the faces in the audience, curious what people were thinking about prayer and healing. Mostly they were quiet, respectful. They didn't seem skeptical, which didn't really surprise me; in Gallup polls, nine in ten Americans say they engage in prayer, and three out of four pray daily. Eighty percent of Americans have prayed for their own healing, and a whopping *90 percent* have prayed for the healing of others.[1] It was likely, based on the stats, that most people in that studio had a deep-seated belief in the power of prayer.

Still, the practice of laying on of hands, of praying over the body, may seem strange to some. And even though I myself grew up in a very religious family that put a lot of stock in the power of prayer, as I watched Nemeh bow his head and murmur over this woman, I felt a familiar kick of disbelief or resistance. In the world where I'd grown up, there were a lot of rules. A lot of judgment. Prayer was about confessing your sins and praying for things you wanted. I'd grown up viewing prayer as another ritual without reason, something we did because we were required to. As I got older, though, I realized that it wasn't that I didn't believe in prayer at all—it was that I didn't believe in prayer the way it was presented to me as a child.

Dr. Nemeh lifted his hands off the woman from the audience. She stood up with a look of relief on her face.

"How do you feel?" Dr. Oz asked.

"It's amazing," she said. "It's gone; the pain is gone."

The audience applauded, so I clapped along, but I wondered if her relief would last. Research into pain, especially back pain, is contradictory. People can have a scan that shows multiple slipped discs or other issues that should be debilitating but report zero pain. Others struggle with chronic pain, but their scans come back clear. I considered that this could be a classic example of the placebo effect—when you get better or, more commonly, simply *feel* better because you believe you will. Patients who believe they're getting a miracle drug, but instead receive nothing but a sugar pill, nevertheless can improve, sometimes dramatically.

The line from mainstream medicine was that placebo was a sort of smoke-and-mirrors effect; people weren't *really* getting better, they just *felt* better. It was mind games, not real medicine. But this journey into the depths of spontaneous healing had already taught me that there were powerful healing resources in the mind and heart that we were leaving untapped. I knew I had to look very seriously at the potential physiological impact of belief on the body. What was the difference between feeling better and actually getting better? Where was the line between believing yourself healed and true healing?

Nemeh's patients cycled onto the stage to tell their stories, taking turns in the spotlight to describe the trajectories of their recoveries. There was Kathy Kuack, who went to Nemeh with lung cancer and a malignant tumor, which had advanced to the point that her doctor was ready to remove the lung. After a visit with Nemeh, the tumor shrank and then vanished. There was Meredith Kreye, incapacitated with Lyme disease—couldn't get out of bed, walk, or see light without a shattering headache—who healed, went back to school, took up horseback riding. And then Leonard DeBenedictus, whose bones were literally dissolving after working for decades with toxic chemicals. Many of his coworkers had died of leukemia and other cancers, he said, and he was on the brink of having to have his fingers amputated. He claimed that when Nemeh told him, "God wants you healed," the pain he'd had for decades evaporated, and his strength and flexibility began to return.

And then Patricia Kaine began to speak. She was the last of Nemeh's patients to tell her story. Sitting across from me on the stage, under the disorienting glare of the hot klieg lights, she seemed calm and cool—straight-backed, hands folded in her lap, fixing each of us in turn with a steady gaze. She was conservatively dressed, with long silver hair parted on one side and a charmingly flat midwestern twang. She was a doctor herself; she'd practiced family medicine for decades. So when she received her diagnosis— idiopathic pulmonary fibrosis—she knew exactly how bad it was. Idiopathic pulmonary fibrosis is a disease of the lungs that's progressive, incurable, and always fatal. Doctors aren't sure what causes it, but the result is irreversible scarring of the lungs, which worsens over time until the patient can no longer breathe. Essentially, your lungs turn to cardboard and you die.

The first question to ask is always: Was the diagnosis accurate? And that's what Dr. Oz zeroed in on, questioning the validity of the diagnosis. The most likely scenario in cases of spontaneous healing is that the disease has been misdiagnosed and that it is not the incurable, fatal illness the doctors think it is. Dr. Kaine nodded. As a physician herself, she had certainly already gone down this line of inquiry.

"They did a biopsy of my lung tissue, and what it showed was fibrosis," she said. "When you're looking at something under a microscope, you can't call it something it isn't."

How could someone have fibrosis—which causes irreversible scarring of the lungs—and now have healthy lung tissues? Medically, it should have been impossible.

Dr. Kaine and the others who appeared on the show all attributed their healing to God working through Dr. Nemeh. They believed that it was his prayer—his ability to channel God's energy—that had healed them. Could they be right? I couldn't discount it. But I was going to have to dig into the research and evidence on prayer and healing, as well as the placebo effect. The two were distinct, of course, but intricately connected by the idea that what you believe can heal you. While those who pray frequently assume that the healing comes from an *external* source (God, or in some people's view, the collective energy of the people praying), placebo assumes an *internal* source (your own mind, beliefs, perception). But what was there in the common ground between prayer and placebo that might yield the next key to spontaneous healing? It was the thread of *belief* that ran through both of them, and it was a thread I needed to follow.

The show wrapped up, and the audience applauded, but it was only the beginning for me. I knew I needed to talk further with Dr. Kaine and with a wider sample of Dr. Nemeh's patients. I was going to have to go to Ohio. It was possible that I'd stumbled upon exactly what I'd been looking for: another unusually high concentration of spontaneous remission cases. Brazil was a place that naturally seemed to collect instances of spontaneous healing because of something particular about the place and the culture, I theorized, and because of the type of person, with a unique approach to health and healing, who felt called to go there—drawing the richest cases of remission all to one place. In epidemiology, when researchers find an elevated level of disease or infection outbreak, they call it a *hot spot* of disease. Ohio, like Brazil, could very well be the opposite: a hot spot of healing.

A HOT SPOT OF HEALING

At first glance, Issam Nemeh's exam room looked like any other. A bit antiseptic, with a paper sheet over the exam bed, medical equipment hanging on the walls, a sink, and a rolling doctor's stool. But little differences stood out, such as the shelves lined with personal mementos from patients who experienced dramatic turnarounds under his care.

In his exam room, Nemeh described what he generally did with patients. Most of it is connection: he talks with them, he listens.

He prays over them, or over a specific body part that bothers them. Appointment lengths are variable. Sometimes people are in and out quickly; other times he'll spend two, even three hours with someone if that's how long it takes. People sit in his waiting room for hours, patiently waiting their turn. He works late into the night, then gets up in the morning and starts again.

At one point, he looked at me sitting in my chair, taking notes, and said, "You've got a back problem."

I did have a back problem. As a kid, I worked hard on my parents' farm, carrying heavy hay bales and five-gallon water buckets. When very young, I had to hold them up high so they wouldn't drag. I'd always assumed my back pain was from that physical labor, that I'd permanently damaged my back through overwork from a young age. I barely thought about it anymore; I'd gotten used to it, accepted it as simply part of life. It came and went but flared up especially badly when I was under stress.

Nemeh looked at my back. Something was out of alignment, he told me. He prayed, a low murmur. It was brief. When he placed his hands on my back, it suddenly felt very warm and pliable as rubber. He moved something into place—or it felt like he did—and the pain was gone.

For the rest of the day, I kept expecting it to return, but it never did. Years later, it still hasn't.

The next day, I began interviews with Dr. Nemeh's patients. In a small conference room at the hotel, I moved some chairs into position and showed the cameraman where he should set up his tripod. He was a volunteer, sent to help out by Issam Nemeh and his wife. I'd asked them to send me patients willing to speak to me about their recoveries. I was explicit about the criteria: I needed people who'd had an incurable medical illness, as well as indisputable evidence of both accurate diagnosis and recovery. I was hoping they'd have at least a few people who met those requirements. Kathy Nemeh, a fiery, outgoing spark plug of a woman and the hyperorganized engine behind Nemeh's practice, sent me *twenty-five*. And there were always more if I needed them, she promised.

People cycled through the conference room over the course of two days as heavy snow fell outside the hotel windows. It was a whirl-wind, with hours and hours of interviews, one stacking onto the next as I took rapid notes and tried to think on my feet to ask the necessary follow-up questions whenever an interview took a sur-prise twist. Back in my hotel room at the end of each day, I went over the evidence. It was tough. They were all fairly strong cases. But some weren't quite as clear-cut as others. With some, I couldn't be completely sure that the person had fully recovered and wasn't simply in a temporary remission that's typical for that particular disease. Lymphoma and leukemia, for instance, are extraordinarily complex illnesses. There are some forms of these diseases that are quickly fatal, but others wax and wane for long stretches of time. In other instances, the diagnoses and recoveries were well documented and real, but the disease in question was obscure and rare. When a disease is peripheral and rarely seen, we don't have a lot of research or data on it, and we can't be sure how it behaves and what's possi-ble. A sudden remission may be in the realm of possibility for the normal course of this disease—we just don't know.

But others leaped out, startling examples of what's possible in human healing. There was Guy, who suffered from severe rheumatoid arthritis, an incurable autoimmune disease that attacks the joints and is progressively painful and debilitating. Under Dr. Nemeh's care, he went from a complete inability to function to leading a normal life. He attributed his healing to Dr. Nemeh but also to forgiveness. He felt that forgiving a close family member who had hurt him deeply decades earlier had "removed a toxin" from his body. And indeed, the way he described it, the process of forgive-ness had seemed to literally loosen his joints.

His story was almost unbelievable, but I knew there was also some degree of scientific basis for his claims; I'd seen multiple studies on the health benefits associated with the process of for-giveness. Researchers theorized that it could dislodge entrenched patterns of stress and anxiety, lessening and rebalancing the stress hormones in the body. *Forgiveness* has been associated with lower blood pressure and lower risk of heart attack; people who are more hardwired to forgive others seem to have stronger, more robust immune responses. *Unforgiveness,* on the other hand, because of the complex mix of hormones and chemicals released by constant negative feelings, can dampen the immune system and make it worse at fighting off viruses and bacteria.[2] Listening to Guy's story, it made me wonder if the science on forgiveness was just the tip of the iceberg. If such strong correlations had been found in controlled scientific studies, perhaps, in certain situations, even more is possible.

And then there was Karen.[3] She and her twin sister had both been born with cerebral palsy, a serious disorder that affects the brain and muscles and can be quite debilitating. Cerebral palsy is a permanent, irreversible condition. And yet Karen had recovered. Before she began seeing Issam Nemeh, Karen had frequently used a wheelchair. At school, she tried to get along without it, pulling herself up the stair railings, but walking was always difficult. Now she could not only walk on her own, she could run. She felt stronger than she'd ever felt in her life.

Startled, I wondered if this could possibly be true, pressing her for more details—and then I remembered my own session with Nemeh, how my back had suddenly felt strange and pliable.

So what did I think about prayer and healing? I still wasn't sure. I could see how the act of praying, in the way that it connects you to others, could launch a praying person into what Barbara Fredrickson called the "upward spiral" of the heart. Feeling connected to others, a sense of community and belonging—those kinds of positive feelings can mitigate stress and activate the parasympathetic. But was there more to prayer? What did the research show? I needed to dig into it. And I still needed to talk to Dr. Kaine, one of those whose story had propelled me out to Ohio in the first place.

"I'LL PRAY FOR YOU"

Dr. Nemeh's patients believed their healings came from God and that Dr. Nemeh was a conduit. He tends to describe himself as an "energy healer" and believes that prayer is, in fact, a form of energy.

But the research on prayer and healing, when I dug into it, was a morass of contradictions and controversy. There's not a lot of hard research to look at—it's difficult to get funding to study prayer—and the research I did find was a mess. A meta-analysis of all major studies done on prayer concluded that less tightly controlled studies obtained positive responses, whereas the tighter, more rigorous studies found no particular correlation between prayer and healing. But they were difficult to evaluate. Overall, there was a pretty even split between studies that found prayer had a positive impact on healing and those that didn't. I wondered about the methodologies, though. In applying the scientific method as it is commonly used, with the classic double-blind, placebo-controlled study design, were we washing away everything that made prayer potentially powerful?

In 2006, Herbert Benson, ever interested in the mind-body connection after his work on meditation and the relaxation response, received a million-dollar grant to run the largest study on prayer ever completed. The study was to look at intercessory prayer and surgical outcomes. *Intercessory prayer* refers to prayer on *behalf* of others. So the question was, could somebody praying in Oklahoma have an impact on the outcome for someone in Ohio who was being wheeled into surgery?

Benson's study was the most rigorously designed study in the history of prayer research. It was randomized, double-blind, placebo-controlled—by official standards, it was watertight. Here's what they did: They took 1,500 people from six hospitals across the United States who were all getting the same surgery, a coronary artery bypass graft. Benson likely chose this particular surgery because he was trained as a cardiologist and because a lot of previous studies on prayer had been done with heart patients. Plus, heart disease is one of the leading causes of death in this country and across the Western world, and this particular surgery is a common one—the year this study was done, more than 350,000 Americans, and over 800,000 people worldwide, received this surgery. That made it easy to get a good sample size.

Patients who agreed to participate were randomly assigned to one of three groups. The first group was told that they may or may not receive prayers during their surgery, and then they did receive them. The second group was told the same thing, but then didn't receive prayer. The final group was told that they would definitely receive prayer, and they did. Typically, about 50 percent of all patients receiving this particular heart surgery are expected to have at least one complication. This was the measure Benson used going into the study to determine whether or not intercessory prayer could have an impact on the success of a surgery—whether or not this number dropped when people were prayed for.

Benson found three prayer groups that agreed to participate for the entire length of the study, which was quite a commitment: the study would run for *three years.* For the duration of the study, Benson's team faxed each group a list of names the night before those patients' surgeries. Catholic prayer group participants at St. Paul's Monastery in Minnesota and the community of Theresian Carmelites in Worcester, Massachusetts, and one prayer group called Silent Unity in Lee's Summit, Missouri, who knew nothing about the people they were praying for except their first name and last initial—*Matthew L., Sarah G.*—repeated the same scripted prayer each time for each name on the list: *For a successful surgery with a quick, healing recovery and no complications.*

The results of the study were distinctly *not* what many had hoped for. The first two groups—those who were unsure as to whether they'd be receiving prayer—had almost identical rates of complications post-surgery, at 52 percent and 51 percent, respectively. This was just a percentage point or two away from the usual rate of complications with this surgery—statistically insignificant. So when people were unsure of whether they'd be prayed for, the prayers they received—or didn't—seemed to have no impact. However, those who knew they'd receive prayer, and *did,* had a markedly higher rate of complications: 59 percent.

What happened there? Why on earth would the prayed-for people have a higher rate of complications? Could prayer *hurt* instead of help somehow?

Benson had a couple of theories. One was that it was a fluke—a 9 percent increase in the rate of complications within a study group could simply be the normal fluctuation of results. It wasn't too far outside the range, and the normal rate of 50 percent is of course an average, compiled from hundreds of thousands of surgeries each year. His other theory was that the study results were complicated by *other* prayers. Study participants were told not to alter their usual plans surrounding their surgeries, to simply continue on as if they weren't being prayed for by strangers in Minnesota, Missouri, and Massachusetts. And many of those people already had friends and family praying for them. Many prayed for themselves. To ask people not to do this, or to forbid friends and family from praying for them, would have been "unethical and impractical."

"Thus," Benson wrote, "our study subjects may have been exposed to a large amount of non–study prayer, and this could have made it more difficult to detect the effects of prayer provided by the intercessors."

It fascinated me that those who knew they were being prayed for had a *higher* rate of complications. Benson's hypotheses about why that happened were certainly valid. But I wondered if there were more to it. Perhaps some people viewed prayer, and God, as something external, something outside of themselves—and so in this case, prayer became a sort of silver bullet. There could be danger in that just as there was danger in viewing medications as a silver bullet. In these instances, nothing in you needs to change—not your attitude or your perspective; you just wait to be healed. Being prayed for, perhaps, is too passive an activity to have an impact on healing. And Dr. Nemeh spoke of prayer as an energy, something that can have different levels of *quality*—but the quality of prayer was a dimension wholly unexamined in this study.

Ultimately, I found that I couldn't take this study—rigorous as it was—as a final statement on prayer. Perhaps it was more of a statement on the design of the study and how studies are run in general. Our studies are rooted in a traditional understanding of science and the scientific method and are designed to measure only things "outside of us," things known through our five senses. Looking at something like prayer, which is infused with mental, emotional, and spiritual factors, is almost impossible for our current conception of the scientific method, which by design washes the individual, with all their uniqueness, their exceptionality, their deeper qualities, out of the equation. With a study like this, we have no idea about the intensity of the prayers and no idea about the level of spiritual development involved.

It was the same way I was trained as a doctor. In medical school, they taught us to block out the context, the individual story, and focus on the disease, the symptoms. We weren't supposed to take into account the patient's feelings, backstory, intensity, or desires. We were trained to cut that out, create a tight circle around their symptoms, and place that small, tight circle on the microscope deck for evaluation. We miss a lot by taking this approach. And so did the studies on prayer. *How* you pray could be an important factor. And what about how deeply people believe in the power of prayer, or if it's more of a social function or tradition for them? Are there ascending qualities of prayer, just like there are levels of capacity between different athletes?

So many of these studies, including Benson's, guaranteed that people were *performing* prayer but didn't examine anything beyond that. I thought of the way that studies on the healing effects of meditation and yoga asked participants to perform these rituals and how we are just beginning to think about how to measure the depth to which people were investing themselves in these activities—or not. There is a difference, it turns out, between meditation studies with untrained college students and advanced meditators. Why wouldn't this also be true for prayer?

Benson's prayer study *was* rigorously designed from the perspective of scientific medical research. His methods were unimpeachable; nobody could have accused him of being sloppy or unscientific. But to me, the study didn't actually tell us whether there was power in prayer when it came to healing. That question had to come down to what the praying person thought, felt, and experienced. Prayer is not yet quantifiable the way a medication is; it can't be evaluated in the same way. You can't say for certain what it's "made of" or what the "dose" is. Perhaps prayer could be transformative, or it could be utterly powerless—*depending on what you believed.*

The same is true for faith. We use the phrase *faith healer* reflexively to describe people like Issam Nemeh, but what do we really mean when we say *faith*? It's a simple word with an enormous amount of weight hanging on it. *Faith* has been defined as "the assurance of things hoped for, the evidence of things not seen." To "have faith" is to be able to hold on to your beliefs, even in the face of adversity or suffering. But just like prayer, *faith* means different things to different people. And if it means holding on to your beliefs no matter what, then doesn't it matter *what,* exactly, you believe in?

Ultimately, both prayer and faith are *expressions* of belief. When we try to dissect whether prayer can heal, or whether faith can heal, what we really need to look at are the belief systems underpinning it all—how we see the world, how we make sense of our lives, what we believe is possible or impossible. In cases of spontaneous healing, was there evidence that what you believe can affect how and if you heal? If so, to what degree? How much is wishful thinking or a psychological solace, but ultimately nothing more than that: something that soothes your suffering but has little impact on disease trajectory? Can what you believe actually affect the biology of your physical body?

On *The Dr. Oz Show,* Patricia Kaine attributed her healing to prayer and to Dr. Nemeh. He'd been a conduit to God, she said. Prayer healed her. But when she went into that conference room months later for the follow-up interview, it turned out that there was so much more to the story.

"MIRACLES ARE REAL"

Patricia Kaine took off her winter coat, sat down, and folded her hands in her lap. She was exactly how I'd remembered her from the soundstage on *The Dr. Oz Show:* cool and composed, no-nonsense, yet with a warm and friendly demeanor. I asked her to tell her story in her own words, in her own way. She paused and took a deep breath.

"How much time do we have?" she said, practical as always.

"As long as it takes," I said, flipping to a fresh page in my notebook.

"You mean you want the *whole* story?" she said. "Nobody's ever asked for that before."

Patricia's sister contracted polio when they were both very young, right before the vaccine came out. The hospital that treated her told the family that it was the worst case of polio they'd ever had where the patient had survived. They were told to expect a lifetime of disability; she would never walk without a brace.

Patricia remembered her sister coming home from the hospital, weak and incapacitated. Her mother would do exercises with her sister every day, trying to strengthen her wasted limbs, even though the doctors had told her there was no point. Patricia's aunt even traveled to Lourdes, the famed healing waters in France, and brought back a vial. Patricia's mother used it to bless her sister's limbs, hoping it would help.

"With my mother's dedication to the exercises, and the Lourdes water, too, she got better," Patricia says. "She walked. She became a nurse. She works as an RN now. But the real importance of this story is that I grew up knowing that miracles are real."

Patricia married young, at twenty. When her husband switched jobs, they moved to rural Appalachia, the area where southeast Ohio meets West Virginia and Kentucky. It was a scrappy, insular, and downtrodden area, beautiful in its own way, with silvery, weathered wooden buildings that stood before a backdrop of forested, sunset-colored mountains. People often lived in those buildings without running water or electricity.

Pregnant with their fourth child, Patricia paid monthly visits to her doctor. She noticed how difficult it was to get care, how wildly the demand for health care outpaced the supply. Her appointment was always the last one of the day. The doctor was obviously exhausted. She'd often be the fiftieth patient he'd seen that day, and yet he still had to muster up the energy, the attention and focus, to review her chart, to listen to her baby's heartbeat, to tell her in a weary voice what she needed to know about prenatal vitamins and the upcoming birth. She felt for him, and she felt for the community, especially the people who didn't even try to visit the doctor because they couldn't pay. There weren't enough doctors to go around.

She realized that this was her calling. She knew she had the intellectual ability to be a doctor. In school, she'd had perfect grades. But she'd set all that aside to become a wife and mother, which was what was expected of girls at that time in her community. When Patricia applied to medical school in the 1970s, only 3 percent of students entering med school were women. She was turned down from school after school, where admissions officers felt that because she was a mother, she couldn't be a doctor. Only two schools allowed her to even fill out an application. Only one gave her an interview. When she walked into the room, all eyes went to her belly; she was six months pregnant with her fifth child. She counted on her fingers right in front of the interviewer and said, "Look, by the time school starts, I won't be pregnant anymore."

She started at Wright State University School of Medicine six weeks after giving birth. She was still bleeding heavily; something was wrong, but she hadn't been able to see the doctor. Her husband was out of work, they had five little kids, and she was now a full-time student, waiting for the loans she'd applied for to come through. She was sitting in the exam room with an infection in her uterus, bleeding into a pad, "stuck in that tiny piece of paper that's supposed to be a gown," when the billing person came in and told her she'd need to pay in full before she could see the doctor. She had to put her clothes back on and leave without getting help. The experience showed her that this was the state of medicine in the United States. This was the reality for so many struggling families.

"I understand what happens to underserved people when they can't get medical care," she said. "I've lived it."

After her first year in medical school, she had only a C average. Technically, that was fine; it wouldn't keep her from graduating or becoming a doctor. But she didn't feel comfortable with her performance or knowledge base. She asked to repeat the year.

"It wouldn't be fair to patients," she said, "to not get the best training."

Wow, I thought. *Now this is the kind of doctor I'd want for myself.*

She graduated after five years with a quarter million dollars in debt, five children, and an out-of-work spouse. She and her husband eventually divorced. After her residency, she returned to Appalachia—the place that had called her to medicine. The vast majority of her patients were on Medicaid or some other form of relief, as she once had been. Some didn't have running water. They'd take their baths in the creek before coming to see her. But from the time the creek froze over until it thawed, there was no bathing. The first year she practiced, she made barely enough to survive and make the monthly loan payments. It was a constant struggle. But every time a patient came in who couldn't pay, she remembered when she'd been in that same position—sitting there, bleeding and sick, in a tiny paper gown, with no money in the bank to pay the bill.

"Looking back, it was all preparation for what I'd go through with my illness later on," she said. "It's not that this one has privilege and deserves care and this one does not. We are all equal in the eyes of God."

After four years of practicing in Appalachia, the government changed their payment structure. Even as she increased the number of patients she was seeing, her income dropped by a quarter. She was sinking. With kids in college and no child support, she couldn't make enough money to pay her loans and support her family. So she took a salaried position in Bellevue, Ohio, up north near Lake Erie. It was right on the highway corridor between Toledo and Cleveland. More people, more patients, better insurance, more money. She could make a living there. Sadly, though, it meant putting her goal of helping the underserved on hold.

And then, in 1995, the first sign of trouble: she was tired, achy.

It's nothing, she thought, *I'm just fighting something off.* But it didn't go away.

For months, she saw specialist after specialist. But she wasn't getting better. At the time, not much was known about idiopathic pulmonary fibrosis; it wasn't really on anybody's radar, not even Patricia's, a dedicated family doctor. Finally, she decided to see an infectious disease specialist she'd worked with and admired during her residency, who ordered a chest x-ray. It turned up an immediate red flag.

In a typical chest x-ray, the two symmetrical shields of the lungs should show up black, while the hard bone of the ribs and spine are white. Patricia's lungs, instead, were fuzzy, almost crystalline, like looking through a shattered car windshield. The terminology in medicine is *ground glass appearance.*

A quick follow-up CT scan showed fibrous tissue in both lungs—the soft and spongy lung tissue was turning to tough, striated scars. A nuclear scan was consistent with this. And then the biopsy confirmed it. Four out of four tests showed only one possible diagnosis: idiopathic pulmonary fibrosis.

Dr. Kaine was already familiar with the disease. In Bellevue, a very small community, another family doctor she knew had also been diagnosed with idiopathic pulmonary fibrosis that very year. And he'd died from it.

Lung fibrosis starts with a tightening along the walls of the lungs as scarring begins. As the disease progresses, the wall of scar tissue becomes harder and tighter, wrapping the lungs like a plaster casing. The lungs become less and less flexible and expansive, and it becomes impossible to take a deep breath. The body cannot get enough oxygen. Patients report extreme fatigue and weakness. Sometimes, caregivers report people passing peacefully in their sleep. Other times, there is chest pain and overwhelming fear as one struggles with oxygen starvation, unable to inflate the lungs and pull in air. But it always ends in death; there is no cure for idiopathic pulmonary fibrosis.

The word *idiopathic* means "of unknown cause." Patricia was diagnosed in 1995; today, doctors still don't know what causes it. In some cases, it could be genetic, although Patricia didn't have a family history of fibrosis. It could be autoimmune—the body turning against itself, the immune system confused. In fact, I found a study from 2015 showing that patients in the acute stages of IPF temporarily responded to autoimmune therapies, suggesting that the root of the disease *is* in fact an immune system gone haywire. However, regardless of the trigger, it's still known to be incurable, progressive, and eventually fatal. And as I researched the disease, I found it was more common than I'd realized; today, it affects over one hundred thousand people in the United States alone, and five million worldwide.

Five years is what the specialists told Dr. Kaine. That's how much time she had, at the very most. And even that was a generous prognosis. The median survival rate for IPF was three years. Less than 20 percent of patients survived beyond five. Patricia wanted to make it into that 20 percent and stretch her time as far as she could. She had grandkids now; there was so much she wanted to do and see. If she was going to die of IPF, so be it, but this was too fast.

Over the next few years, she steadily declined. She got weaker, tireder. She had to go on disability and then on oxygen, carry a CPAP machine around with her wherever she went to help force the oxygen through her ever-more scarred lungs. She was sleeping eighteen hours a day, constantly tired because her body had insufficient oxygen. She tried going to a specialist in Toledo, but she was so wiped out after the drive there and back that she slept for a full twenty-four hours.

When her niece suggested Dr. Nemeh, she shrugged. "Why not?" she said. She'd tried everything else.

Fast-forward a year and a half. Patricia was stronger, more alert, more energetic. She was back to sleeping a regular schedule of eight to ten hours a day. And she was continuing to improve. She went off disability and got back on track with what she'd always felt was her mission in life: to help those who needed it. She went back to work, making home visits to people living in the inner city who had trouble getting to doctors. And she found herself using the CPAP less and less. Eventually, she stopped using it completely. It had become unnecessary.

It was a stunning reversal of a progressive, incurable, and fatal disease. Patricia Kaine shouldn't have been getting better; she should have been getting worse. What sort of sudden magic had Dr. Nemeh performed?

First of all, Patricia said, nothing happened overnight. It happened incrementally, in small steps, over the course of a year and half while she was seeing Nemeh once every two months or so. She would drive out to Cleveland for the visits, where Dr. Nemeh would start with "electro acupuncture," a type of acupuncture he developed that incorporated vibrations and magnetism to target areas of the body in need of attention. He used the machine, and prayer, in every session. It was just Dr. Nemeh and Dr. Kaine in the room. She felt that she was the complete focus. When he prayed over her sick body, it felt to her like energy was flowing from him to her. The sessions could run anywhere from forty-five minutes to two hours—they were scheduled for an hour, but ended up lasting, according to Dr. Kaine, "as long as God wants them to."

"You lose complete track of time when you're in there," she said. "It's like time doesn't exist."

After the sessions, she didn't feel depleted like she had after traveling to see other specialists. She felt calm and energized. She rebounded more quickly. Each of the dozen or so times she saw Dr. Nemeh felt like a leap forward.

"Why do you think that was?" I asked her, scribbling notes.

She thought for a long time. "Every time I would see him," she finally said, "I would leave knowing that I was closer to God."

Finally, a chest x-ray came back with impossible news. Her lungs, those two shield shapes on the light board that had once come up blurry, crisscrossed with scar tissue like a shattered windshield, instead showed clean black. Clear. No evidence of scar tissue.

Even after all the years of hearing these stories, I was still as-
tounded. And Patricia's story was absolutely staggering. How do
you make sense of it? She was diagnosed by biopsy—the gold standard. She was given three to five years to live, with no possibility of
cure. And yet here she was, almost a decade later, sitting in front of
me, breathing easy, vibrant and healthy. But scar tissue in the lungs
does not just disappear.

The case raised some big questions. Patricia hadn't made many
diet or lifestyle changes as so many others had, and so I couldn't attribute her stunning recovery to those kinds of radical life shifts. I
had come so far in my study of spontaneous healing; I'd felt that I
was so close to getting the big picture. But perhaps each of the previous factors I'd isolated—diet, inflammation, immune function,
stress, and even love and connection—all hinged on something
bigger, something deeper, something more fundamental. Each of
these principles had been an important stepping-stone on the road
to understanding, but I was beginning to see that the most pivotal factors were unmeasurables—things that had been left to the
side by science because they simply could not be quantified in a
controlled experiment the way nutrition, inflammation, stress hormones, and even thought patterns could be.

When I asked Patricia Kaine to try to explain what Nemeh
could do, and why, she thought for a while.

"My way of describing it is to think about water," she said.
"If you have to walk ten miles to a well carrying a bucket, you can
bring water back to a community, but it limits how much you can
bring. If you build a conduit, a pipe or an aqueduct, you can bring
much more—unlimited amounts. That's how Dr. Nemeh is, but
instead of water, it's love. And he's the conduit."

A lot of people conceptualize their remarkable healings in this
way: as something separate or external that is poured into them
like a healing drink. They view it as a gift from God, with the
healer working as a kind of conduit. And perhaps there's something
to that hypothesis; there is so much we don't know about this vast
and mysterious universe we inhabit. But as we just discussed, is it

the prayer itself that heals, or the *act* of praying? Is it that healers like Nemeh are truly conduits for some kind of healing energy, or is it that people *believe* with their whole hearts that they are? How much could what you believe truly affect your biology?

I was going to have to dig deeper into one of the more controversial and hotly debated topics in medicine: the placebo effect.

8

The Power of Placebo

In the theory of relativity there is no unique absolute time, but instead each individual has his own personal measure of time that depends on where he is and how he is moving.

—*Stephen Hawking*

The word *placebo* has Latin roots and means *I shall please.* Attentive healers of all stripes have known for eons that belief can play a role in healing, long before the rise of science. But the origins of the term *placebo effect* come from eighteenth-century doctors' attempts to describe a practice they often found themselves engaging in: giving patients drugs or treatments that they knew had no objective medicinal value in themselves in an effort to please or satisfy the customer. It wasn't widely viewed as having significant healing capacities; mostly, it was a way to make stubborn patients go away and maybe give them a little faux relief while they were at it.

But then doctors began to notice that such faux treatments— sugar pills and diluted medications—actually *did* seem to have an effect. In those days, though, physicians weren't typically using what we now call *pure placebos;* the stuff they were giving patients was usually some mild medication thought to be harmless. The medication, often diluted, wouldn't help them, but it also wouldn't harm them. It was a win-win; the physician had already done everything he could, but the patient felt more satisfied. What downside was there? But of course, it was more complicated than that. History is full of stories about snake oil salesmen traveling the country peddling their wares with astounding tales, many of which may have been made up or exaggerated—words an ill person so desperately wanted to hear that they would be willing to part with a few coins for hope.

When patients began to claim improvements from medications thought to be inert or weak, it was initially chalked up to being "just in their minds." And so initially, the placebo response was used to debunk quack medications or treatments. In 1799, an expensive treatment called Perkins Tractors was supposed to "draw disease out of the body" by using "animal magnetism" channeled by a set of specially constructed metal spikes that were held against the afflicted area. Patients claimed relief for everything from pain to boils. A physician named John Haygarth constructed a replica of the Perkins Tractor made out of plain old wood and documented patients experiencing the exact same "miraculous" effects. As many people with rheumatoid arthritis (four out of five) experienced a lessening of discomfort when they used the fake Perkins Tractor as when they used the real one.

But what the experiment proved was not that the placebo effect was especially powerful (it didn't examine, for example, whether people using the Perkins Tractors *actually* experienced recoveries, or if they just believed that they did), but instead served to punch a hole in the claims of snake oil salesmen everywhere. Haygarth's point was that there was nothing special about the Perkins Tractors. It simply preyed upon the *belief* that it would offer a cure.

Pain was, for a long time, the main focus of placebo response research, because it didn't require conditions in the body to actually change—only that the patient's *perception* of those conditions changed. During World War II, Henry Beecher, a field surgeon, ran out of morphine for the wounded soldiers he was treating. He didn't want to have to tell men in excruciating pain that he couldn't help them. In a remote battlefield surgical tent, he rigged up an IV of saline solution, hooked it up to his suffering patients, and told them it was morphine. He figured it might take the edge off a little so they could hold out for the real drug. Their response, however, astonished him; 40 percent of the men reported a "significant" decrease in pain.

Beecher, who went on to become a prominent anesthesiologist and medical ethicist, became fascinated with the placebo response and dedicated years of his career to its study. Since his experience on the western front more than seventy years ago, hundreds more studies on placebo have proven the same thing: it works. Today, going into any kind of research study on the efficacy of a drug, the expectation is that, on average, a full 35 *percent* of participants will experience a strong placebo response—that is, they will receive what is essentially a sugar pill but experience the same effects as those taking the real medication.

It's a stunning statistic. And it's important to remember that 35 percent is the *average*. The range is actually between 10 and 90 percent, depending on the specific illness and the particular medication or treatment being tested.

There's a very common knee surgery that's performed seven hundred thousand times a year in the United States called a *knee arthroscopy*. This surgery alone makes up $4 billion of health-care spending in this country. It's often used to perform a repair on the meniscus, the padding of cartilage that sits on both sides of the kneecap and that provides a smooth cushion for the joint. Meniscus tears are widespread and cause pain with movement, so doctors frequently recommend the arthroscopy to repair it. But when researchers ran studies to compare the outcome between an arthroscopy and a faux arthroscopy (in which the surgeon makes an incision during "surgery" but repairs nothing so that the patient only believes he's had the surgery), it was revealed that there was *no difference* between the actual surgery and the sham surgery. In both groups, people reported relief of symptoms to the same degree. In other words, you don't need a knee arthroscopy to improve your range of motion and mitigate pain. You just need to believe you've had one.

Pharmaceutical companies have profited from the placebo response, noticing that *how* a medication is presented can determine its rate of efficacy. Even with real medications, for example, the color of the pill makes a difference. Blue sleeping pills work better than other colors. Red pills, in contrast, are better at reducing pain. Big pills always work better than small ones; injections work better than pills; and surgeries work better than anything.

So what *is* placebo? Is it just an illusion? Or can it cause actual physical change in the body?

A lot of physicians believe that placebo is simply the expectation of relief causing a physiological response that mirrors that expectation. You expect to feel better, and therefore, you do. Placebo, they say, can't *really* change anything biologically or alter the course of an illness. At Harvard, Ted Kaptchuk, the preeminent researcher on placebo, has looked into the way placebo works along the same neurotransmitters as certain medications, and he's also begun to isolate certain genetic profiles that are, for some reason, more prone to responding positively to placebo. He concludes that placebo is an incredibly powerful force, often underestimated and misunderstood. His studies have proven over and over that placebo can cause real, measurable physiological changes in the body, including to heart rate, blood pressure, brain chemistry, and even diseases of the nervous system like Parkinson's. However, as powerful as he observes placebo to be, he relies on the boundaries of controlled studies to make his assertions and stops short of suggesting that placebo can turn around a fatal disease. "Though placebos may provide relief," Kaptchuk concludes, "they rarely cure."

My question, after reading study after study that hemmed and hawed about placebo, was this: Has the placebo response ever been strongly linked to a case of spontaneous remission? If it's happened even once, that's essential to know.

A *ping* went off in my brain as I remembered a case we'd read about in med school years earlier: an instance where placebo was the only possible explanation for some extreme physiological changes. I remembered a name from that long-ago textbook: *Mr. Wright.*

THE WONDER DRUG THAT WASN'T

I found the story in a clinical report from 1957. The case began exactly as I'd recalled: Mr. Wright, a cancer patient, was dying. He was in the end stages of cancer of the lymph nodes. Tumors the size of oranges had appeared on his neck, armpits, chest, and groin. They were pressing on his windpipe; he struggled to breathe. His doctors had tried every available treatment and had exhausted every option—there was nothing left to do.

Except just then, a new, experimental drug went on the market. It was an anticancer medication called Krebiozen, and the reports on its effects were very optimistic. Mr. Wright had read about the "miracle" drug and begged his doctors to try it.

As soon as the hospital received shipment, on a Friday afternoon, he got his first injection. Three days later, his doctor returned to work on Monday morning to find him up and out of bed, breathing easily, walking around the ward, joking with the nurses. The stunned physician noted in written reports that his tumors had "melted like snowballs on a hot stove." Ten days later, still radically improving, Wright was discharged and sent home.

But a couple of months later, some stories hit the news about Krebiozen not being an anticancer miracle drug after all but a fake quack remedy. When Wright read this, he suffered an immediate and severe relapse. His tumors swelled again, his health plummeted. He was rehospitalized in the same state he'd been in before he'd started on the drug he had so hoped would offer a cure.

His doctor decided to try something unusual with this patient, who was, after all, on his deathbed. He told Wright that the reports were wrong. He told him that he'd just received a new, retooled, "double strength" version of the serum. The first version of the drug hadn't been quite right, he said. But this one was even more powerful.

After one injection, the tumors melted away again. But this time, Wright's doctor hadn't even injected him with actual medication. What was in that plunger wasn't Krebiozen.

It was water.

Mr. Wright enjoyed two months of robust good health. His tumors were gone, he felt great. He went back to his life. And then he read another report in the news: Krebiozen was debunked, definitively, as a treatment for cancer. A group of test subjects had experienced no improvement on the drug.

Wright relapsed immediately. He died within days.

Reading the case study again for the first time since medical school, it reminded me immediately of Nikki, my oncology nurse friend. I recalled what Janet Rose said in her interview—that when she met Nikki, who was in the room next to hers at the *pousada,* Nikki was weak and frail and didn't have long to live. She thought she might stay in Brazil a week or two, at the most.

"But then one day, she broke out into a really high fever," Jan said. "I stayed with her, kept her hydrated. When the fever finally broke, she woke up starving. She hadn't been able to eat for months, and now it was like she couldn't get enough."

The fever interested me—in other cases of spontaneous remission, as Dr. Coley had discovered, people had recovered or improved suddenly after high fevers seemed to activate their immune systems. Of course, there was no way to know now whether a fever had actually played a role in the trajectory of Nikki's illness, but it was certainly worth noting. After that, Jan's version meshed with what I'd remembered about Nikki and her story—that she'd returned from Brazil looking healthy and happy and that she was eating what made her feel good. Jan described how for six weeks after her fever and apparent recovery, Nikki got stronger and stronger. By the end of her stay, she didn't have to use her wheelchair anymore. Jan says that when Nikki left the healing center, she was advised on how to proceed; they told her not to get any diagnostic scans for six months, no matter what. But a few days after Nikki left, Jan got a phone call from her. Nikki confessed to her friend that she'd gone to get the scan. But the machine had stopped working while she was lying on the table.

"What do you think it means?" Nikki had asked Jan.

"It doesn't matter what I think it means," Jan replied. "It matters what *you* think it means."

"I think it probably means I'm not supposed to get the scan," Nikki said. "I just don't know if I can hold out. I'm an oncology nurse!"

Jan heard from Nikki less than a week later: she'd gone back and gotten the scan. The news wasn't good—she still had cancer. She was crushed. She immediately started to feel sick again. She rapidly declined and passed away within weeks, confused and in considerable physical pain.

"I've thought about this so many times since then," Jan said. "In my heart, I believe that if she could have waited those six months, that something could have happened. That she could have healed."

What I remember most about Nikki was her passion, her fierce devotion to her children, and to leaving no stone uncovered in her search for an answer. I've been hesitant to consider that belief could be so powerful, that seeing the tumor still present on CT could cause such a quick decline and death. Would she have died anyway, if she had followed instructions and waited at least six months? I don't know. The physician in me wants to protect her story from being misunderstood, and so I have hesitated to tell it. But the researcher in me knows that what she told me, and what she also told Jan, is important.

Uncomfortable, even complex truths or questions must be faced if we are to improve our understanding of how this all works. Mapping this new terrain will require learning in every way we can. Setting aside our judgments and fears to seek understanding is the only way in. I remembered what Matt Ireland had said about the time after he returned from Brazil: his doctors at Dartmouth had wanted to do an MRI to check the progress of his disease, but he had refused.

"D-day had already passed," he said, referring to the rough time frame his doctors had given him to live. "But I was feeling good. If the tumor had grown, I didn't want the fear, or the thought that the healing wasn't working, to intrude. So I declined the MRI. I really needed to believe in it."

"Faith is a big part of healing, no matter what," Matt said. "If you really have faith and trust and believe in your chemotherapy, maybe that's your answer."

The parallels between Mr. Wright and Nikki were striking. They shared a common theme—a deep faith that the treatment being offered (in Wright's case, the Krebiozen serum; in Nikki's, the healing energy of a spiritual healer and place) would lead to radical improvement. The loss of faith in that treatment resulted in an aggressive resurgence of the illness. Mr. Wright's case has become such a touchstone in medical lore because his cancerous lymph tumors were visible, and doctors were able to watch them collapse and then bloom again, completely in tune with whether or not he had faith in his medication. The effect was immediate and observable to the naked eye. In Nikki's case, we unfortunately don't know what was happening inside her body. She had initially given the appearance of marked improvement, and as advanced as her cancer was, one has to be open to the possibility that she experienced a certain amount of regression. But we just don't know for sure. Perhaps she simply felt better but was still growing sicker and sicker. Perhaps she would have passed away in the same manner no matter what.

There is a dark side to belief as well, which perhaps played a part in both Mr. Wright and Nikki's stories. It's the flipside to placebo, and it's called the *nocebo* effect: you expect to feel bad, and so you do. Studies are able to measure this frequently by looking at side effects. When people are told they'll experience a specific side effect with a medication (everything from headache to vomiting to rashes), there is a measurable spike in the incidence of those side effects.

Some side effect symptoms—like pain—can seem hard to measure. We know that pain has a huge psychological component and that people who are depressed, stressed, or without a strong purpose experience more pain. In fact, as we covered previously, multiple studies have shown that there is no correlation between the degree of actual pathology seen on an MRI with the amount of back pain that people report. So does that mean that pain is sometimes subjective or even imagined? Can the nocebo effect simply be written off as a fluke of perception—a person expects to feel bad and so they do, but nothing is actually wrong with them?

A study run a few years ago in the Italian Alps offers some insight. A team of researchers took 120 students on a trip into the mountains. They spread a rumor among a quarter of the group that the thin air at high elevations could cause debilitating migraines. That group reported the worst headaches by far. And not only that, but an enzyme in the blood that is associated with headaches also spiked in this group. In this case, the nocebo effect measurably changed the biochemistry of the brain and body.

Placebo response research is a rabbit hole of incredible stories like this. In my digging, I also came across an obscure case study from the 1960s in Japan. To test the power of the placebo/nocebo effect, researchers gathered together a group of thirteen people known to be highly allergic to poison ivy. Each participant had one arm rubbed with a harmless leaf, but they were told it was poison ivy. Their other arm was rubbed with poison ivy, and they were told it was harmless. *All thirteen* broke out in a poison ivy–like rash where they'd been rubbed with the harmless leaf. Only *two* reacted to the true poison ivy. I could picture it, that long-ago study: placebo effect on one arm, nocebo effect on the other. It was a small study, but provocative. One body displaying the power of belief to either protect and heal, or to harm.

I thought about the way the placebo response had been presented to us in medical school and how it was viewed by my fellow physicians. We saw it as a nuisance or a distraction, an unfortunate complication to research studies that would otherwise be more clear-cut. You always had to build placebo into your study to make sure that whatever new drug or treatment approach you were testing out could beat placebo. But in medicine, placebo beat the treatment, on average, *35 percent* of the time. And in psychiatry, placebo was regularly outperforming the "real" treatment, with evidence that the strength of the placebo response is growing over time.[1]

The more I read about placebo, the more I began to believe that the term *placebo* only captures a fraction of the true effect that belief has on the body. I could no longer accept the standard line in medicine, that placebo was a sort of superficial nuisance, an example of the mind fooling the body into simply feeling better for a time. What was apparent to me was that sometimes, the body *does* get better. And yet we don't seem to care why.

All of this led me to wonder: What is the truth behind the shifting and powerful interaction between the mind, body, and spirit in a human being? To what degree are our bodies a reflection of the conscious and unconscious beliefs we have absorbed over time? And could the physical body be, in a way, a mirror for something we don't understand yet or are trying to learn?

BEYOND PLACEBO

In 2011, a few years into my work at Good Sam, a patient walked in out of nowhere and became a pivotal case in my spontaneous remission research. Stephen Dunphe arrived late on a Thursday night with back pain. He'd had it for a while but had tried to deal with it on his own. It was only back pain, after all, and he wasn't a complainer. I could tell he prided himself on that. But finally, the pain had become unendurable. He'd driven himself to the hospital.

A CT scan of his back came up with the worst possible news. He had cancer. They weren't sure what specific type yet, but a cancerous tumor had disrupted the bony vertebrae of his spine and was pressing on his spinal cord. Surgery was immediately scheduled for the following week, and he was admitted until then. Further tests revealed that he had multiple myeloma, a cancer of the white blood cells. White blood cells are formed in the bone marrow, and in multiple myeloma, the cancerous cells crowd out the healthy cells and continue to spread, creating multiple tumors and so many abnormal antibodies that the blood can thicken and even clog the kidneys. In Greek, *myelo* means *bone marrow* and *oma* means *tumor,* and that's what Stephen had—a tumor of the bone marrow.

Multiple myeloma is incurable and eventually fatal. Treatment can prolong life, though; without treatment, the average life expectancy is only seven months, but with treatment, that time frame can swell to four and a half years. Overall, though, the treatment options for multiple myeloma are famously ineffective compared to the standard courses of treatment for many other cancers. Often, they give dexamethasone—a type of steroid—but it usually doesn't have much of an impact. It may temporarily reduce tumor size, but it is not expected to cure a disease like multiple myeloma or eliminate the need for surgery.

In Stephen's case, the most urgent task was getting the pressure off his spine. In preparation for his surgery, they started him on a round of dexamethasone on the off chance that it could temporarily shrink the tumor's growth and render the dangerous surgery somewhat safer. Dexamethasone might not have had a great track record with multiple myeloma, but we doctors like to do *something,* and given the stakes, it was unlikely to do more harm and might even help.

The night before surgery, Stephen underwent an MRI, a standard pre-op scan so the surgeons could work using more detailed imagery. He changed into the white gown, lay down on the narrow table, and was slid into the machine. The tube was smooth and white, and he had to lie very still. He noticed the sounds of the magnetic imaging machine as it worked around him: clunks, chirps, and a low hum like a car engine. And then something odd started to happen. A trickle of water appeared, streaking along the inside of the MRI tube, then another, and another. He told himself not to panic—the machine was probably broken; they would pull him out any minute. The water pooled around his body and rose, filling the tube. He felt oddly calm. He was a scuba diver, he told himself—he'd be fine.

At multiple points during the story, I broke in—Stephen was telling me his tale after the fact, and he described it as if it had actually happened. "So, it sounds like you were hallucinating," I kept interjecting, trying to make sense of it. "Or in some kind of altered state." But he would just wave his hand and say, "Yeah, yeah, sure," and go back to describing what he'd experienced as if it were real. Whatever he was experiencing went on for the duration of the scan: he described breathing underwater as the tube filled up; he sensed a benevolent presence standing near. Finally, he heard someone's voice, opened his eyes, and found himself in the radiology suite.

This could easily be laughed off as a strange dream someone had while stuck in an MRI tube for an hour—except for one thing. Impossibly, when the MRI came back, the tumor was, according to the notes in Stephen's file, "nearly completely resolved." The tumor had all but vanished. "It's a spontaneous remission," his surgeon said. Surgery was canceled, and for days, the unit filled with excitement and amazement as nurses, doctors, and trainees cycled through his room, astonished. As there was no longer anything to operate on, he was sent home.

I spoke with both the radiologist and the surgeon. They were flabbergasted, saying they had never seen anything like it. Stephen's surgeon in particular was convinced that we were looking at a textbook case of spontaneous remission, one that could not be explained by any of the other variables (medications, genetics, etc.).

"There's just no other explanation," I remember him saying to me as we stood in the hallway outside Stephen's room, looking at each other in disbelief.

Now, years later, I was still carrying the Stephen Dunphe case file around with me. It stayed in every pile of case study folders that I toted between my home office and the hospital. It was always there, close to the top of the stack, packed with Stephen's tumor scans and white blood cell count readings, notes from the attending doctor. Sometimes I would pull it out just to look at the images: the CT scan of the spine, its normal curve disrupted by the large tumor, and then the MRI from a week later, the tumor vanishing, barely visible. Other cases came and went, but this one stuck—a mystery making my briefcase heavier.

Each step of the way, as I uncovered new potential causes for spontaneous healing, I would pull Stephen's folder out and take a look at his case through that lens—hoping that maybe one of the *other* cases I researched would finally shed some light on Stephen's.

It wasn't diet. He didn't eat particularly healthfully, hadn't made any changes in that department, and certainly the hospital food didn't qualify as healthy. Could reducing stress hormones and getting out of fight or flight have played a role? Doubtful. Stephen didn't describe his hospital stay as restful or restorative in the way that Janet Rose and Matt Ireland, for example, had described Brazil. In fact, Stephen had spent most of the week in his hospital bed looking up grim statistics on multiple myeloma and growing more and more anxious and afraid. He hadn't had a lot of friends and family flock to his bedside; he'd been alone most of the time. He was in pain, confined to a hospital bed, anxiously awaiting a surgery that would not save his life, like so many others who don't experience remission. He'd had the course of dexamethasone, and I knew that some doctors would try to pin the remission on this, calling him simply a "high responder" to the drug. But neither myself nor colleagues I consulted were aware of anything in the literature that described this level of response to dexamethasone. And the term *high responder,* like *spontaneous remission,* can be another black box term where the inexplicable gets packed away instead of examined. If someone is a high responder whose results shatter the upper limits of possibility for a treatment or medication, then the question is why?

I kept trying to work it out, but like a perpetually unsolvable Rubik's Cube, it eluded me. Every question seemed to lead not to an answer but to an equally confounding question. Had the tumor receded gradually over the course of the week, or suddenly during the MRI? Had something—a fever, for example—triggered

Stephen's immune system to finally attack the tumor, or was something else going on? The chart did not reflect the presence of a fever. The unusual thing about Stephen's case was the extremely tight time frame: CT of the back with cancer on Thursday, and MRI demonstrating no need for surgery several days later. Completely inexplicable.

But moments of clarity, or even just the next great question, often come when you're not looking for them. One night, on one of my research trips to Cleveland, Dr. Nemeh took me out to his favorite restaurant. Over some delicious pasta, I asked Dr. Nemeh, who is not only a physician but also an engineer, why, or how, his act of praying has a healing impact on bodies. He thought for a moment.

"Whether it is a laser or love working on the quantum field," he said, "I believe they have the same effect."

It was a startling comment. And it got my mind whirring on the possibilities—especially for the Dunphe case. When I got home, I dug back into the case once again. There were a couple of avenues to explore. They had to do with the altered state Dunphe had described during the MRI and the spinning magnet of the machine itself.

THE QUANTUM PHYSICS OF THE BODY

When Descartes's philosophy of separating mind and body took hold, he ushered in an era where dissections could be routinely performed and we could finally understand the inner workings of the human body. It was a huge leap forward for mankind, but during his time, science was superstitious and highly religious (and not something that we would call *science* today). Scientific reasoning or rational thinking that went against religious beliefs was seen as a threat. Galileo was put on trial when he published his theory—based on years of close observation and study of the stars and other celestial objects—that the earth revolved around the sun instead of the other way around. The idea that the universe did not, in fact, center on humanity was so blasphemous that he was excommunicated from the Church and placed on house arrest. He escaped torture and death by recanting his beliefs—beliefs which we now know to be true.

When the Enlightenment swept in, it set the stage for a rational science, and it was built around elucidating the laws of the physical world. This period brought a sea change that gave us the scientific method and Newton's laws of gravitation and motion, which revolutionized our capacity to understand and explain the world that we can see and touch. We shifted toward a culture where observation, reason, and scientific inquiry were more valued than religious lore and blind faith. Now, at the cutting edge of science today, quantum physics takes the next step, and it's taking us somewhere we didn't expect. Some of the assumptions we've long made about the rules of the universe, and how matter and energy behave, are beginning to unravel.

Quantum physics is essentially the study of the building blocks of matter. It looks intricately at the subatomic particles that make up an atom. Now, I know a little about quantum physics from my time at Princeton, but I'm no physicist. So after Dr. Nemeh's comment about the body's quantum field, I called my friend Andreas Mershin, a physicist at MIT. I knew the basics of how an MRI machine worked, but I needed him to walk me through the specifics.

MRI stands for *magnetic resonance imaging*. It's a form of imaging technology developed from the principles of quantum mechanics. Unlike a simple x-ray, the MRI can provide highly detailed images of soft tissues, everything from the brain to the spinal cord to organs and connective tissue. MRIs are made of superconducting magnets that weigh several tons. The machine creates an incredibly strong magnetic field—about a thousand times stronger than a normal magnet that you put on your refrigerator door—to peek inside the human body. How does the powerful magnet achieve this? It basically "reads" the spinning protons in the water molecules of your body.

The human body is mostly water. In a powerful magnetic field, the protons inside H_2O molecules will become aligned. When you slide inside an MRI, you are entering a solenoid: essentially, a cylinder with a couple miles of superconducting wire wrapped around it.

With an electric current running through it, it's creating a constant electromagnetic field, and what that current is doing is calling out to the atomic particles in your body and forcing the protons inside the nuclei of each atom to align. Meanwhile, as each image is taken, your body is also being washed in pulses of harmless radio waves. Unlike a CT scan, with an MRI, there is no ionizing radiation—just radio frequencies. When the MRI is complete and the pulses stop, all those protons that were aligned with the magnetic field begin to gradually flip back to their usual positions. The radio antennae pick up those flips and record them. And since protons in different types of bodily tissues go back to their usual rotations at varying rates, the MRI machine is able to capture those differences to distinguish between types of tissue. So an MRI can create beautifully detailed images of the inside of your body by essentially playing around with your subatomic particles.

Some researchers are now asking if MRI technology can do more than just imaging: The radio frequency coils of the MRI actually operate at frequencies that can interact with the neurons and cells in the body. Studies have started looking at MRIs as potential treatments for depression, for example—there seems to be something about the magnetic field that under certain conditions can actually influence brain operation. A placebo-controlled study found that people who were exposed to a particular MRI experienced marked improvements in mood,[2] leading researchers to wonder if the spinning magnet was able to change or rewrite brain pathways. And a physicist colleague of mine at Harvard, Dr. Michael Rohan, has also been experimenting with using the fields generated by the MRI as a treatment for depression in bipolar disorder. He happened upon the link by accident, when a research assistant noticed that several patients at McLean went into the MRI depressed and came out feeling much better.[3]

This received quite a lot of attention, including an article in *The Boston Globe.* Dr. Rohan now theorizes that under certain conditions, the electromagnetic field produced by the MRI can manipulate our brains toward health, in this case achieving rapid resolution of depression. Though it's challenging to obtain funding for such an endeavor, the fact that it's rooted in quantum mechanics rather than traditional science is promising. Being on the leading edge of the next era in medicine is not for the faint of heart, as innovators from Béchamp to Benson have found.

At this point, there are more questions than answers about any potential healing effects of a tool like the MRI, and most doctors are skeptical about the topic. I didn't know whether Stephen Dunphe's strange and sudden remission had happened over the course of the days between his CT scan and the MRI or very suddenly in the MRI machine, but I had to wonder if there was a connection. Could the altered state he described have interacted in an unknown way with the spinning magnet of the MRI machine, causing sudden molecular changes to his tumor?

Einstein liked to tell a story about the origins of one of his most famous concepts. When he was a teenager at a boarding school in Switzerland, he had a running thought experiment he liked to lose himself in. Riding his bike down a wooded lane through dappled sunlight, he would picture those spears of light traveling back out into space, moving at the speed of light, a speed at which it was impossible for a human to travel. But he would imagine that he could somehow catch up to those light waves and move alongside them, going at exactly the same speed. He wondered, how would he perceive the light wave? Would it continue to undulate as light waves do, or would his speed—the speed of light—make the light wave appear still or frozen?

I should observe such a beam of light as an electromagnetic field at rest, he wrote later. This thought experiment—this daydream about surfing on a beam of light—led Einstein to some of his most influential concepts, ones that shaped the field of modern physics: the theory of relativity and the equation $E = mc^2$. *Energy equals mass times the speed of light squared.* What does that mean? Basically, it means that all matter in the universe—the chair you sit on, your own body, the earth itself—is a sort of condensed form of energy. It's energy, slowed down. And energy, in turn, is matter, when the atoms begin to move at a faster speed. The difference between something we can touch and feel and something we can just sense is often simply this: *speed*. The physicist David Bohm once said that one way to conceive of matter is as "condensed or frozen light." Our physical bodies, then, in a sense, are frozen light—energy slowed down and given form.

So what are the real implications about healing—about belief and the human body —when we look at quantum physics and the building blocks of matter?

First, quantum physics is showing us that some of the laws of the universe that we thought of as fixed or immutable are, in fact, not. Newtonian physics, it turns out, only represents a small slice of what's out there to know about how our world works. There is still so much we don't know about everything, from why black holes exist to how the subatomic particles of our own bodies behave. And then there was something that Andreas had explained to me on our phone call that had lodged in my mind, making me want to dig even more deeply into the mind-body connection. He reminded me of a foundational study in quantum physics, which in some ways calls into question everything we know about matter and energy and the laws of the universe. It's called the *double-slit experiment*. And it gave us something that may turn out to be another key to the unfurling mystery of spontaneous healing: the observer effect.

THE OBSERVER EFFECT

The double-slit experiment is complicated and has had lots of different iterations through the years. Since its first run, it has baffled most who have tried to figure out what it means, even physicists. But for our purposes, there are just a couple of important things we need to understand about it. It was set up to look at the way photons, or subatomic particles, behave.

"Picture a tennis court," Andreas said.

He invited me to imagine that I was looking down at it from above. Instead of a net in the middle, there was a wall, with two open doorways spaced evenly apart. The court was enclosed, with fences on all four sides.

"So you stand there and start throwing tennis balls at the wall in the middle, with the doorways in it. Some of them are going to miss the doors and bounce off the wall. Others will go through and hit the fence directly behind them. Right?"

"Right."

"So the double-slit experiment basically did this exact same thing, but with an electron beam gun," Andreas explained. He went on to describe how researchers fired electrons at a "wall" with two slits in it, and they saw that the particles that didn't bounce off the wall, the ones that went through the doorways, didn't behave the way they were supposed to. They didn't behave like balls on a tennis court. They should have bounced back at predictable angles; all the tenets of physics and motion tell us that. But they didn't. They took on the properties of a wave. That means they were hitting the "fence" at the back in patterns expected of spreading waves rather than as particles would normally be expected to behave.

The researchers theorized at first that perhaps the particles themselves were interfering with each other, but they behaved this way even when they were fired individually instead of as a group. Finally, they placed a kind of detector—like a video camera for subatomic particles—between the two slits to see if they could get a closer look at what exactly was happening when the particles passed through them. And that's when the strangest thing happened. The particles stopped their wavelike behavior and hit the "fence" straight on, just like the tennis balls would.

"It was like they knew they were being watched," Andreas said.

The double-slit experiment is a tough one to wrap your mind around if you're not a quantum physicist. But the ultimate takeaway from the project was that atomic particles behave differently *depending on if they are being observed and how.* The act of being observed changes the way they function. This is now referred to in physics as the *observer effect,* and it has been proven again and again, in hundreds of experiments. It's hard to believe, but it's true; the act of observing a phenomenon changes that phenomenon. Perhaps, in some ways, we are participating in the creation of this universe; perhaps the "laws" are not so immutable as we believe. If you think about the fact that the atomic particles in our bodies—the very building blocks of all matter—can change their behavior in this way, it opens up all kinds of questions about how the way we *perceive* the world might actually, in some ways, *alter* the world. Or even our physical bodies.

The observer effect suggests, perhaps, that we are each "the observer" for our own ongoing experiment—the way that we "observe" ourselves, our bodies, and the world we move through may actually create the reality that we see and touch. The bodies that we live in, and the way their cells behave, may be more fundamentally fluid and malleable than any of us know.

The implications for all of this are potentially profound and world-altering, especially when it comes to healing our physical bodies. The question then becomes: Why hasn't any of this understanding seeped into the realm of medicine?

Perhaps because we're just not ready for it. As a culture, and as individuals—myself included—I don't believe that we're truly prepared to step into the world that quantum physics tells us is true. It's too overwhelming; it upsets the applecart on most of the assumptions that we have lived with for generations, on which we've built our entire world.

Some physicists try to escape the problem by positing that perhaps the laws at the subatomic level are different from the laws at the macroscopic level, where you and I live. This is an assumption that would be convenient—quantum mechanics at one level, and Newtonian mechanics and the world as it appears to be at another—but so far, every step up the ladder into larger particles has resulted in continuing, indisputable evidence that this world does not behave quite as our traditional scientific canon would have us believe. Just like I was asked to not ask a lot of questions in med school and simply memorize the material, physicists are also taught to rely on the math and not ask a lot of questions. I wonder if some physicists feel as if they've been tricked a bit; they go into physics to understand the physical world, and then the facts tell them that the physical world either doesn't exist—or doesn't exist in the way we think it does.

Quantum physics is a deeply complex, ever-expanding world of research that people spend entire lifetimes working to understand. As American theoretical physicist Richard Feynman famously said, "If you think you understand quantum physics, then you don't understand it." But even just grazing the edges of these concepts, I was beginning to see all the myriad ways that your core beliefs can potentially affect your physical existence. Our minds and beliefs have the capacity to affect our bodies on both the macro and micro levels. By *macro,* I mean how we experience the world around us and how that translates into stress hormones in our bodies. By *micro,* I mean that we can zoom through our cells and into the atoms that make up our bodies and see the potential for change at the subatomic level. To what extent, I wondered, are we creating our own reality?

I went back to Stephen Dunphe's case, the case that had spurred me down this path. I tracked down Dunphe to check in with him—incredibly, years later, he was still doing well. While he is still considered to have multiple myeloma, he has significantly outlasted his prognosis. The sudden remission of his life-threatening tumor had certainly altered the trajectory of his illness, and his life.

I wrote to Henry Stapp, a leading quantum physicist at Berkeley, with the details of the case, hoping he would be able to shed some light on it from the point of view of quantum mechanics. Had Stephen Dunphe somehow become the "observer" of his own physical state, causing the subatomic particles of his body to change their behavior?

Dr. Stapp initially responded with the healthy, careful skepticism of a trained scientist. He wondered about any number of other possible explanations, suggesting that there was probably some other, simpler explanation for the remission. His take essentially boiled down to, "If there are hoofbeats, think horses, not zebras."

But then, unexpectedly, he emailed again. He'd reviewed the case more completely, and after thinking more deeply, had reversed his opinion: quantum mechanics, as he understood it, absolutely supported the idea that the mind had a role to play with physical health—and, even more broadly, with the creation of the world around us. He also admitted that his first reaction, even as a physicist, was to resist the idea. The questions raised by quantum physics are big, deep, and unsettling. But we need to engage with these ideas head-on—not shy away from them. And I certainly agreed with Dr. Stapp's closing sentiment as we signed off our correspondence: that it all demanded much more study.

We haven't figured out how to test the observer effect at a larger scale than the subatomic. But ongoing experiments have continued to support the initial findings, not as theory but as indisputable fact. We will continue as a culture to prepare for the next step forward. And the revelations, for medicine and beyond, could shatter all the boundaries of what we believe about healing and where it comes from. If it's true that the world illuminated by quantum physics is true at the level of the world we see and touch, we will have to forever reconfigure our understanding of the role that faith, belief, and perception play in creating our shared, perceived reality.[4] If the observer has such a profound impact on the subatomic level, then it very well may follow that *you*, as the observer of your own body and experience, can have a similar impact on your physical body, down to its very cells. The details of how this works, I suspect, will continue to be worked out from the blood, sweat, and tears of the people who actually change their perceptions and beliefs and then show us how they did.

Following this, there was one last important thing about belief that I was concerned with. I knew from my own life experience that it's not just what you *consciously* believe that affects your health, your body, your ability to heal. It's what you've been *conditioned* to believe. And those types of beliefs are much harder to both identify and change. Often, you aren't even aware of them. They are hidden, even to you. We call them our *subconscious beliefs,* and we all have them.

WHEN BELIEFS RUN DEEP

Here's a truly shocking thing I found out about placebo: it works *even when you don't believe it will.*

Typically, in placebo-controlled studies, participants know only that they *may* receive a placebo instead of a real drug. But in a twist on the experiment, researchers tried a series of studies where they simply told participants, up front, that they would definitely be receiving a placebo as treatment. And then the study participants *still* experienced a marked improvement in health.

What? The entire basis for placebo, I thought, was that we believe in the treatment, and so it works. This finding threw me into a bit of a tailspin. If placebo is about *belief,* and people who don't believe the placebo will help them are also getting better, then what gives? Does this mean that belief is *not* actually that strong of a factor when it comes to healing?

I needed to look more closely at what we mean by *belief.* Typically, when we use that word, we're referring to thoughts and decisions, the workings of our conscious minds. But as a psychiatrist, I know without a doubt that there are different types and levels of beliefs. There are the ones that you have the power to decide on, that you intentionally adopt as part of who you are and how you move through life. Then there are the other types of beliefs—the deep-seated, often invisible ones that were coded into you when you were young, that you may not even be aware of. We are all a complex composite of beliefs that we have acquired from parents, teachers, friends, peers on the playground, and from interpretations that we have made based on all kinds of experiences, whether wonderful or traumatic. For the most part, though, these beliefs go unexamined.

We humans are famous for not being able to correctly identify our own true beliefs. The philosopher Paul Tillich said that every one of us has one "ultimate concern" around which we organize our entire lives. As a psychiatrist, I can tell you that people often say, and truly believe, that their ultimate concern is one thing, such as their religious faith or commitment to family. But close observers will know that their true ultimate concern is actually something else, whether that be financial security, keeping up with appearances, or gaining the approval of a parent figure (just to name a few). Yes, we are complicated creatures. And we are not good at knowing what we truly believe.

Researchers believe this aspect of placebo taps into a more foundational belief system, one written into our minds and bodies a long time ago. It has to do with the "performance of care." Even when we receive a pill that we *know* is a placebo—and therefore, chemically powerless to help us—we nevertheless will feel better when we take it. Why? Because we feel cared for. We've been conditioned over time to associate certain experiences with feeling better, with healing. It might be everything from the doctor in the white coat dispensing the pill to the sensory experience of being in a doctor's office—the sterile, alcohol-tinged smell, the experience of lying back on the clean, crackling paper of the exam table. Our brains know, logically, that the pill we're swallowing is inert. But there is a deeper, unconscious part of us that feels cared for, and the body responds. Michael Polanyi, the chemist turned philosopher, called this "tacit knowledge," very distinct from explicit or conscious knowledge. Conscious knowledge is you explaining to someone how to change their bike chain. Tacit knowledge is you getting on that bike and riding away. You don't have to think about how to ride the bike—you just do it.

At the beginning of our interview, Patricia Kaine (Dr. Nemeh's patient who recovered from a fatal form of fibrosis) emphasized that after that early experience with her sister's unlikely recovery from polio, she'd grown up "knowing that miracles are real." And I thought about my own childhood, growing up in a rigid and dogmatic environment. As I got older and began to ask more questions, I turned toward science and away from faith. I began to think of faith as a bad thing—a set of blinders that kept you from seeing the world clearly. But I was beginning to see that it wasn't belief itself that was inherently damaging or inherently healing—it was *what* you believed. And it wasn't even what you believed on the conscious level—perhaps that explained the results of Benson's prayer study. It was what you believed without knowing it. Perhaps the body itself could have what we might call "beliefs," right down to its very cells.

We still don't really know how far or how deep the effect we call *placebo* actually runs, but my research into spontaneous healing was showing me that, on some occasions, it appears to be able to flow beyond the box we've put it in. Sure, sometimes people just *feel* better because they expect to; the way that perception and experience interact in the mind is certainly fascinating. But other times there's more. And we should always seek to know where exceptions exist, because these are the treasures where the next discoveries will be found. We *are* seeing the physiological effects of belief in the body, time after time, and spontaneous healing represents a hot spot of these cases. Perhaps those who experience spontaneous healing were either conditioned to be receptive to healing beliefs (Patricia Kaine, for example) or were able to reprogram foundational conditioning that allowed a major shift not only in their core beliefs but in their physical bodies.

It's undeniable that we all have foundational, core beliefs that we aren't aware of, that could be determining our capacity to heal. But how do we identify, and then unravel, beliefs that may be limiting or even damaging?

We think of belief systems as being about God—whether or not we believe in one, or what kind of God we believe in—or about the world and how it works. But spontaneous healing isn't about belief in the way we usually think of it—that you have to belong to a certain religion, or pray a certain way, or even whether or not you are a "believer" or a person of faith. What we are talking about here is something deeper, perhaps even unconscious. It's what you *really* believe about life, yourself, the universe, and the people around you, both consciously and subconsciously; what you truly believe is possible or impossible. At a deep level, the level where all other beliefs are shaped, what do you believe about your value? The friendliness of the universe or lack thereof? Do you matter? Does your life matter? When it comes to belief and its role in healing, the most important question may be: What do we believe about *ourselves*?

9

Healing Your Identity

Guilt results from unused life, from the unlived in us.

—*Ernest Becker*

It was 2015. I had a mic clipped to my lapel and a light sweat under my nice suit. I was about to walk out onstage at TEDx New Bedford and try to convince the audience of scientists, researchers, and other leaders in their fields that spontaneous remission was a black box worth opening.

When the opportunity to give the talk had come up, I'd hesitated. Were people ready to hear about spontaneous healing? Would these cases simply be dismissed the way they had always been before? And most important, what did I actually *know* about spontaneous healing at this point that I could share with the world?

I sat down to put the talk together and realized I knew *a lot*. I knew that spontaneous healings mattered and that we weren't thinking about them or dissecting them in the right way. I knew that many factors came together to make them possible—everything from nutrition to "emotional nutrition"; to how people lived, thought, felt, and connected with others; and perhaps most important, what they believed. And I knew that those who survived from incurable illnesses made big, sometimes radical, changes in these areas.

As I condensed twelve years of research into eighteen minutes, the bigger picture began to cohere: where I'd come from, where I was now, and where I needed to go next. I'd been practicing my speech for days—in the car, in the elevator, in my office. I had it memorized. I reminded myself to talk *slowly*. My name was announced, followed by a brief introduction. Applause. I walked out onto the stage into the blinding spotlight.

"What does it mean when someone survives an incurable and fatal illness?" I began. "Told that they are going to die? The projected time of death comes . . . and goes . . . and then it turns out that the illness is gone. Medicine calls this a fluke. Is it?"

I swept through some of the big concepts about spontaneous remission—the fragmented way we approach medicine, the idea that there is something beyond silver bullets, that cases of spontaneous healing are calling out for us to pay attention. And then I got to the heart of the message I wanted to deliver to the audience.

"The brilliance of Western culture is that when you have a medical problem, you go see a doctor. When you have a psychological problem, you go see a psychotherapist, and when you have a spiritual problem, you go see a priest, rabbi, minister, or sheik. The brilliance of Western culture lies in its capacity to recognize distinctions and analyze the parts of the larger whole.

"In the Eastern framework, however, there is no such sharp distinction between the body and the mind. In Eastern medicine, both physical and mental illnesses are treated by rebalancing the body's energetic system.

"Years later, as I tried to understand what these people with remissions were trying to tell me, I circled back to these ancient theological writings. I was reminded of the teaching that the body is thought to be a metaphor for something that the deeper mind is trying to learn. I began to wonder, are these people able to open a curtain of perception in the deeper mind in some way, and that this then plays a role in their health recovery?"

This was it—the next big question. Summarizing my work for the TEDx talk had allowed me to home in on where exactly to dig next. All this time, while I'd been going from case to case and looking for patterns and clues, I'd been struggling with a fundamental contradiction in what I was seeing. These big, sweeping changes people were making in the way they ate, exercised, thought, worked, lived, and loved were absolutely *essential* to healing. They should have represented all the various areas in your life that you could potentially change or fix. And yet somehow, these various factors just didn't add up—not completely. You could do all these things and still not recover from a disease. You could also *not* do them all (or even most of them!) and still somehow experience a spontaneous healing.

I wanted so badly to understand and to be able to translate the lessons of spontaneous healing to more people—to draw them a map, a straight line that ran from nutrition to lifestyle to stress to love, guiding them to healing. But it was rapidly becoming clear that this wasn't how spontaneous healing worked. While there *were* important repeating patterns and common factors across cases of SR, there were just as many contradictions. The straight line of reasoning I'd been struggling to assemble—one that ran from diet, to inflammation, to fight or flight—wasn't adding up exactly the way I wanted. I'd been trying to work it out like a math equation—*solve for x*—but this problem resisted such a linear approach. "Eat right" plus "fall in love" does not automatically mean you'll get better. In the land of spontaneous healing, two plus two doesn't always equal four.

As much as I wanted to be able to create a sort of instruction manual for radical healing, it was apparent now that spontaneous remission was more than a list of boxes you could check: *eat veggies, exercise, meditate, love your friends and family,* check check check check. How many people do all this—do everything "right"—and still get sick? It wasn't about being perfect or following a prescribed routine. And sometimes, those who rigorously follow the most disciplined approach can be the sickest.

At the beginning, I'd started by looking at the most obvious factors: what people put on their plates, how they lived their lives, how they managed their stress. But I was starting to see that there was something else at the root of it all that allowed these other changes to happen. Something that was harder to talk about—both because we didn't have a standard language for it and perhaps because many people weren't even aware of it on a conscious level. I remembered now that Claire had talked about "getting right with myself." That Dr. Kaine had said that she had to "surrender to a new way of seeing and experiencing myself." I'd been looking for the big changes people made leading up to their unexpected reversals of illness—changes to their diets, their routines, their relationships, their beliefs. Now I wondered if perhaps the biggest and most crucial change was to their very identities.

Initially, these aspects had each seemed so unique to the individual that I hadn't really noticed the parallels. But now the similarities started to emerge. Each person alluded to a process of self-discovery, or self-reassessment, that had somehow helped align and make possible the other pathways to healing I'd been so laser-focused on, such as nourishing the body, changing their relationship to stress, and cultivating love and connection. Perhaps these survivors were all describing the same fundamental experience but using very different language to try to capture it, the way a dozen artists could all paint the same scene, and the results would be wildly different. I'd been missing it, even though it was right under my nose. But now, finally, I knew what I was looking for—the elusive, difficult-to-describe, and very personal process of transformation. It was a way of understanding oneself in an entirely new light that seemed to make all the other changes—from diet, to stress, to love and connection—possible.

THE PERFECT CASE

After my TEDx talk, calls and emails poured in, too many to manage. As I tried to keep up with the influx, my stress levels went through the roof. How ironic, I thought, that my research into how stress could kill you was most likely about to kill me!

Voices spoke up from all over the country, all over the world, clamoring to tell their stories of sudden and "impossible" recoveries. I wanted to investigate every single one and dig out the knowledge that was locked inside, but there were just too many. It was overwhelming. I would have needed an entire team of researchers and interviewers to screen every case pouring in. And while I now had a small platform of legitimacy to work from, I didn't have the bandwidth for that kind of large-scale project. The medical world had opened its door to the idea that spontaneous healing had something to teach us all—but just a crack. I knew I wouldn't be able to convince anyone to fund a longitudinal study on spontaneous healing yet. I was going to have to keep going on my own and do everything I could with what I had. And what I had was this: one man, one desk, and about one thousand emails.

I came up with a triage process for rapidly identifying the most promising, legitimate cases. At the most basic level, to pass into "investigation" territory, a case had to be a genuinely incurable illness and have documented evidence of both accurate diagnosis and clear remission with no complicating factors that could explain their recovery. Once it passed that first hurdle, I evaluated it on a couple of other fronts, one being the specific disease. For whatever reason, there are some diseases that simply lend themselves toward spontaneous remissions much more than others. There are other illnesses that we just don't know very much about; they're rare and not well documented. We don't know how they behave and when they can be considered "incurable." But when Mirae Bunnell's case came along, I felt a hard yank on my line. This one was a big fish.

It was just one of dozens of cases in my in-box one morning when I rushed in to work late, turned on my computer, and scrolled through my email, skimming for anything urgent before I started doing rounds. The subject line was "SR patient Mirae Bunnell," and I clicked on it absentmindedly, intending to file it into the folder of potential cases to follow up on later. But ten minutes later, I was sitting there with my coat still on, reading Mirae's message again. It ticked all the boxes for a watertight case of SR:

An incurable disease. A very careful and thoroughly documented diagnosis. Prestigious doctors at a world-class medical facility. Clearly documented evidence of diagnosis and remission, including scans, diagnostic pathology reports, operative notations from her doctors—everything. And finally, as a self-described "left-brained, analytical person," a "hard-core data geek," she was able to speak with clarity and precision about what she had experienced. But a particular passage in Mirae's email had snagged my attention. She wrote that she believed her healing had coalesced around her process of, as she phrased it, "changing my relationship with myself, and with the world."

The idea of changing your relationship with yourself is big, deep, and nebulous. What exactly did it mean in practice, and could it truly catalyze healing? This was what I wanted to explore with Mirae, if she were willing.

A stroke of luck: Mirae, a software exec living in Saint Louis, Missouri, replied to my request for more information right away. As she and I corresponded by email, the details of her story emerged. By the time I met her in person and she shook my hand with a firm grip and a wide, exuberant smile, I fully understood how miraculous it was that she was standing before me, living, breathing, and thriving.

TOO BUSY TO BE SICK

Mirae noticed the bump in her neck while in the middle of an important negotiation at work. At the time, her work was her life. She was in software sales at a large U.S.-based company and in charge of leading contract negotiations for a client's new multiyear agreement. The deal was important, worth hundreds of millions of dollars, and came with an enormous amount of responsibility. Negotiating the deal would take months. Mirae threw herself into it, working around the clock to get it done.

In her early forties, she was an active, ambitious, independent woman. She loved her little town, a woodsy suburb on the outskirts of Saint Louis. Her longtime boyfriend lived next door, and they got together in the evenings to cook dinner and catch up. They'd been dating for ten years but hadn't married or moved in together—they liked having their own space. Mirae walked every day with her dogs in the dog park that she'd helped create in town. Active with both Pilates and yoga, she was seemingly athletic and strong. But there was more going on, unseen, beneath the surface.

When she was a kid, Mirae got sick from a tick bite. The lymph nodes behind her ears swelled, and she ran a fever. But her doctor didn't recommend any kind of treatment, saying that it was just a "normal reaction" to the bite. This was in a suburb of Saint Louis, where Mirae grew up in a conservative Mormon family. Her mother, a gifted dancer and pianist, set professional career ambitions aside to stay at home and focus on raising the children. Her father traveled and worked long hours, climbing the corporate ladder. He also served as a bishop in the Mormon church. Her parents were very religious and strict, teaching their children to attend all church meetings and services and abide by a very high set of standards. Mirae grew up believing that any deviation from the straight and narrow was a catastrophic transgression. The message was that if you abided by the Commandments, you would be able to stay together forever, even in the afterlife. And if you didn't, you'd be cast out and separated from your family. Forever.

Her older sisters didn't seem to have a problem walking the path. They were obedient and good; they'd grown up talented and were musically gifted but had set aside their career ambitions to stay home and raise children like their mother. To Mirae, it seemed that was what women in the Mormon church were supposed to do. But she had a more rebellious spirit.

"I didn't want things to be mapped out for me," she says now. "I told my parents that when I grew up, I was never going to get married. I was going to have a career. I was going to make a thousand dollars for every year I was old." She laughs. "They just rolled their eyes. But I was determined that I was never going to be dependent on someone else."

She ran away for the first time at fourteen, made friends that

were older, owned cars, and lived in apartments. She was resource-
ful and hardworking, doing odd jobs to start making her own
money. And then, she got pregnant.

Everyone told her to give the baby up for adoption. She refused.

"They kept telling me, 'You cannot keep this baby, it's not fair
to the child,'" she says. "But just like always, if somebody put a rule
in front of me, I was going to break it."

She took her driver's test with all the other sixteen-year-olds,
except she was eight months pregnant. But she was determined not
to let it slow her down. She got her GED and started taking college classes while working full-time. She worked hard; she landed
a better job, and then an even better one. By the time she was in
her early twenties, she was traveling extensively for work, putting
in long hours. She had a young son. She'd accepted help from her
family in caring for him, but she felt conflicted about it. They were
raising him the same way she'd been raised, and she worried that
he would start to cast judgment on her choices and circumstances.
But she didn't feel like she had a choice; she couldn't do it alone.
Plus, she just wasn't feeling well. She was young, driven, and by all
outward appearances, healthy. So why did she feel so depleted, so
dragged down? Life was harder than it needed to be.

Looking back, she feels now that she was always sick, never
healthy. She calls her twenties "the decade of exhaustion." She calls
her thirties "the decade of pain." Joint pain, muscle pain, nerve
pain, seemingly migrating throughout her body without an apparent cause. Signs of a body in distress, a system out of whack. Finally, in her early forties, after seeing doctor after doctor, she got a
diagnosis: chronic Lyme, from the tick bite that was never treated.
By this time in her career, she was in a major role at a software
company. Her work involved managing contract negotiations worth
hundreds of millions of dollars, and she was getting ready to start
negotiations for a new deal that would demand long hours for the
next eight to ten months. It felt like an impossible time to be sick.

Her doctor ordered a PICC line installed in her chest for

dispensing the powerful antibiotics that he hoped would flush the Lyme infection out of her system for good. The central catheter entered her body on the inside of her left arm, a few inches above the elbow, and extended through increasingly larger veins to reach an area near the upper chamber of the heart. She would wrap the external portion of the PICC line to the inside of her arm with a flesh-colored bandage to keep hidden under the sleeve of her shirt. She didn't want anybody to see it or know she was sick. Sickness was weakness; it was failure. As deal negotiations intensified, her workdays swelled to fourteen hours, then sixteen. She'd slip out of the office, sit in her car in the parking lot, hang the IV bag over the rearview mirror, and hook in.

She wasn't initially alarmed by the lump on her neck. It was most likely a result of the Lyme, said the doctors, and would go away as she continued with the antibiotic treatment protocol. Lymph nodes, she knew, wrapped around the neck just under the skin, in a chain like a strand of pearls. Her doctor rolled the lump between his fingers and said, "It doesn't *feel* like cancer." When the lump started getting larger instead of smaller, she was frustrated. She didn't have time for this right now. After years of health struggles, she was starting to wonder, *Why me?* On paper, she should have been a shoo-in for a disease-free life. She had seemingly healthy habits. She ate pretty well, even though she often bolted her food standing up or ate distractedly at her desk. She exercised, working out in her home gym or squeezing in a Pilates class before work. She tried to get enough sleep, but it was hard. Sometimes she needed to pull an all-nighter, fueled by caffeine, to get the job done. But this was life, right? She wasn't doing anything differently from anyone else. In fact, she felt like she was more health-conscious than most, despite pushing herself pretty hard. Why had illness chosen her?

Rebellious as always, she refused to bow to the demands of her body—she would finish this deal, and then she would turn her attention back to her health. She triaged based on priority, and the deal was more important. There was always something or other wrong with her body; she couldn't stop and drop everything each time there was a glitch.

She started pulling her hair over one shoulder to hide the lump, but it had gotten to the point where it was impossible to hide. She was partnered with a dealmaker, a guy who sat next to her with his laptop open, running spreadsheets to figure out various scenarios as she worked the deal. They weren't especially close, just colleagues. But one day, he pulled up a chair next to her, looked her straight in the eyes, and said, "What the *hell* is on your neck?"

She tried to brush off his concerns with an "Oh, it's nothing," but he cut her off.

"I just have to tell you, it's bigger every week. Every time I come back, it's bigger," he said. "You have to do something."

On March 31, she finished the deal, and on April 1, she went in for the biopsy. Two days later, late in the evening, her phone rang.

"You're going to get a phone call tomorrow, and I want you to be ready for it," said her doctor's voice on the other end of the line. "You're going to get some results, and it's gonna be really scary. I want you to get an appointment right away; do not wait until Monday."

She calmly agreed to everything. When she hung up the phone, she sat in silence, stunned. Then she called her boyfriend next door and burst into tears, repeating everything the doctor had just said. Thirty seconds later, he rushed into her kitchen, dropped to one knee, and asked her to marry him.

"Are you kidding me?" she cried. "You're doing this *now?*"

She pulled him to his feet, shaking her head. *No, no, no,* she was thinking. She hadn't absorbed the impact of the news, but she'd seen it in his eyes—it was bad. She wanted to turn back the clock, unwind it all, go back to before.

"This did not happen!" she cried. "You did not just do that!"

Her mind was racing; she wanted to believe that she was about to wake up from some terrible dream. But the doctor's words were echoing in her ears: *metastatic melanoma.*

A TUMOR NAMED "MEL"

In bodies everywhere, every day, a cell mutates and cancer begins. It could be happening to any of us at any time. You go about your day, making coffee, driving to work, completely unaware. But your immune system *is* aware. It flags the site and sends a team of cells (including the natural killer cells that we learned about earlier) to gobble up the mutated cell and flush it out of the body. Good-bye, cancer! You cook dinner, you go to bed, none the wiser. Your immune system has wiped it out before it can gain a toehold and spread like a weed in a sidewalk crack. But a weak immune system *is* that crack in the sidewalk, letting the seed grow; the roots shoot down into the soil and spread. Ineffective natural killer cells and lymphocytes can miss a mutation, and the cancer continues its rapid cell division.

With melanoma, there's usually a primary site where that mutation starts, somewhere cutaneous, on the skin. You might notice an unusual skin lesion or a mole that changes in appearance or bleeds. If there can be anything "good" about melanoma, this is it: its tendency to announce itself. Certain cancers are more lethal simply because they don't send up these kinds of red flags. Pancreatic cancer and colon cancer are two examples of these. By the time symptoms appear, the cancer is already very advanced, less treatable, and deadlier. Melanoma is typically a more "survivable" cancer simply because it's more frequently found early. But when a primary site can't be found, or when it goes metastatic—breaking free of the primary site and spreading through the body—then it's a whole other ball game. Metastatic melanoma is Stage IV cancer, which means it's already advanced.

Doctors searched for Mirae's primary site but found nothing. She scrolled through her memory—maybe there'd been something last year, a scabby spot on her scalp that took a while to heal, but at the time, she'd just assumed she'd nicked it on something. Could that have been the primary site? There was no way to know.

Metastatic melanoma with an unknown primary site (MUP) is rare, and there's not a lot of research on it—outcomes are poorly defined. But in general it's considered to be *not* a good sign. Patients with it have a very low life expectancy, with a median survival rate of about ten months.[1] Things improve a bit if surgery is an option. With surgery, the five-year survival rate rockets to over 30 percent, which is a testimony to how far we've come in treating and managing cancer. *But.* It's important to note here that when we talk about survival rates, we're not talking about remissions. We're simply talking about people who are *still alive* a certain amount of time later. Melanoma is a cancer that a person could live with for months or even years. But once it's metastasized, melanoma is considered incurable. Depending on treatment, five-year survival rates can range from 18 percent to only 8 percent. And if surgery is impossible, that percentage drops even more.[2,3]

Melanoma, Mirae's doctors said, is "the cancer that kills you by millimeters." Worse, the tumor was not resectable. It was tangled up in her lymph nodes, so large that it was deviating her right carotid artery, causing (according to the notes the doctor scribbled on her file), *significant compression and thinning of the right internal jugular vein.* These two vessels—the carotid arteries and the internal jugular veins—are the main vessels carrying blood to and from the brain. The neck is full of vital structures; crammed in a small space are the structures that get food to your stomach, blood to and from your brain and head, air to and from your body, muscles to support and turn the head, and nerves that send messages to your body to do everything from scratch an itch, to run, to breathe. Mirae's tumor was simply too interwoven with these structures to remove. The oncologist, panning over it on the CAT scan, called it "beautifully complex" with Mirae sitting right there. She was shocked, almost offended.

"There was nothing beautiful about it," she says now. "That thing was going to kill me!"

But then, gazing at this image that seemed suddenly very separate from her—not her own body at all, just a picture illuminated on the wall—she could see how it could be beautiful. It was so impossibly big, so unusual. It was amazing, really, that a body could still be working, with that giant mass filling up the neck.

It really was its own entity. They decided to give it a nickname: "Mel," short for *melanoma*.

The immediate concern was the amount of pressure Mel was putting on Mirae's life-sustaining blood vessels and esophagus. Even though the tumor couldn't be removed completely, one doctor wanted to try surgery right away, to take some of the pressure off the vital structures of her neck, which would buy her a little time. Another thought they should try chemo, to shrink it first, and maybe get more. Everyone was looking at her scans—doctors, nurses, technicians—amazed and horrified. One nurse went over to her.

"We were all out in the hallway trying to figure out how you breathe," she said to Mirae. "Can you breathe?"

And in that moment, she found suddenly that she could not take a breath.

For months, she'd been telling herself that the swelling in her neck wasn't anything too terrible, that she'd take care of it as soon as she was done with her deal at work, just like she took care of everything. But now, her mind replayed the images of the "beautifully complex" tumor pressing into her esophagus, and the nurse's question—*Can you breathe?*—echoed in her ears, collapsing her mental ability to stave off the effects of the tumor. As she struggled to breathe and the nurses crowded around to help, dropping her hospital bed flat, tipping her back, and pressing an oxygen mask over her mouth, she tried to process what she was being told—that she would not recover from this cancer.

I looked at Mirae's scans—she emailed her medical file to me, and when I clicked on the attachments and the CAT scan image filled my computer screen, I could see why they'd given Mel its own nickname. I could also see that there were metastases far from the original tumor site, which essentially indicates that the cancer is incurable. At that stage, the median survival rate is about six to twelve months, and treatment is palliative.

The treatment plan they laid out was a gauntlet of thorny odds: there was a fifty-fifty chance that she'd have the right genetic makeup for the drug they wanted to try. Then, if she made it over that hurdle, she had a fifty-fifty chance that she'd tolerate the drug, a powerful and toxic one that many weren't able to continue taking. And *then,* even if she cleared those two previous hurdles, there was only a fifty-fifty chance that the chemo would be able to shrink the tumor by 30 percent, the bare minimum required to make it resectable. The oncologist was honest with her. He put the chances of the drug having any effect *at all* at around 5 percent.

She won the first coin toss, at least: she had the right genetic makeup for the drug.

It's difficult to hear what sounds like hopeful plans for treatment when the long game of that treatment is not actually expected or intended to make you better. It's only expected to extend your life, and maybe improve the quality of the time remaining. Swept up in the language of action and treatment, Mirae used the word *cure* when talking to one of her doctors, who immediately stopped her.

"We don't talk about a *cure* with this disease," she said gently. "We talk about *managing the progression* of the illness."

The reality of her diagnosis had been sinking in incrementally; now it felt like a bottomless abyss. It wasn't a question of *if* this cancer would kill her; it was a question of *when.*

It was surreal, Mirae thought, that one minute you could be sitting at your desk, finishing up a deal at work that you'd thought was so important, and the next, lying on a hospital bed trying to come to terms with your own imminent death. *I'm a smart person,* she thought. *How did I get to the point where I had this thing sticking out of my neck, and I did nothing for so long?* She was overwhelmed with regret. And a part of her wondered if this illness was a message.

"It was as if my body said, *You've been treating me like crap for years. Caffeine, no sleep, eating like a racehorse.* Maybe this cancer was my body saying, 'Screw you. I'm done.'"

They began the drug therapy in May, just as the white-and-pink dogwood trees began to bloom all over Saint Louis. As her body was flooded with heavy daily doses of cytotoxic drugs, she felt exhausted, nauseous, thirsty.

"Why me?" Mirae said. "Sure, I wanted to do things my own way most of my life. But I'm the nicest person I know. I'm considerate. I'm kind. I put everyone else first. If there was a dead animal on the side of the road, I'd stop and bury it if I could. The world is a better place with me in it. *I'm a good person.* Why was God doing this to me?"

She plunged into a dark period, convinced that her illness was punishment for the choices she'd made earlier in life, the ways that she'd gone against the grain. She'd essentially left the Mormon church; she'd gone against her family's wishes time and again. She didn't want to believe everything they believed. She didn't want to wear the dresses her sisters wore or acquiesce to the life she believed she was supposed to want as a woman in the Mormon faith. She'd had a baby out of wedlock, as a teenager. She'd always been the bad one, the wrong one, the mistake. She still had that cold fear that when she died, she'd be alone—excommunicated from everyone she loved.

Before her diagnosis, time had seemed infinite—like an ocean. You could scoop up a bucketful and there was always more. She'd been counting on it—that wide-open sea, the future stretching before her. There was so much still to do. Her son, now married, was graduating from dental school and moving across the country for his residency. She'd spent so many years pouring her time and energy into work—to prove everyone wrong and give him the kind of life that didn't seem possible with a single, teenage mom. Suddenly, now that the future *wasn't* infinite, work didn't seem to matter much at all, even though it was where she'd focussed so much of her attention. How ironic that the things she'd prioritized the most seemed now to matter the least.

"What hit me the hardest," Mirae says, "was that I was out of time to rewrite things."

To rewrite things?

"The story of my life," she replies. "The story I was telling myself about who I was. It was all wrong. And I was out of time to fix it."

THE IMPORTANCE OF YOUR STORY

I've called spontaneous remission a black box that hasn't been unpacked by medical science. With literal black box technology like the kind we use on commercial airplanes, data flows in during the flight and is encoded and stored. If something goes wrong and the plane crashes, investigators can pull essential information out of the black box to figure out what might have happened.

We each have a black box inside of us as well, collecting data on everything that's happened to us over the course of our lives. I'm talking about memories and old emotions, past traumas and losses that have imprinted themselves on our psyches and cells, deep-seated stress and anxiety that can't be accessed by a few minutes of meditation or a change in life circumstances. Griefs and grudges that we hang on to like a security blanket; ideas about ourselves—who we are, what we are capable of, what we deserve or don't deserve—that were recorded during our formative years. Just as the medical community shies away from unpacking the black box of spontaneous healing, most of us do the same with our own black boxes, leaving these subconscious beliefs about ourselves, others, and the world wholly unexamined.

This black box I'm talking about isn't just a metaphor. It's real.

A more scientific term for it is your *default mode network* (DMN). The DMN is basically a collection of loosely connected regions of the brain, both older structures deep in the brain and newer ones in the cerebral cortex, which are activated, or light up, when you engage in certain categories of thinking. I say "light up" because that's what it looks like on an fMRI—areas of the brain glow bright out of the silvery gray like when you blow on embers in a fire.

What lights up your DMN? Daydreaming. Thinking about yourself and others. Getting "likes" on social media. Remembering things that have happened in the past; imagining what might happen in the future. When you become self-reflective or aware of your own emotions. Basically, the DMN is most active when you're not focusing on elements of the outside world but instead are turning inward to a more introspective mode. It yearns for narrative, helping us compose the story of who we are by linking our past with the present and what we consider possible or likely for our futures.[4]

We interpret the things that happen to us in our unique way and "record" events the way we perceived them. When we go back over these events in our minds, as we all tend to do with significant things (especially if they're negative or we experienced them intensely), we activate the DMN repeatedly in the same patterns, creating neural pathways with deepening "grooves" over time. As a kid in school, did you ever write on your desk? I remember the smooth beige wood the desks were made of and how when I started writing, my pencil just skated over the slick surface. But as I pressed into the same lines over and over, the grooves got deeper and more permanent. Pretty soon, all I could do was draw the same shape, retrace the same deepening, darkening lines. This is what happens in your brain, in the DMN, when you go over traumas and stresses and memories and griefs, and all kinds of other beliefs about who you are, over and over.

The idea of the DMN is relatively new in neuroscience, so there isn't a consensus on all the areas of the brain that officially comprise this nebulous yet very important brain system. We do tend to agree that any definition of the DMN should include the prefrontal cortex (the locus of planning, decision-making, and behavior regulation), the cingulate cortex (part of the limbic system, tasked with emotion and memory formation), and the inferior parietal lobe (in charge of *interpreting* those formed emotions and processing language and sensory information). This all comes together to form what an outside observer might call your personality and what you might call "me." Neuroscientists have nicknamed it the *me network*. It's the neurobiological basis of the self; it's *who you are*.

Now, it's important to pause and point out that this isn't *all* of who you are. There is more to identity than just the DMN; the sum total of a person can't be wrapped up in one neurological network. When it comes to radical healing in particular, we'll see that identity runs much deeper than this, but the DMN is an essential place to start. It's the blueprint of the building that you've been conditioned to think of as *you*. Your life, your identity, your sense of self, your story, your method of operating in the world—it's all built based on this blueprint.

So what happens when your sense of self—when your blueprint identity—is built upon ideas that are negative, damaging, or limiting? What do your self-imposed negative beliefs or limitations do to your brain chemistry? To the cycles of stress and fight or flight in your body? To your biological systems, to your cells? To your likelihood of developing disease and to your capacity for healing from it? What's in your black box that could be keeping you from healing or even making you sick?

WHAT'S IN YOUR BLACK BOX?

Back in 1985, a researcher's slip of the tongue launched a study that would reshape the landscape of modern medicine. Vincent Felitti, head of the Department of Preventive Medicine at Kaiser Permanente in San Diego, California, was trying to understand why patients kept dropping out of his weight-loss clinic. The clinic was one of the most successful initiatives at the Department of Preventive Medicine, and yet strangely, it had a 50 percent attrition rate. Participants would begin to lose weight very successfully and would be well on their way toward their stated weight-loss goals, and then suddenly they would drop out and disappear. Why on earth would people be dropping out *just* as they were about to realize their goals?

Interviewing one particular patient who'd been a star of the clinic, dropping almost three hundred pounds over the course of a year before she abruptly quit the program, Dr. Felitti misspoke while reading through a list of interview questions. "How old were you when you became sexually active?" he said—or thought he said. The patient replied, "Forty pounds." Confused, he asked the question again, and she gave the same answer—and then burst into tears.

Felitti suddenly realized that he'd tangled up two questions and transposed phrases. Instead of asking the patient how old she'd been when she became sexually active, he'd asked, "How much *did you weigh* when you became sexually active?" The answer she'd blurted out revealed a truth that she might never have been able to admit otherwise: that she'd been abused as a child. Her first sexual experience was with a family member at the age of four.

It was a revelatory moment. Felitti recalibrated his questions, expanded the scope of his interviews, and quickly determined that people were dropping out of the weight-loss clinic not *in spite* of the fact that they were losing weight but *because* of it. One woman, who regained close to forty pounds in only three weeks after a colleague at work commented on how great she looked and asked her out, said, "Overweight is overlooked, and that is what I need to be." She also had a history of suffering from abuse.

With that slip of the tongue, Felitti had accidentally uncovered the secret to treating his patients. The link between childhood sexual abuse and obesity was profound and, it turned out, widespread. People were gaining weight almost intentionally as a survival strategy in response to the trauma they'd experienced as young children. Therefore, he couldn't just focus on devising strategies for people to lose weight in the present day; they'd have to time travel into their childhoods and heal from that trauma before they could lose weight, keep it off, and get healthy. And when Felitti expanded the scope of his inquiry into childhood trauma and present-day health, partnering with Richard Anda, a leading epidemiologist, to design a massive longitudinal study, they discovered that the issue went beyond sexual abuse and beyond obesity. Far beyond.

Felitti and Anda identified ten types of childhood stress and trauma that they called *adverse childhood experiences,* or ACEs. They screened seventeen thousand study participants over two years, using a combination of physical exams and interviews about their pasts and childhoods. What they found was that strong links between childhood trauma and present-day illness existed across multiple types of experiences and multiple categories of disease. Abuse and neglect, losing a parent, witnessing domestic violence, living with someone who suffered from mental illness or drug dependency, or even just the constant, low-level chronic stress of emotional neglect—all these experiences and more emerged as major predictors for everything from obesity and diabetes to cancer and heart disease. Or, as telomere researchers Blackburn and Epel would put it, for stepping prematurely into the disease span.

So how exactly do these past experiences turn into illness in adulthood?

At first glance, what the ACE study shows us is that trauma and stress from early childhood leads to disease-causing *behaviors*. For example, here's how the CDC explains the pathway to illness established by ACEs: trauma or chronic stress early in life can disrupt your neurodevelopment. In adulthood, the result of that disruption is that we sometimes don't make great choices on everything from what we eat or with whom we live to whether or not we smoke, and thus we put ourselves at risk of developing all kinds of disease, from diabetes to heart disease to cancer. We tend to call these *lifestyle illnesses* because they have their roots in the way we live. Discovering that the root cause of many of our choices and habits can be traced back to experiences from childhood was a huge revelation, one that is finally beginning to reshape the way we screen for and treat these illnesses. I say "finally" because this change was a very long time coming.

Felitti and Anda first published the results of their study in 1998. It should have made every doctor in the country sit up and reevaluate how they were practicing medicine. Instead, most people either ignored or dismissed it. *Correlation does not equal causation,* was the cry from most—a rejection based on the idea that having both trauma in childhood and illness in adulthood was just a coincidence. But the ACE study was so well designed, so well run, and has since been backed up by so many supporting studies that I suspect the real reason it was initially rejected is because the idea behind it was just *too big.* If we believed the results of the ACE study, we would have been compelled to change the way we practiced medicine from the ground up. It's a huge and overwhelming task to think about how to overhaul these systems that we've built an entire industry around.

"Nobody wanted to know this," Vince Felitti says now in describing the negative response to his groundbreaking study. "But it was real."[5]

It's easy to look at the path of progression as laid out by the CDC—the line that leads from childhood experiences to disrupted neurodevelopment to health-risk behaviors—and think, *Oh, ACEs don't apply to me,* because you're not engaging in those behaviors. Maybe you took the ACE screening test and found that you had one or two, but you have healthy habits today. That's great, and what it might mean is that you were able to develop resilience or coping tactics, either on your own or with the help of others in your life. But it unfortunately doesn't mean that ACEs don't impact you. Only *half* of the ACE-related illnesses that people are suffering from can be chalked up to their current behaviors. The other half? It has to do with the fact that stress and trauma can literally rewrite your DNA, recoding your body to be more susceptible to disease and even allowing that illness-prone code to be passed on to your children. As we already know, toxic stress can alter the chemistry and biology of your body, down to your very cells. It's not just that ACEs lead to disease-causing behaviors—they lead directly to disease.

And what if you took the ACE screening test and *didn't* have any ACEs? Also wonderful news. But it doesn't mean that stress, trauma, grief, or other experiences from your past aren't written into your DMN and affecting your health or ability to heal today. The ACE study confirmed that ten types of trauma impact health and cause disease. It doesn't mean other types of stress *don't;* it just means we haven't measured those yet.

At this point in my study of spontaneous healing, I knew I had to look beyond what science had absolutely confirmed to what it was *pointing toward.* The ACE study focused on childhood experiences and proved that those experiences shape your health. But in some ways, the ACE study was a blunt tool; it was a place to start, but it didn't encapsulate the whole story of how our past experiences shape our current identities and also our health. I had to wonder, what about all the experiences we haven't yet studied? Experiences the ACE study didn't look at—like the ideas we receive about ourselves early on about who we are, what we deserve (or don't), what might be bad or wrong about us? What about grief and heartbreak, or the grudges we hold against those who have hurt us? How do these experiences affect us? How do our perceptions and interpretations of these experiences affect us, working their way through the body over the course of months, years, decades? How might they shape the map of our default mode network, determining how we think about ourselves and how we define who we are?

When I first read the ACE study, I felt pretty bleak. When you learn that the best treatment to prevent these experiences from ever taking root and altering your neurodevelopment and physiology is early intervention, it's easy to feel hopeless, especially if you have some serious stuff in your black box. I know I did. I scrolled back mentally through my childhood and teenage years, thinking of all the experiences that had very likely made me more susceptible to all kinds of illnesses borne out of years and years of toxic stress. When I took the ACE quiz, I discovered that I had seven ACEs.

Seven.

It's hard to look at that and not feel doomed to disease. I realize now that my parents were both physically and emotionally abusive. Life was, every day, a war zone. My brother and I were hit. We were forced to endure deprivation in the name of religion. My mother required that I drink and eat spoiled milk and food and created all kinds of other extreme situations to demonstrate that she owned every aspect of my mind, body, and soul. I now believe that she was suffering from her own unaddressed history of loss and, perhaps because of that, had a particularly difficult relationship with me, her oldest child and son. She used to say that the problems between us started when I was two years old, that she went away for the weekend and when she returned, I wouldn't come to her when she called me. She never got over it, and our relationship never recovered. As I grew older, she tried to convince me that there was something inherently bad about me, deep down. And it nearly worked. I didn't realize until much later—after I broke away—that if anyone had known what was going on, my siblings and I would have been removed from the home.

Looking back, I see that I had it the worst out of all my siblings. But now, all my siblings suffer from a variety of chronic illnesses. Studying remarkable survivors, such as the ones reflected in this book, has been one of the most important factors changing my own trajectory; it has been a very personal quest to figure out what genuinely heals a soul. And for me, moving beyond childhood trauma and making sure my body wasn't locked into a cycle of chronic fight or flight also meant getting out of my default mode network.

New experiences are one way to do this; any time you get out of your daily routine and experience something new, your brain exits the DMN, and you get bumped out of your default mode of operating. It's an enormous opportunity both for changing your thought patterns and changing your health. When you get out of the DMN, you have the chance to create and reinforce new neural pathways that can override existing ones.

The term *default mode network,* as mechanical as that sounds, is a much more accurate and precise way of describing what we used to call the *ego.* The ego has been poorly defined in popular culture, but essentially what it refers to is an individual's identity or sense of self—how we integrate our unconscious and conscious selves, our higher and lower impulses, and decide what is true about our lives. But when we talk about the ego, it's often in terms that suggest it's fixed or permanent, when in fact identity is much more fluid than that. And the great thing about the term *default mode network* is that it accurately captures the way that identity is, in part, a function of neural synapses and pathways that can be edited or redrawn, the way a map can be edited or redrawn as a landscape changes over time.

GETTING OUT OF YOUR DEFAULT MODE NETWORK

We rely on thought patterns to live our lives. Imagine if, every time you slid into the driver's seat of your car, you had to think and puzzle through every individual step involved in piloting it to the grocery store: the gas pedal, the steering wheel, signaling, all the micro-tasks that you do unconsciously. You need to be able to perform routine tasks without actively thinking them through. This code that was written into our DMN long ago when we learned how to walk, talk, ride a bike, drive a car, and so on is absolutely necessary if we want to survive and function. When it comes to driving across town, we want to fall back on the programming of our DMN. When it comes to automatically seeing ourselves as damaged, wrong, broken, disempowered, or unworthy, we definitely don't.

Depending on the DMN for day-to-day living and routine tasks makes sense. But letting these patterns and ruts define who we are, doesn't. Radical change—and perhaps, radical healing—can only come when we're able to see and understand ourselves in a completely new light. Perhaps this is why humans have been coming up with ritual, cultural ways of interrupting our default mode networks for millennia—everything from prayer to meditation, from dance to travel to art, can do it. And perhaps this is also why disrupting the DMN may very well play a large role in spontaneous healing.

When she started the chemo for her melanoma, Mirae was more exhausted than she'd ever been in her life. She would lie in bed for twenty hours a day and still felt too weak to even take the dogs out for a short walk. She was constantly feverish, nauseous, and so thirsty that she could drink gallons of water and still want more. Her body ached, her joints burned. Sometimes she couldn't tell if she was shaking from fever or having convulsions. She lost control of her bladder, making her wonder if she'd lost consciousness. And strange, vivid scenes played out in front of her. She started having the same dream over and over: a set of hands appeared in front

of her, big and gentle. She knew them, although she didn't know
exactly how; they just radiated a sense of *home*. In one dream, the
hands showed her a book, slowly turning the pages. It seemed like
she was meant to read it, but she couldn't quite make sense of the
words, and where there were supposed to be pictures, it was just
blank.

She chalked it up to the chemo—all those chemicals were
probably messing with her sleep rhythms. But she couldn't shake
the feeling that there was something to be learned from the dreams
she was having. They were always the same. They were so vivid
and real, unlike any dreams she'd ever had before in her life. She
dreamed of the big hands again, this time flipping through pages
of sheet music she couldn't read. But this time, a voice spoke. "Your
life is like sheets of music," it said. "The frequency of your life sings
a beautiful song that your ears cannot yet hear."

She woke up, grabbed a pad of paper, and wrote that down.
After that, she wrote down everything she was thinking and feeling
when she woke up. She wrote:

- *I was not made with smooth edges or to fit in a box.*
- *This is all part of my plan.*
- *The plan cannot be revealed right now; have faith.*
- *The plan cannot be revealed in fear.*
- *My plan has no pictures because I choose what it will look like and how
  it will show up.*

As she journaled her dreams and what they meant to her, she
started to look at herself, she says now, "in the third person." She
was able to zoom out, seeing the big picture of her life and identity
from above. She'd always felt "wrong," "bad," or "not good enough"
in the context of her family. But for the first time, she could see
herself clearly. In a sense, her whole life had been like a play; she'd
been playing a part on a stage, a role that she and her family had
decided on a long time ago. She'd been cast from the beginning as
"the rebel." Now she saw that she wasn't any of the bad things she'd

always felt; she was simply playing the role that had been given to her. In a sense, it was exactly what her family needed. She was imperfect, but perfect for the context of her family. She was, as she put it, "perfectly imperfect."

She began to understand that she'd been performing for everyone in her life instead of being her authentic self. As independent and ambitious as she'd always been, she'd also spent her whole life trying to please other people—her parents, her bosses, her son—but never herself.

"Whatever those dreams or visions were, they were so healing for me," she says. "Instead of feeling I had done wrong, I realized I was perfect. Perfectly flawed, perfectly suited to my own human experience."

At the same time, she was also making the same big, hard changes that others who experienced spontaneous remissions tended to make in the face of a devastating diagnosis. She changed the way she ate and thought about nutrition. The chemo made it hard to get food in and keep it down, so she narrowed her diet to the most nutritionally dense foods and ate as much of those as possible. She also realized she needed to think about *how* she was eating. To slow down, appreciate the process, and visualize the nutrients flowing into her body. She also radically changed the structure of her life to bring down stress and allow herself to turn off chronic fight or flight by taking a leave of absence from work.

I want to pause to point out something important here. Mirae was lucky to have the support structure in place to take a long chunk of time off work—she had savings, and her workplace, so appreciative of her years of hard work and overtime, gave her a lot of latitude. She had just completed a huge business deal for them, and they told her to take as much time as she needed. Not everybody has this option available to them, and that's important to be cognizant of; for many of us, having to get by and make ends meet means being locked into a routine that might make it harder to heal.

But healing is less about what happens on the outside and

much more about what happens on the inside. You don't have to quit your job to improve your health or even experience radical healing. You don't need to have a lot of disposable income. The wealthiest people can suffer from the worst illnesses, and those with much less can experience dramatic recoveries. There are cost barriers to some of the strategies that people have used, such as yoga, Rolfing, or eating organically, but you can't buy a spontaneous healing. There are no silver bullets; there is no external thing that will end up being the one thing that turns your health around. When you zoom out on the big picture of spontaneous healing, you see that each person finds her own path to the clearing.

Mirae now believes that it wasn't the costlier tactics she tried that made the difference. Taking the time off work certainly helped; it meant time to sleep, rest, and reflect. But at its core, what taking the time off really represented was setting boundaries. She started saying no to stuff that felt overwhelming and unnecessary, that stretched her too far. She stopped apologizing for missing meetings, for not being there every minute. She stopped feeling guilty about it.

"The big thing was realizing that I didn't owe anybody else anything," she says. "I owed my body the time."

Mirae knew what the doctors were hoping for—a shrinkage of 30 percent, just enough to operate—was unlikely. She also knew that any increase in size could damage the vital structures of her neck. So she started tracking Mel's size herself with a cloth tape measure, to check for any change in between scans. She was afraid Mel might start to grow. But then suddenly, Mel started to shrink. Fast. When she called her doctor to report that Mel was disappearing at a rate of a half inch per week, hitting the 30 percent mark and then blowing past it, he didn't believe her until she went in so he could see for himself. He was at a complete loss.

"There must be a lot of people praying for you," he finally said, with no other way to explain what she was experiencing.

BECOMING AN "N OF 1"

The obvious question: Was Mirae simply a "high responder" to the chemotherapy drug?

While responses to chemo certainly do vary from person to person, Mirae's results leaped far over what was known to be possible with this drug, even at the outside limits. Her doctors could not attribute what was unfolding to her course of treatment. As Mirae's tumor melted like ice on a hot stove, they were in uncharted territory.

As the weeks turned to months, Mel had shrunk to the point where it wasn't visible from the outside anymore. Her medical team was astonished and wondering what on earth was going on in there. There was only one way to find out.

The surgeon performed the neck dissection as planned, successfully removing thirty-three lymph nodes from the right side of Mirae's neck. Since cancer often spreads through the lymphatic system, we often remove lymph nodes to assess the extent of spread. The surgeon attempted to remove what was left of the tumor but wasn't able to—because it wasn't there. The pathology report revealed no trace of disease—an impossible result. And the tissue removed from the site of the tumor showed only a faint swirl of black pigment, an inky echo of what had once been there. Mel, that beautifully complex, malignant tumor that had rapidly swelled into Mirae's life-sustaining central arteries, had simply vanished.

Mirae will tell anyone who asks that her doctors at Washington University gave her incredible care. They were highly skilled, compassionate, and dedicated. She emphasizes how grateful she is for everything they did. But she was surprised that they weren't more interested in finding out what she might have done during those intervening seven months, between diagnosis of incurable metastatic cancer and diagnosis of complete remission, that could have played a part in her unexpected recovery. They did marvel at her recovery. They wrote a study on her and published it. At conferences, they give presentations on her remarkable case. When they see her now, they give her a high five and call her by her nick-name: "the Miracle." But they seem content to leave her recovery unpacked. Mirae is simply what they call "an N of 1," which in statistics-speak, means in a class of her own, a data point with no equal.

We can't be sure exactly what happened inside Mirae's body while she experienced her remarkable recovery. We haven't yet fig-ured out how to predict when a spontaneous healing might occur so that we can observe what happens as it is unfolding. All we can do now is put the puzzle pieces together as best we can. And while there are still pieces missing, the picture is beginning to come together.

We know that traumatic experiences like ACEs, and very probably other types of stressful or negative experiences, can be-come part of our default mode network, a brain map that becomes a landscape of limitations. Finding ways to get out of your default mode network can lead to shifts not only in the way you think but also in the way your body functions on a chemical or even molecu-lar level. So while we can't literally rewrite the past, what we can do is change how we experience it and change what becomes part of our default mode going forward.

How? That starts with perception.

Mirae said to me once, "It's the perception that creates the thought that creates the feeling." How we perceive and interpret the world—ourselves, others, events, and so on—determines how we experience and remember the world, how we feel as we navigate it, and ultimately how we respond biologically. The effects trickle down all the way to our cells. We talked about shifting the way we think about stress, changing threat stress to challenge stress, and how it can actually alter the biology of your body. What I'm talk-ing about here is taking that concept to the next level. When you change your lens not just on the stressors in your life but on your life itself—on who you are fundamentally—you have the potential to change your health on a much larger scale.

So how can you get out of your old default modes and change your perceptions? It can start, simply, with experiences. Seeing yourself and the world around you in a new light often begins with the basic first step of doing new things. Breaking your usual routine in some way means being able to see yourself in a new context. It's a natural way to challenge your assumptions about yourself—about who you are and what you're capable of. Some people use meditation or yoga to get out of their DMN. Some use travel. For me, education and pursuing lots of new experiences and ways of thinking have been critical and continue to be. There are probably a thousand ways to do it. However, the key is not just having the experience but making something of it. You have to actively integrate a new truth into your life in tangible ways. Mirae's dreams and new beliefs would have remained only fading memories if she hadn't changed her daily life to match her new beliefs. People who experienced spontaneous healings disrupted the default mode, got out of that rut, saw and experienced themselves in an entirely new way—and then did the work to integrate that knowledge into their lives.

For Mirae, the process was catalyzed by her dreams, which are uncontrollable; you can't make yourself have revelatory dreams. Some of these experiences can't be forced or engineered, but you can ask yourself questions that prompt self-reassessment, such as: What is my story? What is the story I've told myself about who I am? What story do others tell me about who I am? What do these stories get right, and what do they get wrong?

You can also be open to such experiences, to recognize opportunities when they come along and make the most of them. Mirae didn't turn her back on what her subconscious was trying to communicate. Are there ways that your subconscious, your body, or your immune system is trying to get your attention? Mirae paid attention. She learned to listen and then took the messages seriously. She wrote them down, working out her thoughts and feelings through journaling. She was open, at a basic level, to reassessing her fundamental understanding of who she was and what her purpose was in this life.

And then, importantly, she incorporated those lessons into how she lived on the day-to-day level. She began to prioritize taking care of herself, connecting with her partner, making time for the goals and dreams she'd lost sight of long ago, when she'd hooked her sense of self to being "successful" at work. Like Juniper, Jan, and so many others, healing her identity and arriving at a new understanding of herself allowed Mirae to rewrite the rules she'd been living by. She calls that time period "absolutely life-changing."

Perhaps those who experience remarkable recoveries are the individuals who've figured out how to go back to those ideas about who they are—ideas that were forged so long ago, seemingly in steel—and melt them back down. They are still made of the same essential materials, but they've gone back to the core of who they really are, underneath all the stories they've been told, the trauma they've internalized, the stressors or burdens they've carried. They find a way to get beyond their default mode networks and are able to see themselves and experience themselves and the world in an entirely new way.

How will this new version of you see the world? What priorities will you have, what changes will you make in your life to reduce stress and increase joy? How will the body of this new you work chemically when it comes to stress hormones and their impact on your cells? How much more successfully will this new you be able to live deeply, immersively, in the parasympathetic?

When we dig deep into these cases of remission that doctors haven't been able to explain or understand, we see that there is a powerful link between our very identities and our immune systems. Perhaps what ultimately determines the health of the "soil" of your body is how well you know who you really are *at the most authentic level*—beneath appearances, "shoulds," perceived expectations, and all the masks and roles that you assume for yourself and the world. Because the ripple effects that stem from this one deep, central aspect of *identity* flow through everything. It determines the way you think, the way you feel, the way you see yourself. Whether you make time for yourself or not. Whether you move your body and go outdoors and breathe deeply or not. Whether you prioritize putting excellent food in your body or not. How and when and how often the stress response clicks on in your body, and the precise levels of hormones that tumble out, and the way that your specific cells respond to that wash of hormones.

Mirae's doctors admiringly called her an "N of 1," essentially meaning that she's in a unique category shared by no one else—one of a kind. Technically, in medical literature, what the term refers to is a clinical trial where one person is the only subject. Any interventions or strategies tested in such a study are tested on one patient only and are highly individualized, specifically tailored to that person. In some ways, it's as individual and intensively personal as medicine can get. Perhaps what we each need to do, like Mirae, is to make ourselves an N of 1—to run our own clinical trial where we find the individual changes necessary for us and then lean deeply into those changes. And as we move forward, we'll talk about strategies for doing just that—how to conduct your own personal, urgent experiment in health, the way the survivors profiled in this book have done.

We can take the steps we learned about in part 1 of the book to help our bodies regain their natural healing abilities—to bolster and focus our immune systems, to eliminate inflammatory foods and increase nutrient-dense ones, to change the way we deal with stress, and to learn techniques for quieting the chatter in our minds and accessing the parasympathetic. We can do all that, and it will be incredibly beneficial and may even lead to the kinds of remissions that Tom, Juniper, and Jan experienced when they made big, hard changes in their lives. But based on many years researching spontaneous remission, my biggest takeaway is that most of us need to go deeper. We need to dive down to *who we are* at the bottom of it all. Because ultimately, healing your identity may determine whether or not you're able to use all those tools and tactics we've gone through to live in the parasympathetic and support your health and recovery.

Today, Mirae is cancer-free. Since her outcome was so out of whack with her prognosis, she still goes in for regular screenings, although as time goes by, they get farther and farther apart. At first, they were every month, then every six, then she finally convinced them to push it to once a year. Finally, after years of clear scans, her oncologist shook his head in wonder.

"Well," he said. "Looks like I might actually get to use the word *cured* about this disease in my lifetime."

10

You Are Not Your Illness

Everyone is a genius. But if you judge a fish by its ability to climb a tree, it will live its whole life believing that it is stupid.

—*Albert Einstein*

When you look at the picture below, what do you see?

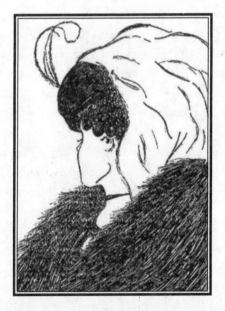

You may see an old woman with her chin tucked into her fur coat, her head wrapped in a white shroud. Her nose is hooked, her eyes small and sad, her mouth turned down. But look again. Focus on the nose, and let it become the curve of a cheek, turned provocatively away. The old woman's eye becomes an ear; her mouth becomes a choker necklace. Do you see the young woman now?

This image was drawn in 1888 by an unknown artist, printed on a postcard, and distributed as a novelty. Years later, a newspaper editor came across it somewhere and, amused, published it in his paper, titling it "My Wife and My Mother-In-Law." *They are both in the picture,* he wrote in the caption. *Find them!*

Now zoom forward to the year 1930, when a psychologist, Edwin Boring, came across the image and scooped it up to use in a journal article he was writing on perception. He was interested in why we see what we do when confronted with an ambiguous image and how easily (or not) we can shift our perceptions. Often, it's difficult for people to see anything other than the first image they perceived—if you see an old woman to begin with, it can feel impossible to see the young maiden. Boring found that viewers needed to somehow experience a "figure-ground shift" to perceive the other image that was right there before them. In a figure-ground shift, we are able to allow certain aspects of the image to fade into the background and for other aspects to become dominant. And then, suddenly, a whole new picture appears before our eyes. We see something that was right in front of us the whole time.

Those with spontaneous healings also experience a figure-ground shift in the way they see themselves. And for many—like Mirae—it feels very abrupt, as if they'd been staring at the picture and seeing the old woman for so long, and then they looked up, and there was the maiden. Mirae described it as "the veil being pulled back," so that suddenly, for the first time, she could clearly see the story of her life, and it was different from how she'd always thought. She experienced a very intense figure-ground shift; it was the same life, the same woman, but a completely new image emerged.

We each need to experience a figure-ground shift in the way

we see ourselves and our illnesses. With the Boring figure, once you are able to perceive both images, you should be able to toggle back and forth at will. But you can only ever see one or the other, the old woman or the young maiden; you can never perceive them both at the same time. So if you see yourself as sick, can you see yourself as anything but?

Karen, the young woman with cerebral palsy whom I met when I traveled to Ohio, is a perfect example of this. Both Karen and her identical twin sister had been living with cerebral palsy since birth. Cerebral palsy, which is typically caused by developmental abnormalities in the womb or oxygen deprivation during birth, affects the body's muscles, movement, and coordination. Some muscles are too contracted, others not enough. Karen had a particularly difficult time with her legs; her heels didn't touch the floor when she walked, and she had trouble extending her legs. During our interview, she described pulling herself slowly up the rail of the main staircase at school while the other kids seemed to fly past her. Life isn't easy when you're a kid who's missing something that everyone else takes for granted.

She finally sought care from Dr. Nemeh, who practiced not far from her hometown. Over the course of just a few visits, she began to experience a shift in how she felt in her body. Some people describe feeling overheated or strange after Dr. Nemeh lays his hands on their bodies; some vibrate, some faint. Karen felt a surge of energy, leaped out of her chair, and ran out of the room. She'd never run anywhere before in her life.

New trials are exploring therapies to treat cerebral palsy, including cord blood and stem cell treatments that doctors theorize might help replace the lost nerve cells in the brain that are the root cause of the condition. But while researchers have hopes for the future, cerebral palsy is currently incurable. Karen, however, is a vibrant young woman who has now overcome most of the debilitating effects she was born with. The last time I saw her, she was happy, healthy, and running two or three miles regularly to build up the muscles she'd been unable to use for most of her life. She's recently enrolled in school to become a physical therapist herself. A new future is rolled out before her like a carpet, one she never thought she'd be able to tread.

Karen's identical twin, who'd come along with her sister, sat quietly in her wheelchair during the interview, listening. She'd of course witnessed the remarkable transformation of her sister's body and life but refused to see Dr. Nemeh herself. She told me, in essence, that she didn't feel worthy of his attentions; she was certain that any attempt she made to improve would fail. She felt too defective and, therefore, unworthy. Hearing this broke my heart, and I will never forget her story. It reminded me that, for all of us, it's just easier to believe the bad stuff. How many of us are living like this, thinking of ourselves as somehow defective, undeserving of real recovery and a great life? And how do we flip the image and go from seeing ourselves as sick or defective to seeing ourselves for who we really are?

THE POWER OF PERCEPTION

I grew up in rural Indiana, surrounded on all sides by wide-open farmland and endless blue sky, yet found the world confining— hemmed in by the rules and judgments of a punitive religious family. I wore handmade clothes that my mother sewed; my brothers and sisters and I got our hair cut at home. We spoke with a rural accent that would probably sound backward and strange to you, even more pronounced than those around us. I'll never forget the day, standing in the church lobby at around seven years old, when my friend said, "Your dad talks like a hick!" This was in one of the poorest counties in Indiana, and yet he thought my father—and not his own—spoke like a hick. But we weren't supposed to care about stuff like that—about how we looked or whether or not we had clothes that were in style. We were only supposed to care about being acceptable to God.

When I realized that the world was bigger and wider and more wonderful than I'd been told, I knew I wasn't going to be able to stay in that smaller, more restricted world. I also knew that if I wanted to achieve my goals of pursuing higher education, getting advanced degrees, and maybe becoming a doctor, I was going to have to change. Just before college started, I exchanged my ugly, plastic-rimmed glasses for contacts, "rebelled" and had my hair professionally cut, and bought modern clothes. When I walked onto the campus on that September day, warm and muggy in the Midwest, the difference was astonishing. It was a palpable feeling, how differently people perceived me. People looked at me with acceptance instead of judgment; they assumed I was like them, instead of some kind of "other." The relief of it almost brought me to tears. I knew I was no different on the inside, but their acceptance helped me find a new way of seeing myself over time.

It has always been helpful to me to understand that, for all of us, there exists a gap—sometimes huge—between who we really are and who we appear to be. This is one of the gifts, among others, of a difficult childhood.

People often think it's shallow to worry about how other people perceive them. And it is critical to know your value, regardless of what other people see. But on a certain level, what people see when they look at you matters. It can affect what job you get or your chances with someone you're interested in dating—and it can affect your ability to heal. We are influenced in part by how others see us, and in fact we teach them how to see us. If *other* people see you as sick or damaged, it can make you feel sick or damaged. It can cement the idea in your DMN that that's *who you are.* If you perceive yourself as "sick" or "ill" or are surrounded by people who perceive you this way, how much longer and harder might your road to recovery be?

We've already seen how intertwined beliefs, physical health, and healing are and how our own individual perceptions shape—from the ground up—how we understand the world around us. Two people can be sitting next to each other in Central Park, for example, but be living in two completely different universes. The first feels oppressed by the constant rush of traffic or frightened by the rapid beat of helicopter blades overhead. People approaching seem menacing—what do they want? The person sitting right next to them will notice other things: a mother lovingly placing a blanket over her baby in a stroller, a couple holding hands and speaking as if only they exist, a shower of leaves raining down from a tree, red and gold in the sunlight. Two different worlds. Extend these radically different perceptions across a period of years and imagine how differently the chemistry and biology of those two people's physical bodies might be.

Perception even affects the senses—what you taste and what you hear. The famous McGurk effect, named after the researcher who first identified the effect in a 1976 paper titled "Hearing Lips and Seeing Voices,"[1] found that what we *hear* is often heavily based on what we *see*. Look it up on your phone or computer just for fun; you'll find a video of a man saying, "Bah, bah, bah," over and over again, who then switches to saying, "Fah, fah, fah." When he switches, the *F* sound is very pronounced. Except the hitch is, the sound file playing hasn't been changed at all. It's repeating the same sound, over and over: *bah, bah, bah.* But we *see* his mouth making the shape of the letter *F,* and therefore, our ears hear it. We manufacture it without even realizing it, a crisp, clear, unmistakable letter *F.*

The same is true for the blind spot in your vision, created by the complete absence of cones and rods at the place where your optic nerve connects with your retina. Yet you compose a sort of "bridge" image over the gap, creating a seamless vision. What isn't there, you invent—without even realizing it.

A study found that people experience *more* pain if they are led to believe that the person inflicting the pain is doing it on purpose. Another study on pain found that if you curse when you hurt yourself, it hurts *less.* Here we can see how our emotions affect our perceptions of pain—if we feel targeted by someone, it hurts more; if we can reject the pain verbally and emphatically, it hurts less. Yet another[2] study shows how truly amazing the science of perception is: a team of maids working at the same hotel, with the same general job responsibilities, were separated into two groups. One group was told that their usual work duties constituted "exercise"—that it actually satisfied the Surgeon General's recommendations for daily exercise. The other group was told nothing. Over the course of the study, the women in the first group became measurably fitter (weight, waist-to-hip ratio, BMI, normalized blood pressure), while the other group experienced no change at all. Perception—in this case, the belief that a certain activity was "exercise"—had the power to change the body.

Here's another good example: most of us, I'm guessing, aren't particularly excited about getting older. As we age, we may begin to think of ourselves as decrepit or diminished; we may fixate on our losses. But this negativity, which is perfectly natural, is also extraordinarily harmful. Research by Ellen Langer at Harvard and Becca Levy at the Yale School of Public Health is discovering that having genuinely *positive* views about growing older improves your health[3] and extends your life, even more so than exercising or quitting smoking.[4,5] Plus, negative thoughts about aging put you at risk for developing Alzheimer's. Why? Researchers found that the chronic stress generated by negative self-perceptions wears down the hippocampus, the small, seahorse-shaped portion of the brain that is responsible for your memories, emotions, and even the beating of your heart.

As we have seen during our foray into physics, our minds are not just passive observers of an objective external reality. The observer effect shows us that our perceptions may have the capacity to shape reality to a certain degree—to change our experiences and sometimes even our physical bodies. And our ability to choose our perceptions strikes at the very core of what makes us human. Unlike animals, we choose how to interpret our experiences, and in so doing are capable of remarkable transcendence. As the philosopher Giovanni Pico della Mirandolo intoned at the dawn of the Renaissance, we are either gods or beasts, angels or demons.[6] We can see what is good and possible, or only what is missing or fear-inducing. And the way you see yourself and your illness can either set hard limits on your potential for recovery or open up unexpected pathways to healing.

JIM BOWIE AT THE ALAMO

In 2014, I received a request from Herb Benson, the developer of the relaxation response and one of the trailblazers of mind-body medicine. It was good, if slightly intimidating, news: Mass General wanted me to give a presentation to the faculty on spontaneous remission. At that point, I'd been on TV multiple times, and I'd been on the TED stage. I shouldn't have been nervous. But I was. I'd be presenting to the toughest, most skeptical audience out there: my own colleagues.

The talk went well. I kept my presentation as scientific and quantitative as possible, and people seemed intrigued. After the talk, I found a page of notes that one doctor had taken and accidentally left behind in the room. She'd written and then underlined, with exclamation marks and a smiley face, something that I'd said: that those with remarkable recoveries are the heroes in self-care, who have achieved something unusual because they see ability and opportunity where others see disability and disease.

The next day, I got an email from the assistant head of psychiatry at Mass General. It was a tip about a spontaneous remission from renal cell carcinoma—a type of cancer of the kidneys that is often deadly, but which for some unknown reason is one of the more likely cancers to spontaneously remit. *Gerald White is an engineer from Texas,* the message read. *He has a remarkable personal story to tell.*

Gerald, who went by "Jerry," was the kind of guy who shouted into the phone. Not in an angry way—he was emphatic. Exuberant. He had a story to tell, and he wanted to shout it to the world. The day I called him to hear his story of illness and recovery, he had another story he wanted to tell first. It was about a wild boar.

Jerry lived in rural central Texas, in a little town on the banks of the Brazos River. The historic downtown, with its brick and awning storefronts, had a Wild West flair, and the big, endless Texan sky was a reminder that the untamed, independent state had once been its own republic. Every year, Jerry participated in a reenactment of the Battle of the Alamo, the last stand of the Texas Revolution. He played Jim Bowie, a legendary frontiersman famous for his deftness with a knife in hand-to-hand combat, who fought to the last even while deathly ill and bedridden. He reportedly shot every bullet in his gun into the approaching army from his bed before he was killed. I quickly realized how appropriate the casting was, as Jerry told me his own story of a legendary standoff in the Texas brush. A wild boar had been getting into his yard, he said, tearing up flowers and grass and generally terrorizing the family and pets. Not one to be cowed by a glorified pig, Jerry, at eighty-five and recovered from two cancers that should have killed him, went after it with an antique pistol.

He emerged from the brush victorious, much like he would emerge from his battle with cancer, as I was about to hear.

"It all started with a malingering yardman," he told me. He'd hired someone to cut the grass, but the man put the project off again and again. Jerry, fuming, finally decided that if you want something done, you'd better do it yourself. He borrowed a riding lawn mower from a neighbor and "tore into the job with a fury." After hours outside in the heat, he had conquered the huge lawn and headed upstairs for a shower. As he was toweling himself dry, he got a shock: his left testicle had suddenly swollen to the size of a grapefruit.

A flurry of medical visits ensued, including a CT scan to get a peek into Jerry's abdomen to see what might be putting so much pressure on his system and causing the testicular inflammation. When the doctor hung the films up, the culprit was immediately apparent even to Jerry's untrained eye. Where his left kidney should have been—on a CT scan, gray as a storm cloud—there was instead a large, gelatinous mass.

His doctor paused for a few minutes, and they both gazed at the scans as Jerry absorbed what he was seeing and then prepared himself for the words his doctor was about to say. Later on, when Jerry thought back to that moment right before his life changed, he felt grateful to the doctor for allowing him that moment of silence and preparation. It was apparent to him that he was at one of life's great turning points—the strange, calm hurricane's eye between *before* and *after.* When the doctor announced the preliminary diagnosis, and Jerry's family began asking questions, Jerry just sat quietly for a while, thinking. His initial response, he says, was denial. He didn't feel so bad. Maybe he could live with it, take it easy, and be generally fine.

He turned to the doctor; his family quieted down. "What if I just do nothing?" he said.

"Then it will kill you," his doctor said.

Now getting over his initial shock, Jerry didn't find this statement too upsetting. In fact, he appreciated the clarity.

"I found his candor refreshing!" he told me.

The diagnosis was renal cell carcinoma, or kidney cancer, and it was advanced, metastatic. Without treatment, his doctors estimated that he had about three months to live. And with treatment, the prognosis wasn't much better. At that time during the 1990s, patients with metastatic renal cell carcinoma were left with relatively few options. Metastatic RCC is known to have low response rates to the traditional therapies that were available then, such as chemo and radiation. More than seventy agents (types of chemotherapeutic chemicals) had been tested at that point, with disappointing response rates of less than 10 percent.[7]

But whether or not Jerry tried any of those iffy treatments, the first and most urgent matter was getting the tumor out, which was putting an enormous amount of pressure on Jerry's renal system. The surgery was done immediately at Baylor University Medical Center in Dallas. The operation lasted seven hours and removed Jerry's left kidney, plus a tumor that Jerry describes as "a twenty-pound honker!"

"I was told that it wasn't the largest tumor of this type *ever* removed," he said, "but I looked, and I couldn't find any evidence of a larger one."

I laughed a little at Jerry's unabashed competitiveness. He sounded so disappointed! The guy who played an Alamo com-

mander, who rushed off into the Texas brush after a wild boar—
this guy wanted to win at everything, even cancer.

Recovery was difficult. It was long and surprisingly painful.
But Jerry got through it by pushing himself to go a little farther
each day on his exercise bike and by reminding himself of what the
surgeon had said after the long surgery: "I got it all."

Except, he didn't.

Jerry, always one to throw himself wholeheartedly into whatever he was doing, had been researching renal cell carcinoma. He'd
discovered that it was one of the more unpredictable and capricious
cancers. It could move fast, spreading elsewhere in the body. A year
after his surgery, a follow-up CT scan found a small mass where
Jerry's left kidney had once been. Although Jerry's oncologist had
told him that renal cell cancer "never comes back in the renal bed,"
the radiologist was of the strong opinion that it was another malignant tumor. A biopsy confirmed it: recurrent renal cell carcinoma.

Jerry was out of mainstream options. He underwent a second
surgery to remove the recurrence, but the cancer would return—
and the only drugs on the market for kidney cancer of this stage
were experimental and controversial. Jerry's son found some interesting research on a new drug, an immunotherapy drug called In-
terleukin-2 (IL-2), that gave Jerry hope. But when Jerry brought
the research to his doctor, the doc was furious.

"He actually leaped out of his chair and pounded on the desk,"
Jerry said. "He shouted, 'Tell your son to quit reading those damn
books! Interleukin kills people!'"

It had been a year and a half since his initial diagnosis of renal
cell carcinoma, and while his surgeons had done well by him, Jerry
knew how important it was to take his health care into his own
hands. After that CT scan had turned up the small mass in his abdomen, for example, Jerry had been the one to demand a biopsy to
check for recurrence; his doctor had been insisting that it couldn't
be malignant. It was.

Jerry was an engineer by training and an inventor who'd filed many patents in multiple countries, and he believed that it's always best to figure out for yourself how things really work. He dug into the research on Interleukin-2 and decided that his doctor was behind the times. The standard cancer treatments (chemo, radiation) weren't very effective against renal cell carcinoma. Interleukin-2, along with drugs like dexamethasone (which Stephen Dunphe had been given), use naturally occurring messenger proteins in the immune system to target cancer cells. It *was* a controversial drug; immunotherapies were in their burgeoning stages in the mid-1990s, and though IL-2 had been approved by the FDA, it had terrible side effects and a relatively low success rate of 20 percent. However, to Jerry, who'd been given a 100 percent death sentence, a 20 percent chance at life seemed pretty good! Besides, he'd never been daunted by long odds before. Remember, this is Jerry White, the Jim Bowie of the Alamo and the walking terror of wild boars. When a follow-up CT scan turned up spots in his lungs, distals (or metastases) that had scattered from the original cancer site and were beginning to grow, his doctor finally caved and approved the immunotherapy.

Jerry described the side effects of the IL-2 as "the worst case of flu imaginable." Fevers, chills, vomiting. As he fought the side effects of the immunotherapy, which had sent his body into an intense inflammatory state in an effort to wipe out the cancer, he decided that he had to do more. Since his diagnosis, Jerry had been furiously researching, reading everything he could get his hands on about renal cell carcinoma, about cancer and treatment options, about survivors and their stories. Nutrition, meditation, prayer—he began to fold it all in, trying to give the treatments he was attempting the best possible chance at succeeding.

One of the toughest parts about the Interleukin treatment was having to receive regular shots of the drug. Most patients had to trek all the way into their doctor's office for the brief procedure, but Jerry's daughter was a nurse, so they were able to arrange for her to give her father the shots in the comfort of his own home. As the months went by, Jerry developed a routine that he believed got his mind and body in the best possible state to receive the immune system—boosting treatment. He took a relaxing bath. He tried to clear his mind, batting away worries or anxieties. He spent a long stretch of time in meditation, working through a program of guided imagery in which he pictured, in very specific detail, his white blood cells rushing through his blood vessels, finding the black, destructive cancer cells, and gouging them out. When he felt ready, his family would gather around his bed and pray with him, placing their hands on his body, sending healing energy that he swore he could feel.

"Even my little grandsons, just four and five, clamored for the chance to pray with everyone," Jerry told me. "Once, one of the little fellows prayed that the shot would be a sword to kill the cancer. I was overwhelmed by that."

The effects of the shot always wiped him out, but still, Jerry found value in the ritual he and his family had created—in fact, those times together as a family on "shot nights" were some of his most cherished memories.

"At the very least," he said, "we managed to take what's usually a cold and impersonal experience and turn it into a thing of beauty."

After eight months, Jerry had had enough. The side effects of the medication were taking a huge toll, and a follow-up CT showed that the Interleukin wasn't having the desired effect. If anything, the cancer was progressing.

Jerry decided to go off the Interleukin before the course of treatment was up. Instead, he decided, he would focus entirely on the meditation and guided imagery he'd been practicing for the past year. It was a radical decision, but Jerry had a feeling that it was his last, best shot.

"It had the effect of elevating the mind-body work to a life-and-death situation," he said. "I think that's what it took for me to give this my full focus and attention."

What did Jerry mean exactly by "guided imagery"? It can

mean different things in different contexts. For Jerry, it meant engaging in intensive visualizations that attempted to, as he described it to me, "communicate from the conscious left-brain hemisphere to the subconscious right brain by use of imagery." Now, I knew that in neuroscience, the understanding of the brain as being divided into "left" and "right" is considered by some to be somewhat simplistic. Yes, there is more to the brain than a left/right dichotomy, but the distinction is still critical, both anatomically and metaphorically, and reminds us that there are very different ways of being in and experiencing the world, and I was intrigued by Jerry's approach. What was important about it was that he was trying to find a way, through intensive, visual meditation, to send signals to his body—signals from his conscious self to a deeper coordinating intelligence within him, capable of altering the functioning of his immune system. Jerry's chosen meditation: to light up the antigens on each and every cancer cell, illuminating them like beacons, so that his own immune system cells—the natural killer cells, macrophages, and T cells—could find them and excise them.

Did he succeed? Apparently, he did! Three months after he abruptly quit treatment and took on his meditative practice, his doctors examined him and declared him "NED": no evidence of disease.

To me, one of the many notable things about Jerry—besides his incredible drive, the engineer's pragmatism and initiative he brought to healing, and the sense of humor that never left him—is how he conceptualized his illness. He kept it separate from himself: an enemy to fight. Looking back over our conversations, the emails he sent me, the long passages he wrote about his illness, I noticed the language he used. He was engaged in a "battle"; his struggle with cancer was a "war." His cancer was "the monster" or "the invader"; it "attacked." It had moved and inspired him when his tiny grandson used the phrase "a sword to kill the cancer."

Many people use war metaphors when talking about dealing

with a serious illness; it's baked into the communal rhetoric we all use to talk about disease. We fight, and we either win or lose the battle. We view disease as an enemy to be conquered, a foe to be vanquished. This approach can certainly be inspiring but might not work for everyone—for some, thinking of their illnesses as hostile invaders could do more harm than good. Take Claire, for example, who thought of her illness as a message from her body, an attempt to communicate with her. For her, listening and *responding* to that message was key. To Jerry, the cancer was the opposing army, slipping into the Alamo, surprising him in his bed. It was that wild boar, digging at the soil in his garden, that he chased out with an antique firearm.

Different metaphors work for different people perhaps because of what they mean. We all use words and metaphors that have slightly varied meanings in the recesses of our own psyches, so what works for your neighbor may not be what works best for you. Whatever you use needs to resonate with you and contain power and life in it; you need to *feel* that power and life. But whether you think about your illness as a message, or an enemy, or something else entirely, the critical thing is that you not think of it as *you*. You are not your illness; it does not define you.

This can be a difficult concept to hang on to and implement when you're in the midst of a serious illness. If the illness you've been living with, fighting against, listening to, and shaping your life around for so long *has* become a part of your core identity, how do you untangle yourself from it?

WHEN ILLNESS BECOMES YOUR IDENTITY

Illness plays a lot of different roles in our lives. Sometimes it can serve as a much-needed respite—something unmanageable or overwhelmingly stressful is occurring in our lives, and our body breaks down, giving us the break we need. For many, illness may be the first time in their lives that they've felt truly cared for, when they've given themselves permission to put themselves first. You don't even have to make the choice or have agency in asking for care; the illness chooses this for you. This can be the hidden gift of illness—it's out of our hands.

But if on some level an illness serves as an ongoing respite for you—a way to opt out of a life that has become overwhelming and regain some semblance of balance—a part of you that you aren't even aware of might resist getting better. If you are so far off the path of the most authentic life for yourself, so busy taking care of and pleasing everyone else that you have long forgotten who you really are and what helps you come alive, then the illness serves not only as a great wake-up call but also as a way out.

Other times, our illnesses can become entwined with our identities and our perceptions of ourselves in a way that can be difficult to untangle. What I see every day in the hospital, whether medical or psychiatric, is that our deepest hopes, fears, needs, and longings are often expressed through our illnesses, and sometimes they are expressed through our illnesses because every other avenue of expression is blocked. It's worth asking yourself: What is this illness holding for me? Your illness might have become a repository for some aspect of who you are—or who you believe yourself to be—so that it seems that letting go of that illness represents a kind of loss of self. Part of healing your identity, then, becomes realizing that you can unhook your identity from illness and remain whole and complete and even carry forward with you the lessons learned from that illness as you shape your new sense of self.

In our daily lives, we all cycle through various identities for the benefit of others or ourselves. Imagine a glass prism: small, compact, and translucent, seemingly simple. And yet, hold it up to the light, turn it just slightly. It turns one color, and then another. Pink, blue, yellow. There are so many different versions of you. You are someone's husband or wife, son or daughter, brother or sister. You are someone's boss; you are someone else's lover, someone else's oldest childhood friend. You are a very different person to your child from how you are to your parent. This doesn't make you less yourself or less authentic—this is simply part of what it is to be human and to be continuously deeply engaged in many distinct relationships with others. Who we are in each moment depends on context.

Sometimes we intentionally rotate the prism to present a certain facet of our identities. For example, I've found that there are distinct times when patients want me to assume the role of an authoritative physician, and to do so boldly, even sternly; in other moments, I can sense their need for me to figuratively lay aside the white coat and speak with them as a person, with my own fears and concerns. Knowing when to do what and to what degree is a skill that I've had to hone over years of practice.

Other times, we shift between identities automatically, without even really noticing that we've done it. For example, putting your children to bed and then descending the stairs to spend time with your spouse, you may switch unconsciously from *mother* to *wife.* In my work with patients, I sometimes refer to this as *switching masks.* These individual facets of our identities can be like masks we wear in that they both reveal and conceal who we are: *reveal* because they highlight that specific slice of our identity; *conceal* because in doing so, they often hide all the others.

Facets of our identity can also feel more like a label that the world puts on you, rather than something you choose. But whether it works for you to think of a facet of your identity as a *mask* or a *label,* it's essential to remember that it's not the whole you and that it may not be the accurate you. Illness—especially chronic, long-term, or terminal illness—can become a mask we get stuck in, a label we can't scrape off. Part of healing your identity is being able to see past the labels and masks, to understand who you are beneath all of them. A prism, though infinitely multifaceted, is ultimately a single, beautiful object. And so are you.

There is a deeper part of us that exists beyond what we see. Spiritual traditions have long tried to capture this with a language of the soul. Renowned neurosurgeon Wilder Penfield spoke about how he would do brain surgery and, with part of the skull removed and while the patient was awake, touch different parts of the brain with a small electrode, eliciting the feelings, smells, memories, sensations, and movements associated with different parts of the brain. He showed how the body looks to the brain from the inside, leaving us with a map of brain function that we call the *homunculus.* But he famously could never locate the self. Of the movements and sensations that occurred when he manipulated specific parts of the brain, the patient always said, "*You* did that, not me."

In this culture, we are consumed with our identities as other people see them. They can end up defining us, but the truth is that we have a whole other identity that is deeper, more complete, more foundational. We aren't what we do. We aren't our past actions. We aren't necessarily the people our loved ones believe us to be. And we certainly aren't our illnesses. The true self exists, invisibly and mysteriously, beyond all these labels and masks. So how do we experience the kind of figure-ground shift that lets us really see and experience this? How do we shift our perceptions to see ourselves for who we truly are, behind all the various masks we wear—especially the mask of illness?

TAKING OFF THE MASK OF ILLNESS

A central paradox of the whole situation is that you can't *force* a figure-ground shift to occur. In so many of the cases I studied, including Mirae's, the way that people described the figure-ground shift they experienced about who they were sounded just as "spontaneous" as their spontaneous healings. But as we've seen, spontaneous healing may not always be so spontaneous; many cases seem to reveal a long process of laying the groundwork for remission.

I was mulling this over in the back of my mind when a patient's mother entered my office for a family meeting with her daughter. She entered and shook my hand. Her smile was bright, her eyes warm. She looked like any other relatively well-off, middle-aged parent: fit, composed, sleekly dressed. While we waited for her daughter, she briefly described her own history. Years ago, she said, she'd been locked into a pattern of destructive behavior—shredding multiple marriages, trying and failing to leave behind her years of childhood sexual abuse, slipping back into patterns of substance abuse, lost jobs—a cycle she couldn't seem to break no matter how hard she tried. She had *adverse childhood experiences* written all over her. She told me that for a long time, she thought of herself as being fundamentally damaged, programmed for unhealthy decisions, doomed to disease and even death. All of it seemed to be so baked into who she was at the core that she couldn't conceive of it being different, even though she wanted so badly to be clean, to be healthy, to be happy. And yet this didn't describe the woman sitting in front of me, who was clearly now composed and thriving.

"What changed?" I asked her, so curious to know what could have caused such a remarkable reversal—one so many of my patients struggled, and failed, to achieve.

To my surprise, she was able to pinpoint a very specific moment when she suddenly realized she'd misunderstood the entire story of her life. I immediately recognized it as the kind of figure-ground shift that so many people had described before.

"I can still remember the exact second that it happened," she told me. "It was in a yoga class. I was in child's pose, with my forehead against the floor, and the realization just swept over me: I wasn't a defective person, which I guess I'd always believed. I wasn't defined by the stuff I'd done, the mistakes I'd made. I was good enough as I am. I was worthy of a good life."

I don't know much about yoga—it's not exactly my thing (at least not yet!). But after the session, I looked up child's pose and discovered that it's the simplest of all poses. You pull your knees to your chest, curl your body over like a child in the fetal position. It makes sense that she was able to change the story of herself while in that pose. She went back to where that story came from and pulled it out by its roots like a weed.

She got up out of that pose, walked out of the yoga studio, and changed her life completely in a way that reflected and honored this new self-understanding. It's been twelve years now, and her life is so different, her past self wouldn't even recognize it. Her career has gone from success to success. Sitting beside her was her husband of ten years, and I could tell he adored her. She may have been the same woman, but in truth she wasn't at all. She'd been able to see past the damaging labels the world had put on her (and that she'd believed), shed the masks that were limiting and disease-creating, that concealed the true her. She reclaimed a core self that she'd lost sight of along the way.

And it hadn't "just happened" in a flash in that moment in yoga class. This woman had laid the groundwork for the figure-ground shift she'd experienced. Sometime before, she'd decided—after years of making excuses—to take her mental and physical health seriously. She tried various strategies to change her habits but struggled and failed. Finally, desperate for change, she enrolled in a yoga class as a step toward health. That was how she found herself in child's pose that day, having that flash of epiphany that ended up changing her life. She wasn't just in the right place at the right time; she'd put herself there.

When I looked closer at so many of my cases, I realized that they hadn't "just happened," either. In every case, from Juniper to Jan to Mirae to Claire and to Jerry, people had been doing a lot of thinking or feeling about what they wanted from life or how they wanted to treat (or not) their illnesses. In some cases, they had made a big life change and were drifting in the wake of that change, which can be a dark and difficult place to be, but also one that allows us to reassess or see something more clearly—to get out of our DMNs.

A pattern was emerging—we can't *force* these flashes of insight and figure-ground reversals to occur, but we can be ready for them. To do that, we have to do the work to cultivate the soil, preparing for them and inviting them in. That might mean, as we discussed in the previous chapter, putting yourself in new situations to get out of your DMN and experience the world, and yourself, from a fresh perspective. It might mean thinking deeply about what your illness means to you—what it's "holding" for you or why you might, in some ways, rely on it. Does assuming illness as your primary identity provide a relief or an escape in some way? What's missing in your life? Are you spending too much of your time taking care of others instead of also paying attention to your own genuine needs and dreams? Or trying to meet the perceived expectations of others instead of living your own authentic life? Where are you not saying *no*? Do you know what your deepest being wants to say a resounding *yes* to? By asking these questions and taking steps to lay the groundwork, you might be able to find a way to put yourself first and live an authentic life that doesn't require you to define yourself by your illness.

Sometimes, to find our true selves, we have to confront the fact that that self is ultimately mortal. Whether we're sick or not, we all have to face this at some point. But for most of us, that's a can we kick down the road until we run out of road—even though looking directly at our own mortality can be powerfully transformative and can help spur that figure-ground shift that is essential to healing our identities.

A couple of weeks after turning down the Whipple surgery, Claire Haser drove to the mall near her house in Portland. She was alone. The last time she'd been there was with her mother, before her diagnosis. They'd gone from shop to shop, talking and trying on clothes. She remembered how she'd evaluated her own reflection in the dressing-room mirror, deciding on a sweater. Now, facing the end of her life, it was strange to remember being able to think so effortlessly about the future—imagining where she might wear that sweater, rubbing the fabric between her fingers to assess how long it might last. Today, Claire was also looking to the future, but in a very different way. She was there to imagine the world without her in it.

An exercise in the book she was working her way through, *A Year to Live,* required her to walk through the world as if she were no longer in it. Claire walked past shops, taking the same route she usually did when shopping for herself or her husband. She ran her hand over a rack of clothes. This same rack would be there when she was gone, she realized, but with different shirts on the hanger. There would still be bored husbands slouching on benches outside of the dressing rooms. The people in the food court waiting in line would be somewhere in the world, going about their days, driving to work and kissing their children and eating ice cream. But she would not. She began to believe that, like a real ghost, nobody could see her, that she was truly already gone. It was a hollow, haunting feeling.

"It brings it home, that the world will go on without you," she says now of the exercise. "Like an arrow to the heart."

It was a difficult experience. But Claire told me that if there was one thing that catalyzed her healing, it was facing and accepting her own death. For many, this is what triggers the figure-ground shift that offers them a new perspective, delivering a blast of clarity that allows them to see finally how they want to live and who they want to be. It's the first domino that sets off a cascade of changes that ripple through their lives, their souls, their bodies, and their very cells.

But it also offers a thorny paradox. How do you truly accept death when what you most want is to live?

11

Healing Death

Physician, heal thyself.

—Luke 4:23

When I was a sophomore in college, I proposed to my girlfriend, my first love. Jane said yes. I remember how I felt—like I was soaring. I'd had a hard childhood. But now I could forge my own family, with Jane, and do things differently.

On the morning of spring break, we piled into an old station wagon with four other students and drove from Chicago to Jane's family home in Connecticut. I sat in the front seat with Jane and the driver. Jane was reading a book I'd just given her, *A Severe Mercy.* It was about a husband and wife's relationship, and I'd found it very moving. I watched out the window as the fields of Ohio slid by, and then, as the sun went down, the dark rolling hills of Pennsylvania. Every so often, there was a square of light in the distance, a farmhouse with someone still awake. It was getting late, and I remember wondering about the people inside those lighted houses— why they were up, if they were alone, what they were thinking or worrying about on a Saturday night.

Just as we went through the mountain pass near Lock Haven,

a tractor trailer jackknifed across an icy bridge directly in front of us. Only a matter of feet existed between the back of the truck and the bridge railing. I remember yelling, "Get to the right!" After that, my memory shatters just like the windshield did.

Afterward, it was eerily silent at first, as if the world were on pause. And then everything came rushing in. The truck driver was out of the cab, swearing and howling, terrified. One of the backseat passengers in our car got out and ran into the darkness, screaming. I could tell immediately that John, our driver, had been killed. Jane was slumped, blood pulsing from a deep gash in her neck. When I pulled her out of the car, her pulse was already fading.

It was freezing, dark. I was hurt, too, but I barely noticed. I wiped the blood out of my eyes and performed CPR on her for over an hour, maybe two. Because of the icy roads, the ambulance couldn't make it to us, and neither could a helicopter. So I just kept going. From my time as an orderly in a hospital, I knew that once you start CPR, you don't stop until help arrives—so that's what I did, robotically, numbly. I kept going until the EMTs finally arrived and pulled me away from her. She was gone.

Later that night, lying in the emergency room, someone reached my parents, only to find out that my grandfather, the one person in my family who I felt truly cared about me, had unexpectedly died that day in Montana of a heart attack. I'll never forget the plastic surgeon stitching up the gashes in my face, flirting with the nurse and joking as I struggled to understand that life as I knew it had just ended. The voices seemed far away, as if I were at the bottom of a well.

Two days later, I barged out of the ICU against doctor's orders and discharged myself against medical advice from the hospital. They made me sign paperwork saying that I understood the risks, that they believed I'd punctured my lung and if it collapsed I would die. I signed it. The only thing that mattered to me then was getting to Connecticut in time for Jane's wake and funeral. I was stubborn, angry, confused, and grieving, and I was going to be at that funeral no matter what anybody tried to tell me. The accident shook me deeply. The fragility of life had become starkly apparent. One moment, Jane was nestled next to me, turning the pages of her book, and the next, I was holding the bloodied book as they took her away.

Why was I still alive? Was there any meaning to any of this? My life had been very painful and confusing up to that point. Why had this happened? Two people I loved, on the same day? Was there any *why* to when we die, or how? Was there any rhyme or reason to the workings of the universe, to the way that life flickered in and then out of it again, energy forming into matter, matter dissolving into energy once again?

The shadow of the accident followed me long afterward like a dog always biting at my heels. Questions swirled. Assumptions I'd built my life on were whisked away, leaving a gulf in their wake. I didn't know what to believe anymore. For a long time, I was numb. I went through the motions of school and work. I presented a stoic exterior, but inside I was frozen. Some people grieve quickly and intensely—I grieved long. But beneath the rote motions of daily life, something eventually began to stir.

For there to be a shadow, there has to be light. If there was something good about that accident—about suffering through the deaths of the two people I most loved and revered in the world, and coming face-to-face with the possibility of my own—it was that it freed me. As I woke from the cold fog of grief, I found that I had ceased to care what others wanted from my life. What did *I* want from life?

I became a serious student for the first time in my life. I had to work hard to recover my mind and focus from the trauma of my childhood. Now I had questions that demanded answers, and I was determined to find them. My questions propelled me onto the Princeton Theological Seminary campus where I found a mentor, pursued my degree in theology, digging into the philosophy of science and the nature of belief; then on to medical school, where I learned the science of the body. I was on my own course now, interested in living my authentic life for the first time ever. The accident, and the deaths of Jane and Grandpa, punched a hole in the walled-in, narrow corridor that had been my life. And through it, a whole other world appeared. There was pain in that world, because it was a world without Jane, and one in which I'd grazed up against my own mortality. But it turned out to be the doorway into *my* life and not someone else's. I was no longer trying to please others. In a very real way, that accident made my whole life possible. It freed me from a cage I'd been unable to escape, that I'd scarcely even been aware of. Death, it turned out, was the doorway into life.

Facing death can be a pivotal moment in life, whether during a serious illness or not. But it's easier said than done.

The denial of death is programmed into us at every level. As Ernest Becker so eloquently said in his Pulitzer Prize–winning book of that title, our civilizations are built on this denial. We build elaborate cultures in such a way that we can defend ourselves on a daily basis against the specter of our own certain death. Some part of us believes in immortality, and we seek this through our religions, our children, our achievements, through the monuments we build and believe will survive our physical selves. As a physician, I see it every day, in the sheer number of people who refuse to sign Do Not Resuscitate orders for their family members, ignoring wishes expressed by their loved ones to not keep doing procedures when the quality of life outcome is awful, or in the number of people who leave loved ones on life support long after it is time to let go. It's easier to put off the inevitable. We do it, too, as doctors: "Not on my shift."

But overwhelmingly, the survivors of incurable diseases I've profiled in this book say that facing their own deaths was a crucial step in their pathways toward healing.

"There are a whole lot of things that happen once you face your death," says Claire. "You're not afraid anymore. You feel like a weight's been lifted off you. You feel free to live your life, however much of it you have left. You're present, you're grateful. There's a lot that flows from that."

Sometimes, to heal your identity and find that authentic self, you need to first pass through the difficult portal of facing and accepting your own mortality.

THE MIRACLE OF DEATH

There's something transcendent about facing death and not backing down. In not skirting around it but walking through it—a fire that burns away everything but the most essential parts of you. It becomes clear, suddenly, what you most want, who you are at your core, what you are meant to do with your time here. It clarifies, like nothing else can, what it means for you to "heal your identity" and create a new story for the rest of your life.

One way to look at it is that there is a kind of figurative "death" of the false self. Many survivors describe it in these terms and in fact tell me repeatedly that their illnesses were their greatest gifts, because they liberated their true selves. By dying, they found life. By facing the worst that could happen and moving through it, they excised the "disease of fear" that binds all of us and then realized that, unexpectedly, they were free to live.

As Claire said to me, confronting her own death was the thing that made it all possible: reevaluating who she was and what she wanted with her time here, living authentically, making radical change. And Mirae said that getting the cancer diagnosis "gave her permission" to stop living the way everyone expected and do what she really wanted.

Confrontation with death allows us to be the person we each want to be and really are, rather than the person others need us to be. It can be the final thing that pushes us to heal our identities, shifting us into authentic, fulfilling lives, moving us more permanently and fully into the parasympathetic. An understanding of our own mortality—sparked for many by a terminal diagnosis—can be the catalyst that causes a major shift in understanding as to who we are underneath it all. It can be the switch that flips, causing that fundamental figure-ground shift. We can suddenly see ourselves clearly for the first time. Other priorities drop away. We are liberated to our authentic selves.

When you shed an old mode of being in the world, it means complete freedom to build or reclaim an identity that is not disease-based or deficit-based. You can build this sense of self on what is right with you, rather than what is wrong.

But there are certainly ways in which a terminal diagnosis can box you in instead of freeing you—people who acquiesce to a prognosis, performing it to the letter. So what makes the difference between accepting death in a way that is limiting, versus accepting it in a way that is liberating? And what exactly is involved in "healing" death? What does facing death really mean?

Let's start with what it *doesn't* mean. First of all, accepting your own mortality does not mean curling up and waiting to die. It doesn't mean acquiescing to a prognosis that isn't true to your specific, unique, and personal situation. Those who experienced spontaneous remissions had something important in common, whether their illnesses were chronic or terminal: something inside them rose up, saying they were people rather than prognoses.

REFUSING TO DIE ON SCHEDULE

It's easy to hear a prognosis—your doctor's best guess of how your illness will progress—and see it as a prophecy. But doctors don't have crystal balls. They can't see into the future.

A prognosis is the most *likely* course of an illness, based on what we've seen and documented in the past. It's far from a sure thing. A prognosis is arrived at by examining all the available data on an illness and taking the mean, or the average, of that data. We home in on the spot on the chart where most of the little dots are clustered, forming a dense little cloud. Meanwhile, more dots stretch on in both directions, representing the full scatter of possibilities: the unlucky who turned out to have less time than expected, and then the exceptional, who vastly outperform our expectations. This chart, upon which all our prognoses are based, doesn't capture the fact that, just as a rain cloud is made up of individual droplets of water, each of these dots is a unique individual. That single black point represents a human life. And many, many of those dots fall outside the mean. A prognosis, by definition, absorbs the exceptional into its averages and obscures it.

The question then is: Do most of us fulfill our prognoses because they truly *are* the most likely inevitable outcome? Or do we fulfill them because we believe them? Do we manifest them because they're what we expect, thereby giving more weight to these averages?

Perhaps we simply continue on the biochemical trajectory we're already on. Our doctors evaluate that trajectory and try to logically predict where we'll land—like watching a ball come off a bat and arc through the sky. You can use your experience as a baseball fan, your knowledge of the game, and your basic understanding of physics and gravity to make a really good guess. But when people like Claire, Juniper, Pablo, Matt, Jan, Patricia, and Jerry introduce deep mental and spiritual change into their lives, this also has biochemical consequences, and it changes their trajectory. Instead of landing in the outfield like they're supposed to, they caught an updraft and went sailing right out of the ballpark.

In the medical world, debates tend to flare up about whether or not telling people their prognoses can actually affect the outcome of their illnesses. Some studies have suggested that giving people a time frame means that's how long they last—that they die "on schedule," as if obediently following orders. As doctors, we tend to err on the side of giving all the information we can—but should we? If hope is medicine, and if belief can change the body's biology, then are we remiss as caregivers when we offer no hope, when our patients believe our guesses that they only have a short time to live?

On a rainy Sunday in April, as I was driving into work to do rounds, I punched on the radio and began flipping stations. I was stuck in traffic, and the squeaky percussion of the windshield wipers wasn't doing much to entertain me. I happened to tune in during an episode of *This American Life,* and right away, I was hooked. The episode was called "In Defense of Ignorance,"[1] and it centered on the theory that maybe, sometimes, ignorance *is* bliss. Perhaps there were times in life when it was beneficial—even lifesaving—not to know something.

Lulu Wang, a filmmaker, told the story of her grandmother, the feisty matriarch of a large Chinese family. Wang described her grandmother, Nai-Nai, as "five feet tall with a full head of permed white hair. She's small, but when Nai-Nai walks into a room, everyone listens." At the age of eighty, Wang's grandmother went in for a routine physical and was diagnosed with terminal, stage IV lung cancer. The doctors predicted she had less than three months to live and recommended that she be hospitalized immediately.

In some cultures—like China, where Wang's story takes place—attitudes toward patients' rights and the involvement of families in care decisions are a little different from how they are in the United States. It's acceptable, even *advised,* to withhold information from a patient about their diagnosis and prognosis if the news is too bleak. There's a communal aspect to decisions like these regarding illnesses and how to proceed, and it's not unusual for doctors to inform the family of the patient first, who are allowed to decide how, when, or even *if* to reveal details of the illness to the patient. In the United States and other Western countries, we take a much more individualistic tack: the patient is the first and often only one to speak to their doctor. Privacy and autonomy are paramount.

The decision to hide a terminal illness from someone might seem shocking and unethical to many. But that's exactly what the Wang family did. It wasn't Wang's grandmother who trekked into the doctor's office to hear the results of her physical—it was her younger sister. And after a family conference, they collectively decided not to tell Nai-Nai her diagnosis.

The doctors were appalled. They insisted that not hospitalizing her was grossly irresponsible—the cancer was very advanced. But there was no way to hospitalize her without telling her the diagnosis. And Nai-Nai's younger sister (Wang's great-aunt, whom she referred to as "Little Nai-Nai") feared that learning this diagnosis would be a blow she might never recover from. She believed that *not* telling her sister she was dying might be a way to prolong her life. "It wasn't just that she didn't want to upset her sister with the news of her death," Wang recounted over the airwaves. "She actually believed that not telling her was a way to prolong her life. Knowing Nai-Nai's personality, Little Nai-Nai worried that her sister would get overwhelmed with fear and depression. She'd stop eating, she'd stop sleeping, she'd lose interest in life. The Chinese believe that mental and emotional health are completely linked to physical health."

The family sought a second opinion, and then a third, hoping that the diagnosis was perhaps in error, but the diagnosis was airtight, and the prognosis was always the same: "Three months, maybe less." So they forged a report from Nai-Nai's physician, whiting out the terminal cancer results, and making a fake photocopy of the test results to fool her. So that their grandmother wouldn't be suspicious about people wanting to see her before she died, they threw a huge party under the auspices of a wedding—the bride and groom had planned to get married the following year, but they bumped up the celebration so that everyone could convene without Nai-Nai guessing why. At the gathering, while everyone put on smiles and secretly, internally said their goodbyes, Wang's grandmother "remained focused on the future—a future she assumed she'd be a part of."

They expected her to decline quickly and pass away. But she just . . . didn't.

A year after her "expiration date" had passed, she was the same. She seemed healthy. She refused to go to her physical that year, saying that she felt good—what was the point? Another year passed, and when she went to the doctor, the diagnosis was the same. Stage IV lung cancer, three months to live. And the next year, the same.

Yet Nai-Nai's body seemed paused in a state of stasis, the disease neither advancing nor regressing. The years went by, and nothing changed. Her body, it seemed, had not gotten the message that it was supposed to be getting sicker. So it just didn't.

As Wang interviewed her great-aunt on the air, Little Nai-Nai told a well-known Chinese joke. It went roughly like this: Two people go to the doctor for a physical. One is healthy; the other has a terminal illness. But the office staff gets the results switched and they each receive the other person's prognosis. The healthy person dies, while the terminally ill person lives.

"Is that really a joke?" Wang asked her aunt. "It's not very funny."

"Oh yes," her aunt replied, laughing.

As I did my rounds that night, I thought about whether it helps or hurts to know about a terminal diagnosis. Are we doing it all wrong? When we offer our well-researched, carefully calibrated prognoses, plucked from the averages on a graph, are we dooming people to that fate?

In my experience as a physician and psychiatrist, I've seen many people feel oppressed by knowing a lot about their prognosis. A terminal diagnosis crushes them. They feel afraid, hopeless, and doomed. But the response is very individual—everyone responds differently. Some people actually seem to feel empowered by learning their diagnosis and hearing their doctor's best guess as to how it will progress. For them, knowledge is power. They know where they stand, see the lay of the land, and can take their health into their own hands. They can map out their own paths. They can confront the reality of their deaths, and then, instead of a wall, it becomes a doorway, and they pass through it.

There's no real consensus that emerges from the research on withholding diagnoses—you can't run a study where you refuse to tell people the truth about their conditions and then see what happens; it's unethical. And even the cultures where such an approach has been widespread are beginning to push toward more agency for patients and to put more information in the hands of the individual. Ultimately, the answer is not withholding information from patients and keeping them ignorant of their condition—in none of the cases of spontaneous remission that I studied over the years did ignorance or avoidance help anyone. At the very least, people should be afforded the chance to know that their time here may be more fleeting than they'd assumed and to live the way they want in the time they have left. At the same time, we in the medical profession need to do a better job of giving prognoses in ways that empower people rather than constrain them. We need to stop being so afraid of offering "false hope" that we put hard limits on what's possible.

Stephen Jay Gould, a prominent evolutionary biologist who taught at Harvard for many years, was diagnosed at age forty with mesothelioma, an especially deadly form of cancer that affects the abdominal lining. He was given eight months to live. That, his doctors told him, was the "median," so it was what he could reasonably expect. He was devastated—until he started doing his own research and realized that the "median" only represented *some* of the possible outcomes. Yes, there were more cases clustered there, around the middle, but there were many others scattered on both ends of the spectrum.

Realizing that the possibilities were in fact much more fluid, that there was more hope than any of his doctors had suggested, he penned an essay, a call to arms, for others facing such prognoses, titled "The Median Isn't the Message." *I am not a number,* Gould insisted in his essay. *I am not a statistic. I am a human, and my life does not follow a course charted on a medical graph.* Gould decided that good, rational reasons existed to support the idea that perhaps he was on the side of lengthened life, more than the median. He recovered completely from the mesothelioma, living another twenty years before dying from unrelated causes.

Perhaps it's less about withholding information about your prognosis and more about what *kind* of information we offer. Do we offer the median, constraining people to what's "average"? Or do we offer hope? Will this person be empowered by knowing what is "average," or more by a range of possibilities? Can we be honest, clear, and realistic, while at the same time offering people the opportunity to become exceptional?

In 1954, the world record for running the mile was four minutes and two seconds. For almost a decade, nobody had been able to improve on that time. In fact, some doctors didn't think that breaking the four-minute mile was physically possible. But that year, Roger Bannister, a medical student, broke the four-minute mile on a cinder track at Oxford University. It was a major moment in sports—newspapers all over the world published the photo of Bannister crossing the finish line at three minutes and fifty-nine seconds, his face awash with relief, his body limp with exhaustion. But he wouldn't hold the record for long. Forty-five days later, someone else broke the four-minute mile, improving on Bannister's time by a second and a half. After that, even more were able to achieve it—to date, over five hundred athletes have run a mile in under four minutes. As soon as one person demonstrated it was possible, more were able to follow in his footsteps—what was thought to be a physiological barrier proved to be, in the end, a psychological barrier.

Lulu Wang's story is powerful and compelling and certainly worth folding into our developing understanding of why diseases sometimes progress and sometimes remit. But I don't believe that the answer is keeping people in the dark about their diagnoses. Besides making unilateral decisions for people that we shouldn't be making, we'd be robbing them of a potentially transformative experience: facing death can be a catalyst for radical life change. It is an opportunity to gain the kind of clarity that only death can bring. It has the potential to turn not only our health but also our lives around. And when we look at the big picture of spontaneous remission and look for patterns, we don't actually see ignorance or denial as a major factor across the board. In fact, we see the opposite; we see those who experienced remissions actively engaged with their own mortality. We see them facing it, wrestling with it, coming to terms with it. In a counterintuitive twist, running away from death can hurt us more than turning toward it.

HOW RUNNING FROM DEATH RUNS US DOWN

In Western culture, we aren't great at dying. I don't mean that we don't do it—of course we do! We all do it, eventually. What I mean is that we live in a culture that tends to push thinking about death to the side or delay thinking about it. And it's only once we get to the end of our road that we realize we haven't had a chance to think about not only what kind of death we want but what kind of life we want.

We don't have a lot of conversations about death. *Not yet,* we say to ourselves. *I don't have to think about this yet.* We are a culture that fetishizes youth and beauty, where death is spoken about in hushed tones, privately. Even our mourning rituals have become distant and impersonal. Most of us die in hospitals, and someone else—someone we hire and don't actually know—comes in to take care of things, taking the body away, preparing it for burial or cremation. In many cultures, the death of a loved one involves very intimate rituals intended to both honor the deceased and, at the same time, help the family members through the shock and grief of having lost someone. Washing the body before burial, for example, is a ritual that many cultures have preserved, yet we've cast it aside. Our ancestors participated in grieving rituals that kept them up close and personal with the reality, and the physicality, of death. But in Western culture today, there is a widespread cultural disconnect, a mass denial. Instead of dealing with death, we outsource it. We might think we're sparing ourselves unnecessary pain and anguish, but what are we missing out on? What collateral damage are we doing to our bodies and souls?

When we think we have all the time in the world, we are less likely to take advantage of the time we really have. Not only can our inability to face death keep us from living the life we truly want and need to live, it can also harm our physical health. Take, for example, the conundrum of hospice care. You may read the word *hospice* and have an immediate negative connotation; it probably makes you think immediately of death. And indeed, hospice care is end-of-life care. It can occur at a nursing home or other type of facility, but it often occurs at the patient's home. In a nutshell, hospice means that your illness is terminal and you are no longer trying to treat it. Instead, the focus is on comfort. For a lot of patients, this means pain management, and hospice care providers are fluent in the language of pain relief. But hospice care is often much more than that. It's not only helping patients be as comfortable and feel as well as possible given the circumstances, it's also helping them make the most of the time remaining. Sometimes hospice involves therapy and goal-setting. It incorporates attending not only to the urgent physical needs of the patient but to the urgent emotional and spiritual needs as well.

It might not come as a shock, then, to learn that hospice care can actually *extend* life. While a specter of hospice persists—a person on his or her deathbed, on a morphine drip—the reality is quite different. A few years ago, *The New England Journal of Medicine,* one of the most prestigious medical journals, published a study that proved that terminal lung cancer patients who started hospice immediately after diagnosis lived three months longer than the control group on average. (That's "on average," so again, let's remember that some people will be far outside that range.) And not only did they live longer on average, but they enjoyed a better quality of life for that extra time.

When I looked at the study, there didn't seem to be any true cases of spontaneous remission. However, the fact that the progression of disease slowed and that the well-being of the patients improved was significant. It was a clue. It told me that there was something important—essential, even—about coming to terms with death. Perhaps it brought peace and lessened anxiety. Perhaps it freed people from others' rules and expectations. As all the survivors of incurable diseases had been telling me, there was something transformative and freeing about truly understanding the brevity, the preciousness, of your one life. And perhaps the unique approach of hospice, which is highly individualized and very patient-centered, plays a massive role.

Hospice, when you really look at it, is a wonderful model of care. Of course, not all hospice care is created equal—philosophies and providers can vary widely in approach and skill. But hospice care represents a unique area in medicine where we often don't just treat the mask of illness—we treat the person behind the mask, their body, heart, and mind. We find a way forward based on this unique individual, with all his or her specific needs and desires and goals. Now, imagine if we applied the principles of hospice to medicine *across the board.* Imagine if it were the default in medicine to consider a person's specific and unique situation, their goals for treatment, their hard-line deal breakers for when the side effects are too much, their deep anxieties about illness and death, their hopes and dreams for their time here. What we would end up with is a patient-centered philosophy of medicine that takes into account the whole person instead of homing in so tightly on the disease that we lose the bigger picture.

Here's the catch about hospice, though: to qualify for it, your physician has to attest that you have six months or less to live.

Now, as we've learned, a doctor doesn't know for sure what a patient's time frame is. All they can say is that based on the normal progression of this particular illness, and on the data, six months is average. And then boom, you qualify for hospice.

But some people won't move to hospice—they won't take the spot available to them. As wonderful as hospice could be for them, as much as it could extend their life and buoy their quality of life and well-being, they can't bring themselves to admit that they have six months or less to live. That they are really going to die.

What a cruel paradox: you can have a shot at more time, but to get it, you have to face and accept your imminent death. For a lot of us, it's just too hard.

The earlier you enter hospice, the more it can extend your life and improve your quality of life. But in a 2012 survey, more than *half* of the people who finally chose hospice had only twelve days or less to live by the time they entered. Many only had a few days. Claire Haser talked about this in one of our many phone chats. "I was good friends with a hospice bereavement counselor," she told me. "She said, 'Claire, most people won't go there. Even if they're on their deathbed, they won't go there. They won't even accept hospice until they're so sick that they have days to live.'"

We have a lot of work to do, in both medicine and as a larger culture, when it comes to talking about death and understanding what it can tell us about life.

In 2004, Bernard Crettaz, a Swiss sociologist, hosted an informal gathering at a restaurant in his home city of Neuchâtel. He had recently lost his wife of many years and was horrified by what he saw as a "tyrannical secrecy" surrounding death in Western culture. His idea for the gathering was that it would be a kind of open salon at a public location, such as a restaurant or café, and anyone who wanted to could come. There would be no set agenda or specific topic. People could just come and talk about death—if they had lost a loved one, or were facing death themselves, or if they simply wanted to explore the concept before they found themselves in one of those positions.

"I am never so in tune with the truth as during one of these soirees," Crettaz writes in his book on the death café movement that he founded. "And I have the impression that the assembled company, for a moment, and thanks to death, is born into authenticity."[2]

No matter where you are in the arc of your life, facing death is an essential part of figuring out who you are and what you want to do with your time on this earth. And of course, those who experienced spontaneous healings aren't immune to having to grapple with mortality.

EVERY STORY HAS AN ENDING

It's easy to forget that *spontaneous remission* doesn't mean *cured forever.* In medicine, a spontaneous remission refers to any unexpected cure or improvement from a disease that usually progresses. When a progressive or incurable disease goes backward instead of forward; when an individual performs far outside the mean, becomes an outlier, becomes exceptional, then we are looking at a spontaneous remission.

Remember Mr. Wright? His strange yo-yo remissions, fueled by his belief in the Krebiozen he was taking, followed by the relapses he experienced when his faith in the drug was shaken, still qualify as spontaneous remissions. Even though Wright eventually died from his disease, he's still a stunning example of spontaneous remission, one that serves as a powerful reminder of what's possible. He's also an example of the power of hope (and of hopelessness), one that we are still looking at and unpacking, trying to learn from it. I also believe that Janet Rose's recovery from end-stage lupus qualifies as a spontaneous remission, even though she still sometimes feels the effects of the lupus on her heart. She interprets it as a message from her body to slow down, reduce stress, and prioritize health. She came back from the brink of death, improbably, has healed beyond what any doctor thought was possible, and has learned to use signs of relapse as a tool for keeping herself healthy.

If we're chasing a cure that lasts forever, we're looking for something that doesn't exist. For as long as humans have been around, we've chased immortality like a mirage. Myths and storybooks are full of tales of people who set off looking for it: the Spanish conquistadors hunting for a fountain of youth; the emperor of ancient China who sent fleets of boats onto the sea to hunt down the "elixir of life"; the story of Gilgamesh, the warrior king of Mesopotamia, who saw his friend die in battle and became aware, for the first time, of his own mortality and tried to figure out how to cheat death. Even today, people have themselves cryogenically frozen, hoping they will be woken up in a future where technology has progressed to the point that they can be revived and healed.

But quests for immortality never seem to work out. That emperor from China, for example—he took mercury pills under the advice of doctors who claimed they would extend his life. But he took too many and killed himself. And literature is full of stories of characters who achieved immortality, only to want the opposite: a life that comes to an end at some point is a life that has meaning. Quests for immortality always seem to end the same way: the searchers never find what they're looking for, though they waste much of their precious lives trying.

Had I been on my own quest for immortality? All these years, I'd been running around, researching, flying here and there, scouring long emails for the signs of a true spontaneous remission. How many hours, days, weeks had I spent filling up notebooks while people spoke? Perhaps there was a part of me that wanted there to be a way to cheat death. If I unlocked the secret of spontaneous healing, I could use it for myself if I were to get sick—a kind of GET OUT OF JAIL FREE card I could keep at the ready if death came calling in the form of an incurable disease. Was this all just another search for the elixir of life?

One of the amazing lessons that has come out of doing this work for so long—about seventeen years at this point—is that I've been able to see how the stories of the people I encountered along the way have progressed. Patricia Kaine, for example, still shows no signs of fibrosis. As a way of expressing gratitude for how the illness changed her relationship with herself, she has focused her medical work on those in need. She sends out a weekly newsletter called *Doc's Daily Chuckle,* filled with jokes, stories, and quotes meant to make people laugh and feel uplifted. She believes that laughter is medicine, that gratitude can heal, that being of service to her community gives her purpose in life and something to live for, and that this helps her stave off disease. I subscribed to her newsletter, and it does make me laugh. Here's a joke from a recent one:

> *Mickey sat in the doctor's office and kept up a strange litany.*
> *"I hope I'm sick. I hope I'm sick."*
> *Another waiting patient asked, "Why do you want to be sick?"*
> *Mickey answered, "I'd hate to be well and feel like this!"*

Pablo Kelly and Matt Ireland, the young men stricken with the incurable brain cancer glioblastoma multiforme, were still in remission as of this writing, raising their young children, hoping for more years of health and grace, all the while knowing that it might not last forever. These weren't shallow quests for immortality, I realized, and neither was mine.

It's humbling to hear all these stories, shared with me so generously by the people I spoke to—humbling in the same way that car accident all those years ago was humbling. You realize that you can do everything "right" and still get sick. Or you can make apparent "mistakes" like we all do and still end up with a remission. And like some of the people I spoke to for this book, you can even experience spontaneous remission and then struggle again with illness later on. There is so much we don't know yet, so much we don't control. On the other side of healing, there is life. But along with life comes its shadow, ever present—that someday, it will come to a close.

Every story has an ending. Claire Haser, whose story introduced this book, retired to Hawaii as she'd always wanted. She and her husband bought a house near Honolulu. Their daughter and son-in-law moved onto the property as well. They were musicians who booked gigs all over the city; in the evenings, when Claire and her husband settled out on the lanai, the sound of their rehearsals floated up from below.

Claire had ten healthy, happy years in Hawaii with her family after the terminal cancer diagnosis that should have ended her life. And then, in early 2018, one of her regular scans found a lesion on her lung. It looked suspiciously like a cancer metastasis.

It was small and static—not growing—which confused her doctors. A metastasis, especially if it was somehow related to her original pancreatic cancer, would be odd after all these years and wouldn't really behave this way. But when they biopsied it, it turned out indeed to be adenocarcinoma—from the pancreas.

It was bad news, and strange news. After a ten-year reprieve—not a trace of disease—the cancer had returned. But when Claire wrote to tell me, she also said this: *The silver lining for me is that my new doctors do truly believe I had pancreatic cancer now. My oncologist, my surgeon, and doctor all scoffed at my diagnosis—they said I was misdiagnosed, that I read the pathology report wrong, that I'd had something else, not pancreatic cancer—all this was said to me. This time, when the surgeon read me the pathology report—that I had pancreatic cancer mets on my lungs—I felt such huge relief that I would at last be believed and not dismissed. Being dismissed by doctors is a bitter pill to swallow. I've some-times felt like the doctors were my enemies as much as the cancer.*

It should come as no surprise that Claire has decided against aggressive treatment. She's seventy-three now, and another scan is pending. She thinks she may be headed toward the end of her life, but as she says, "I've been here before." Once again, she's decided that given her diagnosis, prognosis, and treatment options, she doesn't want to spend her remaining time in treatments that will make her feel worse in the hopes of tacking on a few more months. This is an individual, incredibly personal decision that everyone needs to make for themselves based on their specific circumstances, illness, and treatment options. But for Claire, more time isn't worth much to her if it's full of chemo side effects, hours spent lying on a radia-tion table, the fluorescent lights of a doctor's office waiting room.

"I'm sure that's the right decision for someone else," she says. "It's not for me."

She went through a bad patch recently where she felt sick and depleted. The fatigue really got to her. And a surgery on her lungs that was supposed to help get a more accurate diagnosis made her feel worse. But now, she says, she's feeling okay. As always, it's trial and error. She tried a medication that was supposed to help her breathing, and when it didn't, she went off it and felt better. Some days are hard, and some days are easy, graceful. She still has stage IV cancer. It's not easy, facing death. She writes to me that she's seeing a therapist "to get my mind around it." She's gone back to the same book she used ten years ago, *A Year to Live.* She calls it "her Bible."

"It's not the dying part that's the stumbling block," she tells me with a wry laugh. "It's the getting there."

For a long time after the accident that took Jane, I wondered if I was properly reckoning with death—hers and my own. I think perhaps I had the wrong idea about what facing death really means.

It doesn't need to be terrible. It doesn't have to be morbid or depressing. There is no one way to come to terms with your own mortality. But what I do know is that after that accident, I became interested in authenticity for the first time in my life. Just as Mirae said, when she realized that she'd misunderstood who she was and what her life was meant to be, it felt like "a veil had been ripped away." I saw myself, and my future, very differently. I no longer felt compelled to live my life on anyone else's terms but my own.

Facing death doesn't mean you succumb to death. You can accept your own eventual mortality and still fight to live. You can face death and still choose life.

CHOOSING LIFE

After her diagnosis of incurable metastatic melanoma, Mirae Bunnell had plenty of dark nights of the soul. She wrestled with what to do, how to proceed. There was a part of her that didn't want to fight it. The doctors said she would die, so that's what she figured would happen.

"I sat at the kitchen table with my boyfriend, and I remember saying to him, I remember this exactly, I said, 'I feel like I have a choice. I know it's up to me and that it will be really hard work. I'm not sure I want to do it,'" Mirae says. "He was very hurt by that."

Mirae says now that there was something attractive about giving in to it. About accepting the fact that she was going to die in a few months and then "going gently into that good night." Her boyfriend was upset by what she said because "he didn't experience it," she says now. "He didn't know. But for anyone who gets close enough to touch it—death—it feels like home."

Over the course of the next two nights, she sat up into the wee hours, acutely aware of her own mortality. Finally, she made her decision. She wasn't afraid of death anymore, but she chose life.

Pablo Kelly, who lives in a state of inexplicable remission that baffles his doctors, also lives with the reality that his glioblastoma multiforme could return at any time. It might stay away forever. Or it might be back tomorrow.

"I don't think about dying as a problem anymore," he tells me on a muffled, crackling phone call from the UK. "I was supposed to be dead ages ago."

The way that Pablo has chosen life is evident in the way he lives now. He decided early on not to undergo the standard treatment for glioblastoma multiforme because of the side effects—the major one being infertility. Pablo had always thought about having children someday. But the choice presented by his doctors crystallized the answer to the question that hadn't even been asked yet. The treatment that might save his life would also render him unable to have children. It didn't take him long to decide to decline.

"If I was going to live, I wanted to have a life, and I wanted to have kids," he says. "If I couldn't do those things, then what's the point?"

Pablo is still in remission. He still eats the strict diet that he believes has kept him in remission. It can be difficult, when everyone else around you, your whole community, operates on a different set of rules. He tries to make the conscious choice every day not to focus on fear. He eats the way he does not because he's afraid of death but because he wants to live.

His daughter was born in June, healthy and perfect.

"I cried my eyes out," he said on the day he wrote to tell me he'd become a father.

Thinking about Pablo, something that Bernard Crettaz, the founder of the death café movement, once said surfaced in my mind. In a last interview, he revealed that he was ceasing to host any further death cafés—up to that point, he had hosted them religiously for over a decade. When the interviewer asked why, he said that it was painful to stop, a huge loss. But after hearing so many others wrestle with death, he'd decided that it was time to think about his own. After internalizing a lot of messages about death and sin from religion when he was a kid, he needed to heal death for himself. The death café movement, he said, was inspired by that—a reaction to the negative connotations he'd learned as a kid. When he founded the movement, he said, "I went back to the

Greeks, and the Greeks said, 'Live each moment of your life as if it were your last,' and that's it. Be the maximum of your being."[3]

Be the maximum of your being. How many of us could say that we were really doing that?

Crettaz died, at the age of eighty, two years after he gave that interview, after he stepped down from the death café movement to attend to his own life and death. Before the interview concluded, he told the journalist that it didn't matter to him how, or when, or where he died. "It doesn't matter," he said. "If you put all the intensity of yourself in this moment, then you live."

There is a level of intensity, of dedication, among those who spontaneously healed, that is unparalleled. The comparisons to great athletes are apt; these are the high achievers, the ones who do what we've all decided is physically impossible. People who break physical records are people who dedicate themselves completely to their training, pushing themselves as far as they can go—and then farther. In some way, were survivors of incurable diseases doing the same?

12

Burn Your Boat

I had the feeling that there was no harm, no shame, no judgment if I wanted to be done. But also that if I wanted to, if I chose life, it would be hard work.

—*Mirae Bunnell, metastatic melanoma*

If I had followed the laws of medicine, I should be in the grave fifteen years by now.

—*Patricia Kaine, idiopathic pulmonary fibrosis*

I accepted the diagnosis, but not the prognosis.

—*Juniper Stein, ankylosing spondylitis*

I know there's something beyond medicine. They gave me up for dead. And here I am, fifteen years later.

—*Matt Ireland, glioblastoma multiforme*

Remember that if you don't take charge of your healing, someone else will, and you probably won't like the outcome.

—*Jerry White, renal cell carcinoma*

In 1519, Hernán Cortés, the Spanish explorer and conquistador, arrived on the coast of Mexico near Veracruz, intending to claim the land occupied by the Aztec empire for Spain. He had eleven ships, thirteen horses, and five hundred men. The Aztec empire at that time stretched from the Gulf of Mexico to the Pacific and was the largest and most powerful Mesoamerican kingdom of all time. Its population numbered over five million. Its fighting force, which was famous for being fierce and unbeatable, was many times larger than Cortés's small army.

Cortés wasn't even supposed to be there. His commander had revoked his order to sail to Mexico, but he went anyway. Landing on the beach at the edge of the Gulf of Mexico, Cortés had an army that was too small for the task before him and no support behind him. The fleet of eleven ships that sat anchored in the bay was their only backup plan if they failed, which was the probable outcome given the odds. But once all the soldiers were on the beach, Cortés gave a shocking order: burn the boats.

As a military tactic, this one doesn't seem particularly smart right off the bat. But think about what Cortés was doing—he was leaving his men no other option than to win. When he burned the boats, he burned any possibility of retreat.

"We take the city or we die!" Cortés is said to have shouted to his men.

I don't identify with the conquistadors of that era, who ran roughshod over indigenous cultures. But the story of Hernán Cortés and his army, so much smaller than the fierce and legendary fighting force they were going into battle against, has always stuck in my mind. It's Cortés who always gets the spotlight in this story, but I want you to imagine yourself as one of the soldiers. You have your own life, family, goals, and dreams. And then you find yourself on that beach, watching the boats burn in the bay, eleven distant bonfires. Your escape plan going up in smoke. Imagine what it must have felt like to realize that the only way to go is forward, with a choice of risking everything or ending up with nothing.

The story of Hernán Cortés burning his boats in the Gulf of

Mexico resonates[1] because on some level, we all know that it's possible to overcome an impossible situation—but *only if you leave yourself no other option.* That's what "burning your boat" has come to mean—giving yourself no escape hatch, no backup plan, no other option but to press forward into adversity.

When I think of burning your boat in the context of healing, I think of Tom; when I asked him if he ever cheated and ate anything outside of the nutrient-dense diet he'd settled on to cure his diabetes, the answer was "never." I think of Juniper Stein in yoga sessions, pushing her body deeper into the poses, into the pain, snapping the calcifications that cemented her joints, knowing it was working, now one of the healthiest and most vital people I know. I think of Jan, letting go of her children so that she, and they, could be free—a heartbreakingly difficult thing for a parent but something that seems to have saved her life. I think of Mirae, sitting at her kitchen table, deciding whether or not she wanted to fight for her life. When each of these people figured out their own personal key to health, they doubled down on it.

Most of us, whether we realize it or not, leave ourselves an "out": a pathway back to old behaviors, habits, belief systems, or ideas about ourselves. We make a new plan, a new resolution, but leave an escape hatch in the back of our minds—a boat in the harbor—so that when the stress gets high enough, we can always go back to our old life, our typical ways of perceiving and thinking. A boat floating in the bay can be a comforting habit. It could be alcohol or drugs, for some. It could be a relationship, romantic or otherwise, that you know isn't good for your stress and health. It could be food. It could be sitting back and letting other people—doctors, family members—chart a course for your life and health instead of charting your own. It could be as simple as just staying with the status quo because it initially feels incredibly hard to make big, sweeping life changes—the kind you may need to make to have a life that supports health and vitality.

Survivors of incurable diseases don't leave themselves an out. Once they realize what big changes help them feel better and heal faster, they rapidly get rid of any pathways back to old habits or old ways of being in the world. That can look like everything from throwing away all the pro-inflammatory, nonhealing food in your pantry, as Claire did to begin her journey, to leaving a relationship that's keeping you from being your most authentic self, as Jan had to in order to heal. To recover from end-stage lupus, she had to cut herself free from her old life completely, leaving a toxic marriage, a stressful job, financial difficulties, and fraught relationships with her older children, who had never known her except as someone who was ill. She flew to Brazil, dropping abruptly out of her life as if parachuting out of a crashing plane. And when she tried to return to that life after getting better, she relapsed. To experience radical healing, she had to create a radically different life.

Everyone I've profiled in this book developed their own unique approach to healing. They found their own way toward healing their identities like explorers blazing their own paths through the forest but arriving at the same clearing. And once there, they left themselves no option to go back. They burned their boats.

TAKING CONTROL OF YOUR HEALTH

One of the problems that has plagued the research into spontaneous healing is a failure to quantify the degree to which people truly participate in various treatment methods. Millions of studies look at *whether* someone participated in a particular treatment program, but not *how* or to *what extent*. People apply themselves to tasks in radically different ways—some as if their life depends on it, and some because they'll get fifty dollars at the end.

The scientific method allows us a standardized approach to experimentation that makes sure there are consistencies across studies so that we can draw important comparisons. It creates an essential template for science and research that we use to measure the efficacy of medications, treatment methods, lifestyle changes, and so on. But not everything is measurable in this way.

The traditional scientific method as it is typically practiced is only designed to study things that we can see and touch. When we do a study that measures the impact of a medication, we know exactly how many grams are in the pill that a participant swallows. But when we do a study that measures the impact of something like meditation, we approach it similarly. We track how many times a week participants meditate and for how long. We can record that Jane Doe meditated three times a week for twenty minutes each time; we can compare her data to a control group that didn't meditate at all. However, there's so much we don't know about Jane. How intensive were her sessions? To what degree was she personally invested in it? How effective were her meditation techniques at calming fight or flight and initiating the relaxation response? How deep did she go? What did her meditation practice mean to her? Was she simply waiting for the time to be over, or did she engage with the process with intensity and an open heart?

There are so many nuances, so many internal factors that are invisible to our carefully controlled, quantitative studies. We are leaving too much unexamined because it doesn't fit inside the narrowly defined sphere of the scientific method as we have currently formulated it. Our study design can tell us that Juniper Stein practiced yoga for two hours every day, but it wouldn't reveal how much more intensively she engaged than the woman doing the lotus pose right next to her. It can tell us that Patricia Kaine prayed for a certain number of hours, but not what those prayers meant to her.

Looking at spontaneous healing, it becomes apparent that *degree of involvement* in a treatment tactic may be of the ultimate importance, and yet most studies ignore this or simply aren't able to account for it. We see all the time that people receiving an intervention—anything from chemo to diet to meditation—vary enormously in terms of their response. It occurred to me that the relevant independent variable might not be the presence or absence of a particular intervention but the use that these individuals make of it. Before I went off to college as a young man, I remember people saying to me, "College is what you make of it." What they meant was, I couldn't simply sit in a classroom and expect to get the depth and breadth of learning and knowledge that might really change my life. I had to do that part myself.

So the question becomes, how deeply do people immerse themselves in these various pathways to healing? And how much of a difference does that really make?

Medicine is in the early stages of accepting—albeit grudgingly—the role of the mind in healing the body. Some doctors are finally beginning to recommend stress-reduction techniques, as they've come to realize how large a role fight or flight actually plays in creating a disease pathway. But something holds us back. Most of us, both doctors and patients, are still trained to look for silver bullets; we look for an easier treatment than changing our lives. But what spontaneous healing has taught us is that waking up to a deeper awareness of our value and strength is capable of changing our physiology. If we assume that the mind is powerful and capable of altering disease progression, it follows that a *significant* mental change may be capable of precipitating a significant physiological change—in some cases even a remission.

In the late 1980s, a study[2] done at Stanford University by David Spiegel showed that women with breast cancer survived eighteen months longer, on average, if they attended group therapy twice a week. The study got a lot of press and attention and is still repeatedly cited and viewed as a landmark study today. But when others tried to replicate the study, they couldn't.

And then Alastair Cunningham gave it a try. Cunningham, a professor and psychologist whose main passion was the intersection between behavioral medicine and health psychology, designed a study to investigate that very same link between therapy and survival. In the 1990s, he was running a cancer clinic at the University of Toronto. At the age of forty-seven, he himself had been diagnosed with stage III colon cancer and given a 30 percent chance of survival. Dr. Cunningham is unusual for a few reasons, and it's these unique characteristics that made me sit up and take notice. Unlike the tradition where psychologists, trained as they are in the study of the mind, have little to do with medicine, and vice versa, he was a psychologist working in a medical clinic for cancer patients and also a professional at treating cancer who himself had been diagnosed with cancer. This wasn't just an abstraction or a professional interest for him; it was personal.

Cunningham ran a study[3] in 1998 that contradicted the Spiegel study, failing to find the same link between therapy and recovery or longevity. Group therapy, Cunningham concluded, did not have a significant impact on disease course or survival rate.

But Cunningham noticed something interesting. A very small slice of the study group actually *did* show significant improvement after therapy. Seven women in the intervention group lived significantly longer than the others; and two of the seven were still alive eight years after the start of the study and appeared to be in remission. It was too small a sample to be statistically significant; Cunningham's overall conclusion still had to be "no significant effect found." But after reviewing those patients' accounts of their experiences of participating in the study, Cunningham began to suspect that a person's level of involvement in therapy had something major to do with the outcome.

Here's what he discovered about those seven survivors: they actively sought out other approaches to healing in addition to the therapy that everyone else participated in. Those who lived longer were doing a number of things on their own, not dictated by the study. They were personally invested, and it showed. They reported intensive meditation, dedicated yoga practice, journaling, intentional gratitude, and more. Basically, they exhibited not only a pattern of taking responsibility for their own treatment but also a willingness to radically change habits, routines, and even the larger scaffolding of their lives. Admitting that other interpretations were possible, Cunningham theorized that a "get up and go" attitude might be related to survival or remission.

He didn't expect to find this in the study and certainly wasn't looking for it. But Cunningham couldn't ignore what he'd seen— that the people who lived longer or achieved remission were the ones who took it a step further, who dedicated themselves to their own care.

Cunningham then designed a more focused prospective longitudinal study[4] to investigate the link between what he called "psychological work" and longevity in patients with metastatic cancer. *Psychological work* is a term that casts a fairly wide net, and into that net we can place a lot of the pathways used by the survivors in this book. Cunningham certainly would have included therapy and other forms of self-help; I think immediately of the deep work on the self done by Mirae, Patricia, and others—the profound reassessing of identity, goals, and desires. This time, Cunningham zeroed in on highly motivated patients who had shown a prior interest in self-help techniques. He found a significant relationship between "involvement in self-help" and survival duration. His next study attempted to zoom in even closer. What did "involvement in self-help" mean to participants?

Cunningham's 2002 study, *Fighting for life: a qualitative analysis of the process of psychotherapy-assisted self-help in patients with metastatic cancer,*[5] was an unusually intensive effort to go deep and figure out what was really going on, both quantitatively and qualitatively, in patients' lives when they participated in these types of studies. Though small, it was very carefully done, with over one hundred hours devoted to the study of each participant. Few studies have ever invested anything close to this degree of effort. Cunningham found that nine patients, whom he classified as "highly involved," were the ones who devoted regular daily time—often several hours—to meditation, mental imaging, cognitive monitoring, journaling, or relaxation activities. Of those nine, eight enjoyed a high quality of life and lived at least two years beyond their original prognoses. And out of those eight, two had complete, unexpected remissions, which remained years after the time of publication.

At the other end of the spectrum, Cunningham singled out eight subjects who were significantly *less* involved than the average participant. By their own reporting, they were either unconvinced that self-help would really do anything to change their disease trajectory or were hampered by issues such as diminished self-esteem. In other words, feeling unworthy of the efforts. In this group, none had a good quality of life. Only one lived more than two years after diagnosis and was therefore on the low end of the curve, though her medical prognosis was no more unfavorable at the onset of therapy than for the "high involvement" group.

Overall, Cunningham found that people who were highly involved with what he took to calling "self-help therapies" lived nearly *three times longer* than those with low involvement. And it's interesting to note that the self-help therapies that Cunningham identified track very closely with the kinds of spiritual, psychological, and life-changing work done by those who experienced spontaneous remissions.

Cunningham distilled his research into a basic framework that distinguished conditions or characteristics associated with poor survival outcomes versus longer survival, and here's what he came up with:

Conditions associated with poor survival outcomes:

- Inflexibility associated with low self-esteem or fixed worldview
- Skepticism about self-help techniques, or a limited ability to apply them
- Other activities seemed more immediately appealing
- Meaning was habitually sought outside the individual, from some external source
- Strong, contrary views about the validity of spiritual ideas

Conditions associated with longer survival:

- Strong will to live
- Actual changes in habits of thought and activity

- Relaxation practices, meditation, mental imaging, cognitive monitoring
- Becoming involved in a search for meaning in one's life

Were survivors psychologically different from their peers who did not survive? What made the difference?

In a study[6] that attempted to clarify this question, Cunningham found that survivors tended to display a much higher degree of early involvement in their psychological self-help than others. Another series of studies into the effects of yoga on cancer recovery found that the small number of people who actually experienced recoveries had a very different, and much deeper and more significant, relationship to the practice than those who did not. The results of these studies, plus the others leading up to it, convinced Cunningham that engaging in this sort of "identity healing" work was potentially a major factor in recovery. But because such a small slice of subjects truly engaged in it, it was difficult—if not impossible—to get this across in the published studies. Studies, by design, look at averages, and the average results washed out the exceptional, making the effect of the interventions tested by Cunningham seem "minimal."

As hard as Cunningham tried, he still couldn't overcome the core problem with traditional approaches to scientific studies—that their very design preemptively negates the exact question he was trying to answer. How you relate to the activity makes a huge difference and, as Cunningham found, designing a study that truly incorporates the degree of involvement of participants is almost impossibly difficult. It would rely entirely on self-reporting and transparency and would be subject to the vagaries of language and perception.

Alastair Cunningham was a uniquely suited person to tackle this problem. He's now retired but still runs groups for those seeking to take treatment into their own hands. Crucially, he's been on both sides of the desk—as a psychologist *and* as a patient.

What Cunningham saw, through the research that has spanned the bulk of his career, is that how fully we immerse ourselves in these healing pathways can have an enormous impact on the course of an illness. It's common sense, really. We certainly expect that the amount and quality of effort has a payoff in sports, but we have lost this perspective when it comes to our health.

It's important to point out that taking responsibility for your healing process is not the same thing as taking the blame for your illness. Certainly it's true that when we know better, we do better. But it's also true that you have little say about the family, cultural programming, and genetic structure into which you were born. Part of the resistance to "mind-body medicine," on the part of the medical mainstream, is the belief that this approach to healing "blames" the patients for their illnesses. The overriding theory is that the downsides (that people will feel that they brought illness upon themselves through something they did or didn't do) overwhelm any potential benefit. And while I disagree, I also have to admit that there's some truth to it. Some people do feel blamed and over-whelmed by the idea of taking ownership of health and healing. And the mind-body medicine movement isn't always great at un-tangling "blame" from "ownership."

BEING SICK IS NOT YOUR FAULT

One of the good things about our current medical model is that you can often just go in, get your illness treated, and not feel judged or pressured. Sometimes, you just want to let your cold be a cold, or your heart disease just be heart disease. Or have your alcohol problem or bipolar disorder be understood simply as a disease. And there's an important place for that. Marcia Angell, in an article for *The New England Journal of Medicine,*[7] presented the argument suc-cinctly. While she admits that there is some value to exploring the link between disease and the mind and that there may be some-thing real there, she believes that it's not worth exploring because the potential damage when people blame themselves for their ill-nesses is too great.

Dr. Angell comes down hard on illness as a reflection of the psyche. She gives a great example from history about how tuberculo-

sis was assumed to have a psychological cause until it was discovered
to be associated with mycobacterium tuberculosis and susceptible to
treatment with rifampin. The same could be said about the treatment of syphilis or gonorrhea, historically viewed as moral illnesses,
but actually bacterial in nature and now easily treated with antibiotics. But a biological basis does not always indicate a biological cause.
In other words, just because the biological level is involved does not
mean that the biological level is always the primary cause.

Angell's dismissal seems to have less to do with whether there's
anything valid to explore and more to do with a concern that people
will blame themselves for their illnesses. Her stance that people not
blame themselves if they don't get better is valid and essential, but
it exists outside of the question about the role that our deep beliefs
about ourselves and the world play in our health and illnesses. We
can't confuse the two. We can, and *should,* take the stance that we
are not to blame for the illnesses that come our way *and* that we have
more power than we know when it comes to healing from them. As
Maya Angelou says, "When we know better, we do better."

The case of Dr. John Sarno is a perfect example. Sarno, who
died just a few years ago at the age of ninety-three, was a doctor at
New York University whose approach to treating chronic pain was,
to say the least, controversial. He believed that most chronic pain
was psychological at its root. He understood this not as blame but
as opportunity. He was able to take on the patients whose pain had
not responded to traditional modalities; he often said that some
80 percent of them would go on to get better.[8]

His obituary in *The New York Times* detailed how colleagues
at NYU would "belittle him behind his back in lunchtime
conversations . . . even as some would visit him privately for their
ailments." I've experienced this dynamic; it's tragic—and contrary
to the true spirit of scientific inquiry—that the politics of health
cause people to take such a public position. But it's also important
to understand that there are a lot of smart closet professionals who
want more freedom to talk about these issues.

And now, after his death, Dr. Sarno is being proven right.

Studies are emerging,[9] after all those years of doubt and skepticism, showing that there often *is* an emotional basis for chronic pain. Ahead of the research, without any "gold standard," double-blind studies to pass the test of the establishment, Sarno forged ahead, knowing that his patients experienced radical recoveries when chronic pain was approached through the lens of emotion and anxiety. And he was right.

I believe that as doctors, we need to listen more to our patients—and I don't just mean in the exam room. I mean listen to the larger messages, the many voices whispering all across the country and around the world, trying to tell us what they know intuitively about their bodies, and illness, and healing. So many people wrote testimonials to John Sarno, expressing how his methodology had saved their lives. And the response from the medical community was, "The studies don't back it up." Well, now, finally, they do.

I remember a patient of mine saying to me, in the context of a larger conversation, "I know that I hang on to injuries longer than other people." It stuck in my mind, and now I realize why—it perfectly encapsulates the way so many people can know something intuitively, instinctually, about how their bodies heal or hang on to injury and illness, and medicine just isn't equipped to hear them.

If we want to make radical progress in the field of health care, we have to start looking for the whole truth, instead of half-truths that fortify our own biases and skepticisms. From mainstream medicine to mind-body medicine, we've gotten too polarized to be productive. Each side demonizes the other, unable to acknowledge what's *right* about each approach to healing. When we are too nervous to explore the truth about high achievers in healing because we worry that people might feel blame, we do everyone a disservice.

So who has the power to change this dynamic?

You do.

Over the years, I've seen that change comes slowly, even as technology advances by leaps and bounds. We have incredible new resources at our fingertips, from wearables that utilize big data to give us a window into the inner workings of our bodies, to the vanguard of immunotherapy, where researchers reprogram cells from our own bodies and then rerelease them as new, improved cancer fighters. All of this is exciting and holds incredible potential for revolutionary new approaches to health and healing. But will we take this opportunity? The kind of change we need means reevaluating the very structure that medicine is built on. It means questioning some of our basic assumptions about how we practice medicine and how we approach disease. The drivers of change here will not be doctors and other practitioners—they will be people like you and me. People who decide they aren't going to wait for the experts to come up with the solutions they need. Those who feel the pull of something higher are the drivers of progress—your choices have the power to shape not only your own health and vitality but also the field of medicine.

If anything you hear makes you feel blamed or responsible for your illness, rather than empowered, you should ignore it. Set it aside—it's not for you, and that's okay. Not every message is for every listener. Not everything will resonate or inspire. And not everything has to happen immediately. Sometimes we do need illness as a respite—a time to recalibrate, to rest, to reassess. Sometimes we aren't ready to say goodbye yet to a part of ourselves that is holding us back. Sometimes, like Mirae, like so many people who experience spontaneous healing, we need time. Give yourself that time. There is no set schedule for any of this. This should feel like an opportunity, not a burden. If it feels like a burden, it might not be the right time to burn your boat—and that's okay. This is your path. No one else's.

To move forward without feeling judged, blamed, or responsible, it's important to remember that ultimately, it's not about the illness. It's not about right or wrong or about specific things that you do or don't do that will heal you or not. It's about getting a life that's meaningful, where you understand and experience your own worth, and where you know what your purpose is and what you want from this life—however short or long it may be.

Sarah, thirty-eight years old, was manic when she was admitted to McLean. She'd been struggling with bipolar disorder most of her life and more recently, relapses of alcoholism. She was living at her mom's house, had lost her job, was ripping through money. Her family had bailed her out financially over and over and checked her in at the hospital when her symptoms got out of control. She was on multiple medications, but they didn't seem to be working as they once had.

Sarah's identical twin, Theresa, asked me for a family meeting. She, too, had been diagnosed with bipolar disorder as a teenager; she, too, had struggled with it for years. She understood exactly what Sarah was going through and wanted to help. When the day came for the meeting and Theresa walked into my office, I was stunned. I could barely see the resemblance between the twins. Sarah struggled with physical ailments that are often the by-product of mental illness and depression. Bipolar disorder can affect body health in many ways, from obesity to heart and thyroid disease, perhaps triggered by the cocktail of stress hormones bombarding the body's cells and tissues during flares. Sarah appeared many years older, and the many mixed episodes of hard living, depression, and mania had taken their toll on her body.

Theresa told me her own story. She and her sister had spent their twenties with an apparently similar trajectory, seeing the same psychiatrist, who would put them on one medication, then pull them off and try another. They never seemed to be able to get their symptoms under control. She began to notice that other approaches tended to keep her more stable: staying away from alcohol, for one, and watching what she ate and if she went out at night or stayed in and slept. When she turned twenty-eight, she decided: *Enough*.

"I just decided I was done—done with the cycle of never-ending medication trials, of talk therapy, of relapse," she said. "I took control of my life."

She cut out processed foods, immersed herself in a Buddhist meditation practice. Meditation, of course, isn't a magic pill that can fix a serious mental illness. But for Theresa, it was the linchpin that grounded her, around which all the other changes spun. And with the level of dedication and commitment to learning that she brought to it, I don't doubt it had profound effects on her brain and, following from that, her body.

It was hard to make real change, sometimes agonizingly so. The first two years were difficult. But Theresa's meditation practice opened the door to other big changes and led to a fulfilling career and a loving marriage. Now, she feels that self-care has built up her reserves so that setbacks don't knock her for a loop anymore. She's been healthy, happy, and off any form of medication for the past eight years. "You can do this," she said to her sister. "You just have to decide to." The sisters sat side by side, looking like they had come from two different worlds. They were sixty seconds apart in age but years apart in health.

These twins illustrate how biology is not destiny. The DNA of identical twins is 99 percent the same. And yet, their physical health does not run as parallel as their genes do. Sarah's and Theresa's health profiles are now so different that looking at them on paper, a physician would probably never guess they were sisters. Theresa had a "burn your boat" moment, while Sarah never did. Their lives diverged sharply from that moment on.

Relying on old habits, routines, or ways of thinking or being in the world isn't a character flaw. It's part of being human. As we've already examined, our DMN makes life efficient and more manageable, but it can also sabotage us despite our best intentions. Even people who are making lifesaving changes, who are on the pathway to health and recovery, will leave themselves an out. It's often an unconscious choice—a safety valve that you leave in place, a pathway back to unhealthy behaviors that, for whatever reason, help you get through difficult or stressful times. If you have a boat floating out there when stress is low and conditions are optimal—when you're winning the fight—it's probably okay. The problem occurs when things get tough. When it seems like you might lose. When you question your choice to fight. That's when you fall back—if there's a place to fall back to. The body is comfortable with the old homeostasis.

To attain the life you want, especially while ill, you have to identify any boats you have waiting in the harbor and burn them down for good. Earlier, we talked a little about what a "boat" can look like—how it could be a habit, food, or substance. An addiction, such as to alcohol or tobacco, would be an obvious example, but anything you're attached to that causes a stimulus-reward response in your brain falls into this category. Foods, activities, routines, even people can activate your dopamine loop and keep you stuck in ruts you know don't ultimately work for you. But boats can be even harder to see. Often, they look like "reasons why not."

When faced with a sweeping or difficult change, we can look for reasons why the change won't work, or why it's not worth the effort. Talking yourself out of making the changes you know you need to make is a type of boat. Relationships can be boats, in unexpected ways—sometimes, even a rewarding relationship with a friend or lover or family member can become a way out of necessary change, when we worry so much about the impact that change will have on the relationship that it keeps us from moving forward. And it's true that sometimes, people in our lives can struggle when we make radical change. Other people's emotions and expectations then become a boat—a seemingly valid reason not to move forward with radical change, because you are too afraid of what you might lose.

It's easy—effortless, almost—to come up with reasons why not. One way to identify your boats is to try to become aware of those reasons why not that fly into your mind, without really trying, when you picture your life once you make the change you know you need to make. Do you worry about someone's anger or disappointment? Are you afraid of the unknown? Do you picture your life without a routine you rely on and feel resentful and resistant?

Sometimes, when we make radical change, we do experience loss. When I left home to pursue the life I knew was right for me, I lost a lot. I lost my home, my community, and much of my family. I lost a version of myself that I left behind in that small town in the cornfields. But I gained so much more. In the story, Cortés's army loses a fleet of ships but gains an empire. What we often need to do to find the courage to light the match is to focus not on what we stand to lose but what we stand to gain.

LIGHTING THE MATCH

People find motivation to make radical change, and stick to it, in all kinds of ways. Claire Haser told me that at first, she was motivated primarily by fear. In the early days of her diagnosis, when she was nauseous with terror at the thought of dying so soon, she came across some studies online that said that salt was found to have a causative effect with pancreatic cancer. "I *love* salt," she said. "But I was amazed at how fast I got it out of my diet." But fear, as motivation, can only take you so far.

Fear got Claire started, but fear is a fuel that burns hot and fast. It can't sustain us through the long journey of fighting a chronic or incurable illness. For Claire, the work she did to confront death, to decide what kind of life she wanted to have with the time she had left, made that fear evaporate and gave her a more renewable source of motivation and power. She started to ask questions like, "What is this cancer trying to teach me?" "What's the message of this illness?" "What is the opportunity?" For Claire, she found the motivation to be uncompromising in her pursuit of the life she wanted by listening to her body, becoming more in tune with it, and by moving toward ways of being and thinking that made her feel better in her body, mind, and soul.

Juniper Stein was the one who said, "I accepted the diagnosis, but not the prognosis." She accepted that she would have to live with this disease—what she did not accept was the expectation about *how* she would live with it. She did not want to be a young newlywed in a wheelchair. She didn't want to be physically held back. She didn't want to be a burden on her family. She had a vision of what she *did* want: a family, a body that worked, that could carry her through the world and accomplish everything she wanted to do, and to be able to live without the constant distraction of debilitating pain. As she pushed through the hardest, most painful days of her yoga practice, she kept that vision in her mind: what she wanted.

Mirae Bunnell said it was easy to understand the changes she needed to make but hard to get her mind on board. It resisted, stuck in its own feedback loop of stimulation and reward, the chemical pleasure pathways that reinforce old patterns with hits of dopamine and serotonin. "It's like a negotiation," she says now. "My physical body was telling my mind what it needed to heal and stay healthy, but my mind balked at the discipline required to fulfill that."

When stress is high, we fall back on old, engrained ways of coping. The science of how the brain works is clear on this; under pressure or in the moment, the brain will play a trick on us and convince us that the right thing to do is to use the old behavior, the familiar path. "Just this one time," we tell ourselves, and we believe it. The mind is powerful in this way. We see it most easily with addiction—the neural pathways that arc toward immediate pleasure and comfort—but it plays out in all kinds of scenarios that affect health and our capacity for radical healing. We talked earlier about addictions—to alcohol or drugs and also to foods, habits, routines. Even certain ways of thinking can be addictive. A negative or limiting thought pattern, for example, can become addictive and prevent you from developing mental circuitry that's more healing. And it's just as difficult to break and rewrite those old thought patterns, habits, and beliefs as it is to overcome an addiction. Your biology and neurology will do anything and everything to keep you from making change.

So how do you make radical change and stick to it when you're up against this kind of nefarious opponent—your own mind and body?

Some people mark change with a ceremony. Some make big changes all at once—Jan, relocating to Brazil. Pablo, rapidly switching his diet and never going back. Others, like Claire, do better with a process of learning how to gradually meet their deeper needs so that the old, unhealthy, or out-of-date behaviors begin to fall away on their own. They "fill the hole in the soul" that this belief or habit was trying to assuage until they simply don't need them anymore.

When your back is up against the wall and you're in danger of falling back into old habits, beliefs, or choices, it can be hard to make the right decision in that moment. It's important to make a plan ahead of time for what you're going to do in that situation, because your mind (DMN) will trick you when you're in the moment, feeling the pressure. Here are some things to ask yourself now:

- What are my triggers? In what situations or circumstances do I struggle the most to stick to my guns? Can I avoid these or prepare better for them?
- What is the vision I have for my life—something so inspiring, I would sacrifice immediate pleasure to attain it? What will help me to achieve that? What might prevent it?
- Who can I trust to counsel me in this situation? Who can I call who'll support instead of undermining me?
- What "reward" can I give myself for following through? Make it meaningful and immediate. Contact with someone you care about? Play a favorite song? Something that makes you feel great.
- What will help me understand my value and worth and see the importance and goodness that I bring into the world?
- Why did I decide to make this change in my life? Remember your reasons. Recall your vision of the life, the healthy body, you really want. Let yourself feel it.

Our minds are wired in certain ways that keep us from truly burning our boats and going all in. Those long-standing synapses pull us toward habits, routines, and beliefs that can be damaging and that can stunt healing and hold us back. Why would you hack a new path through the forest if there's already a well-trodden path? Imagine water running through riverbeds, the deep grooves carved into the earth. Thoughts—which manifest as electricity in the brain—take the path of least resistance, just as water will do as it finds its way across a grooved landscape. Over time, those riverbeds get deeper and deeper, the stream more and more difficult to divert. We already know that your DMN can lock you into patterns of thought and habit that can come to define your life and health, writing a map for your future that you don't even realize you're following. But we also know that the DMN can be rewritten.

Forging a new neural pathway is a leap of faith. The good news is that our brains are not hardwired; we can create new neuro associations that link pleasure and reward with healthier habits. But it's not easy. It means burning the boats of those old neuro associations so we can create new ones. Picture Indiana Jones, making his way through the temple of deadly obstacles at the end of *Indiana Jones and the Last Crusade*. He comes face-to-face with a wide, un-crossable chasm. The only way to proceed is to step into the abyss, with no idea what will happen. He does—and a solid bridge meets his foot. It was there all along, camouflaged but present. When your brain creates new synapses, the transmitters in your neurons do a similar leap, reaching into an abyss to connect, build a new bridge. When Indy gets across the gap, he tosses a handful of sand to outline the path and make it easier to see next time, faster to cross. Neuro associations in your brain work the same way, making the path easier and more familiar the next time you need it.

It takes forty-five days to create a new neural pathway. Forty-five days: a month and a half. When you think about it that way, in the span of a whole life, it's not so long! But when you're in it, doing the day-to-day, trying to change a habit, a thought pattern, a belief you've held on to all your life, it can feel endless.

To get through those forty-five days, treat yourself like Pavlov's dog. Your job now is to neuro-condition yourself like you're your own lab rat. What you want to do is give yourself massive instant pleasure when you do anything that's keeping you on that road to healing. Anything from recognizing a negative or limiting thought pattern to choosing a healing food over an inflammatory one is worth rewarding. Make your own list—what is rewarding for you?

And remember through it all that what you are doing is creating an entirely new map. It's hard going when you're laying a new path. It's frustrating. But you're moving forward. You've left the beach; the harbor is far behind you. There's no boat waiting there anyway. Turning back is not an option. *We take the city or we die.*

You can do anything for forty-five days. Because after those forty-five days, there will be the rest of your life.

Over the past fifteen years, I've seen a lot of stunning recoveries. And as we've covered over the course of this book, they are each unique. There is only one story exactly like Claire's; only one like Mirae's. But it's in the personal that we find the universal—and, I believe, the way forward. For medicine to take that next important leap, we need to act on some of the most urgent lessons of spontaneous remission, which tell us that to reach new depths of recovery, we have to heal the following: our diets, our immune systems, our stress responses, and our identities. It's these four threads that run so brilliantly through the fabric of nearly every story of recovery I've examined and which could lay the groundwork for a revolution in medicine. But first, we can accomplish this revolution on a smaller scale, for ourselves, as the survivors profiled in this book have done—if we burn our boats.

When I left for college, I left home for good. For years, I'd been living a kind of half-life, trying to compromise between what my family wanted and expected from me and what I wanted out of life—what I *needed* to be a healthy, thriving person. They were locked into a model, based on punitive rules and narrow beliefs, that I couldn't bear to exist in anymore. At the same time, it was painful to leave, because the stakes were high; if I left, I couldn't go back. I would be excommunicated. I would be dead to them.

It was one of the hardest things I've ever done. And it turned out to be one of my most important gifts, because after I made my choice, they didn't leave me any avenue back. I was the one who left the boat to go to shore; they were the ones who burned the boat. A difficult time in your life—like an illness—is often a time when people choose to burn their boats. But look at the Cortés story: he gave the order; the soldiers didn't make that choice. Sometimes, illness burns your boat for you. The question is: Do you lie down on the beach, or do you move forward?

None of us know how much time we have here. There is no key to immortality—not even spontaneous healing lasts forever. What the survivors of incurable illness in this book found was a way to move forward that accepted this: that there would be an end, but that in the meantime, they were going to live the best, most authentic and fulfilling lives that they could. They were going to find those big, deep changes that made them feel better and more alive and lean into them as hard as they could. If it meant restructuring their lives, they did it. If it meant letting go of limiting relationships, they let them go. They looked at themselves in the mirror and asked, *What is the story I've been telling about myself, and how is it wrong?* None of them embarked on this journey halfway or with the idea that they would cheat death; they set forth with the mission to claim the life that was theirs for the time they had. In doing so, they healed. They healed the way they treated their bodies. They healed how they responded to the stresses and challenges of life. They healed their toxic or damaging beliefs about the world and what was possible. And finally, they healed the story of who they are, so they could find the freedom and the capacity to make lifesaving changes.

"It was foremost a struggle of the mind and spirit," Mirae said of her recovery. "The body followed."

CONCLUSION

A Medicine of Hope and Possibility

> Out on the edge you see all kinds of things you can't see
> from the center. Big, undreamed-of things—the people
> on the edge see them first.
>
> —*Kurt Vonnegut*

COASTAL GREECE: 300–350 BC

Let's travel back in time to another era. Imagine, just for a moment, that you live in ancient Greece. You live in a small village in the countryside, in a house made of bricks, with wooden shutters to keep out the Mediterranean sun in the heat of the day. There is a courtyard where your children play knucklebones—a game like modern jacks, but with cleaned and polished goat or sheep bones to pick up. Your family gets their water from the courtyard well and bakes cakes with honey and figs in a clay oven inside.

You come from a family of farmers or fishermen. You go to bed when the sun does. You work hard; your life is not easy. If you get sick or hurt, a local physician might prescribe herbs or prayer. You might visit a temple and leave an offering of gold or silver—probably more than you can afford—to Asclepius, the god of healing.

If you're very ill, you might make the difficult pilgrimage to one of the great temples farther away on the coast, called asclepeions.

Named after the god of healing, the asclepeion is the center of healing in Greek society. It integrates emotional, spiritual, and physical care. As soon as you arrive, you are taken to "incubation," where you sleep overnight in a dormitory with other patients. In the morning, you meet with a priest and report your dreams to him. This priest-physician will create a prescription plan for you. It usually begins with a period of purification, or Katharsis, marked with a switch to a clean, nutrient-dense diet and a healing trip to the baths. You may even be prescribed art therapy—a process of purging or processing emotions through creating. The priest-physician might create a personal prayer or mantra for you to carry in your mind and repeat, to help you maintain a positive outlook. And if a more serious treatment needs to happen, even a surgery, it will happen here, at the asclepeion. Under a kind of anesthesia made with opium, you'll be put into a dream state, and the procedure will be carried out by trained surgeons. Your name might even be etched into a marble slab, preserving forever a record of where you came from, the nature of your illness, and what the treatment consisted of—marble slabs that would be found thousands of years later, by people looking for a better way to heal.

It's fascinating to me how close some of these ancient rituals are to the steps taken by so many who experienced spontaneous healing. The immediate, radical diet changes. The soul-searching. The removal from the stress and grind of ordinary life to a place of healing, a community that was, as a whole, striving for physical and spiritual health. The acknowledgment, present in the utilization of dreams and prayer and meditation, that healing often begins beyond, or deeper than, the physical body.

I'm not advocating for a return to ancient times. This is not about going backward. There was so much about the body, and about disease, that we did not yet understand at that time. People used to toss coins into sacred springs, wishing for a cure. I'll toss a penny into a fountain and make a wish, but I don't think it will cure me. But it's worth asking if, in our haste toward progress, we left anything essential behind. What would medicine look like if we could reach back in time, reclaim that forgotten knowledge, and weave it into the incredible tapestry of science, innovation, and technology we possess today? The medicine of the future no doubt will reclaim pieces of that lost past—to reach new levels of possibility in healing, it will have to.

HONOLULU, HAWAII: 2049

Good morning, Claire. Welcome to the Wellness Clinic. How are you feeling today?

The woman steps into her reserved room at the clinic, and visual sensors scan her face, recognize her, and immediately pull up her entire medical history. The data is gathered from a variety of sources: culled from trackers, sensors in the environment, wearables, apps, digitized data in her medical record, and more. As the AI greets Claire warmly as if she's an old friend, it is simultaneously—at a speed a million times faster than human synapses—assembling all that data into a detailed portrait. This AI knows and remembers more about Claire's health and health history than she—or her doctor—possibly could. It knows that she has a family history of cancer—her great-aunt, whom she is named after, died of the disease before she was born. Today, cancers are much rarer. In the years since the overhaul of the medical system, the numbers on what used to be called *lifestyle illnesses* like cancer, diabetes, and heart disease—and other chronic illnesses like autoimmune disorders and depression—have been plummeting so fast, it's hard to keep accurate stats on hand.

As Claire settles in, the AI's soothing voice guides her to change into a robe. Meanwhile, using a unique algorithm, the AI is aggregating Claire's data, searching for points of connection between health vulnerabilities and opportunities for a more flourishing life, effortlessly connecting the dots that used to take people *lifetimes* to figure out. It knows her habits and what changes she's made or is trying to make. The recommendations the AI will make are based on this superhuman ability to connect hundreds of thousands of data points about how to improve Claire's health. It can correlate those data points with emerging scientific data that has just been published; the AI grabs new peer-reviewed studies as soon as they hit the internet and tucks them into the file for any patients they might pertain to.

The AI also knows how its past recommendations have worked for Claire or not. It knows if she's followed through on those recommendations, or if she wasn't quite able to stick to them, and it can tailor new recommendations, or analyze the data and come up with a new pace or plan that might be more attractive or possible. It is completely nonjudgmental. Besides, by the time Claire walks into the clinic, the AI already knows everything; data has been flowing into her file for weeks, effortlessly incorporated into the big picture of her health profile. She doesn't have to reveal or confess anything. It's already there. This is the job of the AI—to be the ultimate impartial, impeccable observer. It exists only for you and for helping you develop a vital, healthy, flourishing life.

But wait—where is Claire's doctor in all of this? Have AIs replaced human doctors?

Not at all.

In 2049, AIs have freed physicians to truly *be* physicians. The word *physician* is a kind of Latin and old French mashup. *Physica,* from Latin, means *things relating to nature,* while the old French *fisicien* can be translated as *the art of healing.* Today, in 2049, physicians are true artists of healing. And they are absolutely indispensable.

Claire could have met with the AI from the comfort of her bedroom, by pulling up the portal on her laptop, but today is a day for an in-person clinic visit. While the AI that beams into her home is great for check-ins on her nutrition and goals, her stress levels, and to get a quick sense of how much time she's been able to spend in the parasympathetic, today she needs more than a check-in. Today, she needs the intensive, in-person presence of her longtime health coach, who knows her and cares for her in a way that feels very different from the benign, informational presence of the AI.

Claire doesn't know a lot about the great-aunt she's named for;

her mom was close to her, though, and used to talk about her. Her great-aunt had been a kind of warm, constant, guiding light for their family, someone who always seemed to have her priorities straight, who would be real with you, no BS. She left behind a guidebook for recovering from pancreatic cancer that has become a kind of sleeper hit. Originally self-published online as an ebook pamphlet, it consisted of short articles pulled from her great-aunt's blog. Refreshingly straightforward and honest, it laid out the steps and decisions her great-aunt had made while navigating a fatal disease, thinking she was in the last months of her life. And then came the twist ending: she didn't die. The cancer vanished for over a decade. Doctors were baffled and, in an effort to explain the inexplicable, discredited her diagnosis. But she knew her body; she knew it was real. And when the cancer eventually returned, after an impossibly long remission, she was finally validated. The medical community had to start taking her seriously.

And it wasn't just Claire's case. Voices from across the country, from all over the world, had been growing louder and louder. People were no longer accepting the standard line, that they were simply an outlier, that there was no explanation for their astounding recoveries. They were determined to tell their stories so that others could benefit from their trials and errors, and hopefully, their stunning successes.

And it worked. The path Claire's great-aunt blazed has now become a well-trodden one. A lot of people have followed in her footsteps, and many of them have found radical healing in the way she did all those years ago. It's easier now. Back in the early 2000s, there wasn't much support for the road Claire was walking. She was alone when she pushed her way through that wilderness, encountering skepticism and resistance with every step. But as more and more people demanded a different approach to healing, the medical world gradually began to change.

Technology has been changing, too. It's been rapidly moving forward—nanobots can now be easily inserted into the bloodstream to find and eradicate burgeoning cancer cells, to repair the walls of blood vessels, remove senescent cells, repair an ailing thyroid or heart, and so much more. And it's becoming more accessible. Wearables that collect essential data, recording blood pressure and oxygenation and stress levels, have become affordable and ubiquitous. Like the computers and apps of her great-aunt's day, capacities have skyrocketed and costs plunged as the digital laws of dematerialization and demonetization have continued to work their magic.[1] Algorithms, once created, can be reproduced billions of times for no cost, so their services are no longer out of reach for people.

These technologies are lightweight and unobtrusive,[2] integrating invisibly into Claire's life, and they know, even when she doesn't, whether she's operating in the parasympathetic or in fight-or-flight mode, and for how long. They know what sorts of situations help her to shift into the parasympathetic and which do the opposite. And they can even prompt her to reframe stress she's experiencing from threat stress to challenge stress. When Claire taps the app icon on her phone over her morning coffee, a visual calendar fills the touch screen, the events of the day color-coded to indicate whether they will offer an opportunity to shift into the parasympathetic (a lunchtime walk through the neighborhood near her office to meet a friend) or an opportunity to use stress as a challenge (a meeting with a contentious colleague who always puts down her ideas).

All week long, Claire's AI downloads grocery lists and meal plans onto her phone, ready for her to send to the grocery store so it will be packed and waiting for pickup or even delivery as she heads home to meet her kids. Throughout the day, reminders to drink water and take relaxation breaks vibrate from her wristband. She's prone to headaches, and for her, staying hydrated and managing her stress is the best way to prevent them and avoid the need to chase them with medications.

When Claire's doctor walks through the door, she feels that rush of oxytocin that happens when a close friend or loved one appears. She really enjoys her meetings with her doctor, which usually happen about once every few months and last as long as they need to (or at least it seems that way!). Claire remembers being a little girl at the doctor's with her mother, how she spent most of her time with nurses who weighed her and measured her and ran down endless checklists. When the doctor finally entered, rushed, with only a few minutes, the first thing he looked at was the computer screen—not her.

With her doctor, Claire has a real connection. This woman, who was there for the birth of Claire's children, has guided her through so many rough patches, health-wise. She is well versed in the arts of human connection; this has become a major part of the curriculum at all the top medical schools. Claire describes her concerns—a lot of work anxiety lately, a business deal that has turned out to be very challenging, and a feeling that her body isn't responding well to the stress. Digestion issues, trouble regulating her temperature, difficulty falling asleep. As a woman at this age and with her family history, she's at risk for developing an autoimmune illness, and she's worried these are early warning signs.

"They might be," her doctor agrees. "Stress can be a trigger for a lot of autoimmune diseases, especially if you're genetically predisposed. But let's do everything we can to turn that trigger off."

The doctor has already been alerted by the AI that Claire's cortisol and adrenaline levels have been high and that her sleep has been disrupted most nights. A quick swipe on the tablet she picks up off the counter (for most of the visit, she hasn't needed it, since her main goal is to sit and connect with Claire) shows her that Claire's last telomere check, an easy cheek swab that only takes a few seconds, showed nice length and preservation. And that her fitness age, a better measure of her real age than chronological age, is actually pretty good. But if a major stress pattern is emerging; it's good to address it now. When patients don't, it can lead to a spiral where they end up in a life they don't want, feeling trapped, experiencing major dysfunction in the body.

For the rest of the session, Claire and her doctor talk through the data and conclusions assembled by the AI and make an action plan for Claire. It involves talking to her husband about the issues at work so he's clued in that she needs more support. It means shifting back to an anti-inflammatory diet, which has worked amazingly well for her in the past, and making time in the mornings for a swim or a yoga class or even just a quick walk through her neighborhood, things the AI has found always drop her cortisol levels immediately and tend to keep them more balanced even on the most stressful days. With a few taps on the touch screen, the doctor fine-tunes the AI to monitor Claire's stress levels and inflammatory markers going forward, so they can catch anything that might be starting before it becomes damaging.

Decades ago, we used to wish for a system of medicine that served as a guardrail at the top of the winding cliffs of life, keeping people healthy and safe on the roads. Instead, we developed a system that parked ambulances at the bottom of the cliff and waited for people to fall and then rushed them off to the hospital. We saved lives, sure, but didn't touch the major killers and causes of suffering. But a revolution in medicine, fueled by technology, hope, and the shining example of high achievers in health, has finally gotten us there. Claire's doctor, and the entire system of medicine working behind her, has been that guardrail her entire life.

In 2049, the tending of the body and mind is completely integrated due to an invisible, seamless connection of the physical and AI worlds. Algorithms know us better than we know ourselves. They can detect the causes of our feelings and concerns that we typically don't notice. They tell us which relationships and interactions leave us feeling stressed and exhausted and which leave us energized and at peace. It is easier now to cut through the noise of the "shoulds," the pressures, the desires of others, our own desires to please. We are constantly reminded, gently, of our responsibility to our mental, physical, and spiritual health.

Doctors today are no longer burdened by the impossible task of staying caught up with reams of medical research on a myriad of diseases and treatments and can instead focus directly on the person. AI does all that mind-work for a physician—it *is* her mind—so that she is free to listen and serve as a compassionate counselor and coach. She had been accepted to medical school not for her ability to memorize vast reams of data but for her compassion and interest in human behavior and communication. She is not the expert on Claire's body any longer—*Claire is*—but she is a beloved coach, and it's not too much to say that there is a measure of love that exists between the two. Claire feels seen and loved in a warm, objective, professional, nonjudgmental sense, and she always walks out of the room feeling like she's just been with someone wise, who has clearly spent years developing a deep sense of human behavior and a respect for human choice and empowerment.

Once it was proven that the care and attention of the physician was found to be transformative, even at the subatomic level, the values of the medical world shifted dramatically. No longer are doctors expected to be repositories of information—this is the AI's job, as essential assistant. The doctor's job is to connect, to understand, to see the entire tapestry of a patient's life, and to compassionately tailor their care to their specific experience in the world. The AI has not replaced the doctor; it has freed the doctor to really listen and connect, to innovate, to be a friend and a coach, to truly practice the art of medicine. It's an art that involves weaving together the four pillars of medicine today: healing our diets, healing our stress response, healing our immune systems, and finally, healing our identities. We have reams of research now that support that fourth pillar as the most essential, and doctors today write more prescriptions for actions, experiences, and big life changes than they do for medications.

Most important, we've figured out what the AI can do brilliantly and where its skill set ends. All the AI in the world cannot provide the one thing that really heals: love.

AI can detect and organize vast reams of data in the direction of improving physical and even mental health; it can uncover issues and sources of ill health and distress better than the mind of even the most experienced expert. But it cannot love. Technology may introduce us to a world of unparalleled physical comfort and to revolutionary treatments, but there are places where only love can go, where only nonjudgmental compassion, validation, and connection can go. The world of love and the higher realms it allows us to access are perhaps synonymous with the world of healing. And under certain conditions, which we admittedly do not understand very well yet, the physical world bows to its laws and is even shaped by them. When this occurs, an illness can melt away.

When Claire leaves the clinic, her course is corrected. She won't be sliding down that cliff today or any time soon.

BOSTON, MASSACHUSETTS: PRESENT DAY

I have two documents up on my office wall. Patients often notice them the first time they visit, and that's my intention. They are the Declaration of Independence and the Emancipation Proclamation.

We hold these truths to be self-evident, that all men are created equal, that they are endowed, by their Creator, with certain unalienable Rights, that among these are Life, Liberty, and the pursuit of Happiness.

I keep them there as a reminder, to myself and my patients, that often what we truly need are not medications or even talk therapy with a person like me (though of course these can help at times) but to throw off the chains of whatever is oppressing us so that we can make a life where we can be the best, highest, and most authentic version of ourselves. "Thank God psychiatrists weren't at the Boston Tea Party!" I sometimes tell my patients to make them laugh. "They would have written those people a prescription and sent them home. But they didn't need Zoloft. They needed to throw off the chains of oppression and get a life—a life of freedom, respect, and dignity. They needed to make a world that was better, where their true potential could be realized. Where they could bring their unique light into the world."

The Declaration of Independence was, in so many ways, a story. All revolutions are stories. They help us to see what is possible that wasn't possible before. They paint a vision of a better future, and that is why they come to pass: because when we see it, we can realize it.

We need another revolution now. The revolution of stories.

Stories of remission, and recovery, and life after illness. Stories of how people got there.

All the survivors of incurable illness whom I interviewed for this book talked about the drive they felt to share their stories with the world, as painful and personal as those stories are. It is not easy to share these types of stories, to bare your soul to the world. These survivors opened up to us the soul searching they went through, the humbling and terrifying process of facing death and discovering their true selves. And they did it because when they were sick and facing a terminal diagnosis, they felt alone, without a way forward.

When Claire Haser was first diagnosed, she searched and searched for stories of people who had recovered from pancreatic cancer at her stage. She couldn't find any. That's why she decided to share her story, in such depth and detail. She wanted the next person who went looking for a story of survival to find one: hers. She, like so many who reached out to me, did so with the hope that she could help people. She wanted to give back, recognizing that her healing from pancreatic cancer was not just about her—it was about creating a window of possibility for others and for the world.

The people in this book made themselves N of 1: the single subject of their own intensive study. And in this lies the critical piece of a new science and a new medicine as we move forward, shifting away from an exclusive reliance on randomized studies that may or may not be relevant to you in your lived life, and toward actual data about *you*. And just as we've learned from the people in this book, what's most personal is most universal. Your healing is about more than just you or those you love who might be struggling with illness. We are all part of a story of human health, one far greater than our own pain or mortality or recovery, one that started thousands of years ago, and one that will continue on, long after we all are gone. And our contributions to this ever-changing human story will help determine what directions it takes in the future.

We need hope in medicine. Lucky for us, it's already there.

It's there in the stories of those who overcame incurable diseases. It's there in the doctors and nurses and surgeons who *are* practicing a medicine of hope—as hard as it is for them to work within and against a system that seems bent on magnifying disease, on treating with silver bullets instead of growing health from the ground up. It's there in the scientific studies—obscured by averages, but still there. Look for the outliers. Look for the scattered dots at the far edges of the chart. Don't let the law of averages bury them. They are there, and there are more of them than we think. Believe that you can be one of them if that's something that you really want. And push your health-care providers to help make that possible.

Change doesn't just happen. It doesn't happen when it *should*. It happens when people get loud. When they refuse to be ignored anymore. When they shout their stories from the rooftops. Help us sound the revolution. Share this vision of medicine with those who are ill and suffering, who need a different story about their health. Share it with your health-care providers, who have the power to begin to shift this narrative from inside the system. Share it with your loved ones who may not have had to yet face a difficult illness—maybe they will never have to. My hope, and the hope of every contributor who shared their own life story of recovery, is that their stories, and all of yours, will finally be so loud, everyone will have to stand up and listen.

AUTHOR'S NOTE

When I started this research in 2003, I felt alone. In recent years, however, others are also forging ahead with this line of inquiry as our culture begins to shift toward more openness to the study and consideration of well-being. It's important to be aware of the important work of others as this effort gains steam.

Kelly Turner's excellent book, *Radical Remission* (2014), looks at spontaneous remission as it applies to cancer and, more recently, she has started a network for those who want to improve their health. In *Mind Over Medicine* (2014; revised edition 2020), Lissa Rankin discusses the topic of spontaneous remission, expands on that in her new edition, and overall provides an outstanding, whole-person guide for those seeking to introduce a different level of self-care and well-being into their lives. A number of others have helped pave the way in recent years: Caryle Hirschberg and Mark Ian Barasch with *Remarkable Recovery*, Bernie Siegel with *Love, Medicine, and Miracles,* Kenneth Pelletier's *Mind as Healer, Mind as Slayer,* and Louise Hays with *Heal Your Body*. These works have each advanced the conversation in their own important way.

Also in 2014, the National Cancer Institute announced the development of an "Exceptional Responder Initiative," and gathered tissue samples to analyze from more than a hundred patients.

Finally, in 2018, Dr. Isaac Samuel Kohane, chair of the department of bioinformatics at Harvard Medical School, rolled out an exceptional responder network, and seeks to become the first national registry for patients who beat the odds and respond to treatments that failed to help others. The project hopes to gather data that eventually reveals patterns to explain what went right.

The research discussed in *Cured* started in 2003 and therefore has been able to follow the trajectory of many of its subjects for years, which is particularly important when it comes to spontaneous remission. It seeks to establish the importance of examining spontaneous remission not only in cancer but across the entire spectrum of illness. My hope is that these initiatives, among others, herald a new era of scientific inquiry and exploration that will allow us to truly understand and utilize the lessons of spontaneous remission.

Please visit www.drjeffreyrediger.com for a guided program of exercises and prompts that aim to inspire a deeper, personalized journey toward health and well-being.

ACKNOWLEDGMENTS

First and foremost, words cannot express my profound gratitude to all those who so generously brought me deep into their lives, sharing with me their medical files and stories of remarkable recoveries, often allowing me to follow them for years. I am irrevocably changed as a result—a different person and a much better physician.

I also am indebted to all the patients at McLean and Good Sam who, over the years, have shared with me their most private stories, usually at the most extreme moments of their lives. In so doing, they continue to reveal to me what really makes us tick as human beings, and also illuminate for me just how completely the mental exists in the physical, and also how much physical resides in the mental.

I am more grateful than words can express for the team at Idea Architects. Alyssa Knickerbocker, in particular, was so smart, so capable, and throughout this long project maintained such an impossible level of equanimity, even in the context of childbirth, sleepless nights, and my writing errors, that she can only be described as brilliant at what she does. I also benefited more than words can say from the extraordinary guiding hands and perennial wisdom of both Doug Abrams and Ellen Stiefler (Transmedia Agency), as well as many others at Idea Architects: Boo Prince, for her insightful, brilliant coaching, Ty Love, Lara Love, Janelle Julian, and others, all of whom were more than patient and thoughtful, wise and tactful as the situation required.

My heartfelt gratitude and love also extend to the entire team at Flatiron Books. Principal among them are Bob Miller and Sarah Murphy, to whom I owe an immeasurable debt and whose character and wisdom have left an indelible imprint upon me. Many others at Flatiron also did their work tirelessly and with such kindness and dedication that I was repeatedly touched and impressed. It is a great privilege to be associated with individuals of such consummate skill and high caliber.

This book would not be what it is without the support and wisdom of Jill Bolte Taylor, who has become not only a dear friend but also a wise counselor about remaining true to one's core beliefs and what it takes to navigate the world of writing and speaking. Ever the impromptu genius of memorable language, she said, when we first met, "I've been waiting for you for twenty-two years. In twenty-two years, not one doctor has ever asked how I had a full recovery from my stroke." That is of course, remarkable, a statement exactly about what I'm hoping this book helps assuage.

I also want to thank my colleagues and friends at McLean Hospital, Harvard, and Good Samaritan Medical Center, all of whom have provided indispensable support and friendship over the years. The leadership team at McLean, in particular, has stuck with me through the highs and lows of this project, including Drs. Scott Rauch, Joe Gold, Gail Tsimprea, Duncan MacCourt, Simona Sava, Lisa Llanas; and also Mark Longsjo, Darlyn Scott, and Rich Silva. And I could never forget our support staff, including MaryAnn Betts and Sue McPhee, who gracefully take care of more details than anyone can imagine, and also Ruth Byrnes, who has been a constant source of support and encouragement. In addition, I want to thank the leadership team at Good Samaritan Medical Center, including Drs. Marisella Marrero, Kenneth Lawson, as well as Mathew Hesketh and Matthew Cotti for their patience with my hours and days away for writing and speaking. Finally, Drs. Karim Malek (oncologist, ImmunoGen), Kaushal Mehta (neuro-radiologist, Good Samaritan Medical Center), and Chris Katavolos (senior hospitalist, Good Samaritan Medical Center) provided critical insights. And Drs. Andreas Mershin (MIT), Henry Stapp (UC Berkeley), and Michael Rohan (McLean/Harvard) did the same as physicists. Any mistakes in this text, however, are mine and mine alone.

Many of us owe a profound debt to the teachers in our lives, and for me that is certainly true. Incomplete as it is, I will restrict myself to expressing gratitude to just a few: Dr. Richard Butman, Kenny Dodd, and Jerry Root at Wheaton College, the late Drs. James Loder and Diogenes Allen at Princeton Theological Seminary, and the late Drs. Les Havens and John Mack and also Dr. Ellen Langer at Harvard, all of whom have deeply influenced my intellectual and personal trajectory with their humanity and vision.

I am also grateful for the tireless patience of Dr. Issam and Kathy Nemeh over the years, as I struggled to come to terms with how people heal, and with the factors associated with such recoveries. Quite a team and with a lovely family, they have dedicated their lives to the healing and well-being of others, and continue to be a model of inspiration for me. The same is true for Miguel Coll, who continues to be a bright star in my life, showing me a living example of resilience and dedication, and also Anne Cuvelier and the Newport group, all of whom have enlarged my understanding of how mysterious and wondrous this human journey really is. This work has also benefited from the generous research support and friendship of Bill Hanes and the wise counsel of Kim Schefler.

I also want to thank members of my family, many of whom have also made sacrifices so that this book could be born. My children, Landon, Bryn, and Simeon are chief among them and are brilliant, special lights in this world. Then there's David, my brother, and friend. We live in different worlds, he and I, surrounded by people and media with very different perceptions of the world. He helps me see that, among other things, we all really want and need the same things, and that at the very bottom things are not nearly as polarized as the current media and political din and distortions would suggest.

I want to give special acknowledgment to Rachael Donalds, my colleague and best friend. She inspires and galvanizes my life and actions in more ways than I can count, and her work as the founder of Biosay has been particularly influential, created as it is out of a vision that seeks to give people the tools they need to take radical charge of their health and well-being. It inspired some of the ideas in this book and her work will help lead us, I believe, into a new world where we increasingly see that health and vitality depend not so much on a new medicine as on a new way to engage with our health collaboratively, and also on a new state of mind (www.biosay.com). I believe in this mission, consider it a workbook for *Cured,* and have invested in it. If you want to download the Biosay app and join this wellness community, scan the QR code below:

Finally, I also want to thank David and Neri Donalds for simply being who they are, outstanding supports and wise counselors, helping me navigate the waters of diverse worlds and ideas gracefully and wisely. I am especially grateful for Neri, who manages so many details of my life, ranging from contracts and all manner of personal and professional details, all with great aplomb, attention to detail, and vast prodigious skill.

NOTES

Introduction

1. Caryle Hirschberg and Brendan O'Regan, *Spontaneous Remission: An Annotated Bibliography,* Institute of Noetic Sciences, 1993.

1. Into the Impossible

1. To that end, the reader will notice that a few illnesses resurface repeatedly in this book. I maintained this commitment for years with research in Brazil and elsewhere. The illnesses studied were the most incurable illnesses known and therefore have served as the best site for my skeptical exploration.

2. William B. Coley, "Contribution to the Knowledge of Sarcoma," *Annals of Surgery* 14, no. 3 (1891): 199–220, www.ncbi.nlm.nih.gov/pmc/articles/PMC1428624/?page=1.

3. Carol Torgan, "Immune System Shaped by Environment More Than Genes," National Institutes of Health, February 2, 2015, www.nih.gov/news-events/nih-research-matters/immune-system-shaped-environment-more-genes.

4. S.M. Rappaport, "Implications of the Exposome for Exposure Science," *Journal of Exposure Science and Environmental Epidemiology* 21, (2011): 5–9.

2. Natural-Born Killers

1. Inspiration for this visual was drawn from a poem published in the *Iowa Health Bulletin* in 1912: "The Fence or the Ambulance," by Joseph Malins.

2. Robert Langreth, "Six Miracle Cancer Survivors," *Forbes,* March 2009.

3. "White Blood Cells Can Sprout 'Legs' and Move Like Millipedes," Science Daily, May 4, 2009, www.sciencedaily.com/releases /2009/05/090504094424.htm.

4. Charles W. Schmidt, "Questions Persist: Environmental Factors in Autoimmune Disease," *Environmental Health Perspectives,* June 2011.

5. Marc Ian Barasch, "Remarkable Recoveries: Research and Practice from a Patient's Perspective," *Hematology/Oncology Clinics of North America* 22, no. 4 (2008): 755–766, www.academia.edu /20207816/Oncology_Hematology_Article.

6. Ibid., 756.

7. M. K. Bowers and C. Weinstock, "A Case of Healing in Malignancy," *American Academy of Psychoanalysis Journal* 6, no. 3 (1978): 393–402. Can also be found in the spontaneous remission database at the Institute of Noetic Sciences, https://library.noetic.org/library /publication-bibliographies/spontaneous-remission, Appendix 2, 541–542.

8. Over a century ago, Sigmund Freud defined mental health as the capacity to both love and work—the capacity to give and receive love at a deep level and to also work productively and meaningfully over a long period of time. So it's no surprise that Daniel's recovery was reflected in dramatic shifts toward increased competency in both of these domains.

9. And now, finally, scientists are turning to the effect of positive emotions on the immune system. For example, Jennifer Stellar, Dacher Keltner, and their team reported that positive emotions were associated with lower levels of pro-inflammatory cytokines in healthy individuals in two separate studies (J. E. Stellar, N. John-

Henderson, C. L. Anderson, A. M. Gordon, G. D. McNeil, and D. Keltner, "Positive Affect and Markers of Inflammation: Discrete Positive Emotions Predict Lower Levels of Inflammatory Cytokines," *Emotion* 15, no. 2 (2015): 129–133, www.ncbi.nlm.nih.gov /pubmed/25603133). We know from other research that sustained levels of cytokines are associated with diminished health and with a wide range of illnesses, such as heart disease, type 2 diabetes, and autoimmune illnesses.

10. James McIntosh, "What Is Serotonin and What Does It Do?," Medical News Today, February 2, 2018, www.medicalnewstoday .com/kc/serotonin-facts-232248.

11. Jessica M. Yano, Kristie Yu, Gregory P. Donaldson, et al., "Indigenous Bacteria from the Gut Microbiota Regulate Host Serotonin Biosynthesis," *Cell* 161, no. 2 (2015): 264–276, www.ncbi.nlm .nih.gov/pmc/articles/PMC4393509/.

12. Paul Enck, "Spore-Forming Bacteria Regulate Serotonin Biosynthesis in the Gut," Gut Microbiota for Health, June 22, 2015, www.gutmicrobiotaforhealth.com/en/spore-forming-bacteria -regulate-serotonin-biosynthesis-in-the-gut/.

13. Mary Longmore, Ian B. Wilkinson, Andrew Baldwin, Elizabeth Wallin, *Oxford Handbook of Clinical Medicine*, Oxford University Press, 2014, p. 417.

14. Such an idea makes bacteria a cofactor rather than a cause of disease. We are all surrounded by millions of bacteria at all times, both inside and outside our bodies. They can only become invaders when something essential has broken down in our immune systems.

15. This story bears some similarity to the story we saw earlier with Daniel, who was helped to experience the unconditional love of his beloved grandmother in a way that became an enduring presence for him. This dynamic surfaces repeatedly in stories of SR.

16. H. Foster, "Lifestyle Changes and the 'Spontaneous' Regression of Cancer: An Initial Computer Analysis," *International Journal of Biosocial Medicine* 10, no. 1 (1988): 17–33.

3. Eat to Heal

1. Emily Boller, *Starved to Obesity: My Journey Out of Food Addiction and How You Can Escape It Too!* (New York, Post Hill Press, 2019).

2. Though type 2 diabetes is not technically an "incurable" illness, it is commonly treated as incurable. Wood's doctors did not treat it as reversible and were shocked when he did recover.

3. *Global Report on Diabetes* (Geneva, Switzerland: World Health Organization, 2016), https://apps.who.int/iris/bitstream/handle/10665/204871/9789241565257_eng.pdf;jsessionid=0F963002F4841769C45 5B12790BD8BDA?sequence=1.

4. Ibid. The percentage of people worldwide with diabetes has nearly doubled since 1980, rising from 4.7 to 8.5 percent among adults. And prevalence has been increasing faster in recent years, not only in adults but now also in children. This increased prevalence is increasingly impacting not only the quality of life and finances of individuals and families but also the economies of nations. The rising rates of obesity are thought to have an important relationship to this increasing prevalence.

5. D. W. Nyamai, W. Arika, P. E. Ogola, E. N. M. Njagi, and M. P. Ngugi, "Medicinally Important Phytochemicals: An Untapped Research Avenue," *Research and Reviews: Journal of Pharmacognosy and Phytochemistry* 4, no. 1 (2016): 35–49, www.rroij.com/open-access/medicinally-important-phytochemicals-an-untapped-research-avenue-.php?aid=67696.

6. Claire Haser, *Living with Pancreatic Cancer,* www.livingwithpancreaticcancer.com.

7. B. Chassaing et al., "Dietary Emulsifiers Impact the Mouse Gut Microbiota Promoting Colitis and Metabolic Syndrome," *Nature,* March 2015.

8. T. Colin Campbell, "Nutrition, Politics, and the Destruction of Scientific Integrity," T. Colin Campbell Center for Nutrition Studies, August 16, 2016.

9. T. Colin Campbell, *The China Study* (Dallas, TX: BenBella Books, 2017).

10. Campbell Appleton, "Effect of High and Low Dietary Protein on the Dosing and Postdosing Periods of Aflatoxin B1-Induced Hepatic Preneoplastic Lesion Development in the Rat," *Cancer Research* 43, no. 5 (1983): 2150–2154.

11. Banoo Parpia, Cornell-China-Oxford Project videocast, Cornell University. www.cornell.edu/video/playlist/the-china-project -studying-the-link-between-diet-and-disease.

12. Two hundred years ago, in the early 1800s when sugar was limited mostly to the wealthy, the average American consumed about 2 pounds of sugar each year. This represented less than 1 percent of caloric intake. That number has steadily increased over the past two centuries to the point where the average person now consumes approximately 152 pounds of sugar (and corn syrup) each year. And each country, as it adopts the Western diet, tends to follow this trend, especially in the large cities where the Western diet is most prevalent. This level of sugar consumption is so high that conversations about adopting a "balanced approach" often make no sense since what we call "normal" is itself wildly skewed. "How Much Sugar Do You Eat? You May Be Surprised!," New Hampshire Department of Health and Human Services, www.dhhs.nh.gov/dphs/nhp/documents/sugar.pdf.

13. Lily Sanborn, "Sugar Cravings: Evolution, Addiction, or Both?," *Frontiers: Washington University Review of Health,* April 20, 2015.

14. "2019: The Year for Nutrition," *Lancet* 393, no. 10168 (2019): 200, www.thelancet.com/journals/lancet/article/PIIS0140 -6736(19)30080-7/fulltext?utm_campaign=tleat19&utm_source =HubPage.

15. I experienced something similar to the power of food and community when, at the invitation of a friend, I spent some time in the Greek islands. Here, as they have done for many centuries, people sit outside during the evening for hours, enjoying one another and conversation, eating nutritionally dense meals consisting of vegetables, fish, and wine (the Mediterranean diet). It's tragic that in the large cities like Athens, a public health disaster is unfolding as people flock to the fast-food restaurants, regarded as "cool" because they are Western and American. Rates of heart disease,

diabetes, cancer, obesity, and other illnesses aren't just increasing; they are skyrocketing. We can do better and need to do so, not only in the United States but also in terms of worldwide leadership. Leaders gain the authority to lead to the exact degree that we genuinely help and don't hurt.

4. Shut Down the Disease Superhighway

1. John A. Dodson, Andrew Petrone, David R. Gagnon, et al., "Incidence and Determinants of Traumatic Intracranial Bleeding Among Older Veterans Receiving Warfarin for Atrial Fibrillation," *JAMA Cardiology* 1, no. 1 (2016): 65–72.

2. "The Top 10 Causes of Death," World Health Organization, May 24, 2018, www.who.int/mediacentre/factsheets/fs310/en/.

3. B. A. Glenn, C. M. Crespi, H. P. Rodriguez, N. J. Nonzee, S. M. Phillips, et al., "Behavioral and Mental Health Risk Factor Profiles Among Diverse Primary Care Patients," *Preventative Medicine* S0091-7435(17)30495-4, December 22, 2017, doi:10.1016/j.ypmed.2017.12.009. B. Bortolato, T. N. Hyphantis, S. Valpione, G. Perini, M. Maes, et al., "Depression in Cancer: The Many Biobehavioral Pathways Driving Tumor Progression," *Cancer Treatment Reviews* 52, January 2017, 58–70, doi:10.1016/j.ctrv.2016.11.004.

4. Noha Ahmed Nasef, Sunali Mehta, and Lynnette R. Ferguson, "Susceptibility to Chronic Inflammation: An Update," *Archives of Toxicology* 91, no. 3 (2017): 1131–1141.

5. Ibid., 1131.

6. There is a common myth that high levels of fat in the bloodstream cause cholesterol to stick to the walls of the arteries and that this then causes atherosclerosis. But we now know that this is a misunderstanding. Without damage to the endothelium, the development of a plaque cannot occur. Robert P. Hoffman, "Hyperglycemic Endothelial Dysfunction: Does It Happen and Does It Matter?," *Journal of Thoracic Disease* 7, no. 10 (2015): 1693–1695. See also: E. P. Weiss, H. Arif, D. T. Villareal, E. Marzetti, and J. O. Holloszy, "Endothelial Function After High-Sugar-Food Ingestion

Improves with Endurance Exercise Performed on the Previous Day," *American Journal of Clinical Nutrition* 88, no. 1 (2008): 51–57.

7. Nasef, Mehta, and Ferguson, "Susceptibility to Chronic Inflammation." Terrence Deak, Anastacia Kudinova, Dennis F. Lovelock, Brandon E. Gibb, and Michael B. Hennessy, "Neuroimmune Mechanisms of Stress Across Species," *Dialogues in Clinical Neuroscience* 19, no. 1 (2017). Ruth A. Hackett and Andrew Steptoe, "Type 2 Diabetes Mellitus and Psychological Stress—A Modifiable Risk Factor," *Nature Reviews: Endocrinology* 13, no. 9 (2017): 547–560. Petra H. Wirtz and Roland von Känel, "Psychological Stress, Inflammation, and Coronary Heart Disease," *Current Cardiology Reports*, September 20, 2017, 111.

8. "Autoimmune Disease List," American Autoimmune Related Diseases Association, www.aarda.org/diseaselist/.

9. F. G. Hage, "C-reactive protein and hypertension," *J Hum Hypertens* 28, no. 7, (2014): 410–415.

10. Amit Kumar Shrivatava, Harsh Vardhan Singh, Arun Raizada, Sanjeev, and Kumar Singh, "C-reactive protein, inflammation and coronary heart disease," *The Egyptian Heart Journal Review* 67, no. 2 (2015): 89–97.

11. J. Watson, A. Round, and W. Hamilton, "Raised inflammatory markers," *BMJ* 344, no. 454 (2012).

12. A. Nerurkar, A. Bitton, R. B. Davis, R. S. Phillips, and G. Yeh, "When Physicians Counsel About Stress: Results of a National Study," *JAMA Internal Medicine* 173, no. 1 (2013): 76–77.

13. P. H. Wirtz and R. von Känel, "Psychological Stress, Inflammation, and Coronary Heart Disease," *Current Cardiology Reports*, September 20, 2017, 111.

14. Ljudmila Stojanovich, "Stress and Autoimmunity," *Autoimmunity Reviews* 9, no. 5 (2010): A271–A276.

15. L. Stoianovich and D. Marisavlievich, "Stress as a trigger of autoimmune disease," *Autoimmune Review* 7, no. 3, (2008).

16. "How Stress Influences Disease: Study Reveals Inflammation as the Culprit," Science Daily, April 2, 2012, www.sciencedaily.com/releases/2012/04/120402162546.htm.

17. Nicole D. Powell, Erica K. Sloan, Michael T. Bailey, Jesusa M. G. Arevalo, Gregory E. Miller, et al., "Social Stress Up-Regulates Inflammatory Gene Expression in the Leukocyte Transcriptome via β-Adrenergic Induction of Myelopoiesis," *Proceedings of the National Academy of Sciences* 110, no. 41 (2013): 16574–16579.

18. M. Østensen, L. Fuhrer, R. Mathieu, M. Seitz, and P. M. Villiger, "A Prospective Study of Pregnant Patients with Rheumatoid Arthritis and Ankylosing Spondylitis Using Validated Clinical Instruments," *Annals of the Rheumatic Diseases* 63, no. 10 (2004): 1212–1217.

19. Jose U. Scher, Andrew Sczesnak, Randy S. Longman, Nikki Segata, Carles Ubeda, et al., "Expansion of Intestinal *Prevotella copri* Correlates with Enhanced Susceptibility to Arthritis," *eLife,* November 2013.

20. S. Dimitrov, E. Hulteng, and S. Hong, "Inflammation and Exercise: Inhibition of Monocytic Intracellular TNF Production by Acute Exercise via β2-Adrenergic Activation," *Brain, Behavior, and Immunity* 61, March 2017, 60–68, www.ncbi.nlm.nih.gov/pubmed /28011264.

5. Activate Healing Mode

1. Theodore M. Brown and Elizabeth Fee, "Walter Bradford Cannon: Pioneer Physiologist of Human Emotions," *American Journal of Public Health,* October 2002.

2. Walter B. Cannon, *The Way of an Investigator* (New York: W. W. Norton, 1945).

3. H. Benson, J. A. Herd, W. H. Morse, and R. T. Kelleher, "Behavioral Induction of Arterial Hypertension and Its Reversal," *American Journal of Psychology* 271, no. 1 (1969): 30–34.

4 Anne Harrington, *The Cure Within: A History of Mind-Body Medicine* (New York: W. W. Norton, 2008).

5. S. W. Lazar, C. E. Kerr, R. H. Wasserman, et al., "Meditation experience is associated with increased cortical thickness," *Neu-*

roreport. 2005; 16(17):1893–97. www.ncbi.nlm.nih.gov/pmc/articles /PMC1361002/.

6. Rachael Donalds, *"Digital" Determinants of Health,* TEDx New Bedford, February 23, 2018. https://youtu.be/89CjV6tqIAM.

7. Sian Yong Tan and Yvonne Tatsumura, "Alexander Fleming: Discoverer of Penicillin," *Singapore Medical Journal,* July 2015.

8. E. S. Epel, J. Daubenmier, J. T. Moskowitz, S. Folkman, and E. Blackburn, "Can Meditation Slow Rate of Cellular Aging? Cognitive Stress, Mindfulness, and Telomeres," *Annals of the New York Academy of Sciences* 1172, August 2009, 34–53.

9. E. S. Epel, E. H. Blackburn, J. Lin, F. S. Dhabhar, N. E. Adler, et al., "Accelerated Telomere Shortening in Response to Life Stress," *Proceedings of the National Academy of Sciences of the United States of America* 101, no. 49 (2004): 17312–17315.

6. The Healing Heart

1. "The Inflammatory Reflex: A New Understanding of Immunology," SetPoint Medical, https://setpointmedical.com/science /inflammatory-reflex/.

2. Barbara L. Fredrickson, Michael A. Cohn, Kimberly A. Coffey, Jolynn Pek, and Sandra M. Finkel, "Open Hearts Build Lives: Positive Emotions, Induced Through Loving-Kindness Meditation, Build Consequential Personal Resources," *Journal of Personality and Social Psychology* 95, no. 5 (2008): 1045–1062, www.ncbi .nlm.nih.gov/pmc/articles/PMC3156028/.

3. Barbara Fredrickson, *Love 2.0: Finding Happiness and Health in Moments of Connection* (New York: Hudson Street Press, 2013).

4. Bethany Kok and Barbara Fredrickson, "Upward Spirals of the Heart: Autonomic Flexibility, as Indexed by Vagal Tone, Reciprocally and Prospectively Predicts Positive Emotions and Social Connectedness," *Biological Psychology* 85, no. 3 (2010): 432–436.

5. Nicole K. Valtorta, Mona Kanaan, Simon Gilbody, Sara Ronzi, and Barbara Hanratty, "Loneliness and Social Isolation as Risk

Factors for Coronary Heart Disease and Stroke," *Heart* 102, no. 13 (2016): 1009–1016, https://heart.bmj.com/content/102/13/1009.

6. Julianne Holt-Lunstad, Timothy B. Smith, Mark Baker, Tyler Harris, and David Stephenson, "Loneliness and Social Isolation as Risk Factors for Mortality: A Meta-Analytic Review," *Perspectives on Psychological Science* 10, no. 2 (2015): 227–237. See also: "Loneliness Has Same Risk as Smoking for Heart Disease," Harvard Health Publishing, June 2016, www.health.harvard.edu/staying-healthy/loneliness-has-same-risk-as-smoking-for-heart-disease.

7. See: Jane E. Brody, "The Surprising Effects of Loneliness on Health," *New York Times,* December 11, 2017, www.nytimes.com/2017/12/11/well/mind/how-loneliness-affects-our-health.html. N. J. Donovan, O. I. Okereke, P. Vannini, R. E. Amariglio, D. M. Rentz, et al., "Association of Higher Cortical Amyloid Burden with Loneliness in Cognitively Normal Older Adults," *JAMA Psychiatry* 73, no. 12 (2016): 1230–1237. doi:10.1001/jamapsychiatry.2016.2657.

8. Tim Adams, "John Cacioppo: 'Loneliness Is Like an Iceberg—It Goes Deeper Than We Can See,'" *Guardian,* February 28, 2016, www.theguardian.com/science/2016/feb/28/loneliness-is-like-an-iceberg-john-cacioppo-social-neuroscience-interview.

9. Karin Brulliard, "A Woman's Dog Died, and Doctors Say It Literally Broke Her Heart," *Washington Post,* October 19, 2017, www.washingtonpost.com/news/animalia/wp/2017/10/19/a-womans-dog-died-and-doctors-say-her-heart-literally-broke/.

10. Abhishek Maiti and Abhijeet Dhoble, "Takotsubo Cardiomyopathy," *New England Journal of Medicine* 377, October 2017, e24, www.nejm.org/doi/10.1056/NEJMicm1615835.

11. Neeta Mehta, "Mind-Body Dualism: A Critique from a Health Perspective," *Mens Sana Monographs* 9, no. 1 (2011): 202–209, www.ncbi.nlm.nih.gov/pmc/articles/PMC3115289/.

7. Faith Healing and Healing Faith

1. J. Levin, "Prevalence and Religious Predictors of Healing Prayer Use in the USA: Findings from the Baylor Religion Survey,"

Journal of Religion & Health 55, no. 4 (2016): 1136–1158, www.ncbi
.nlm.nih.gov/pubmed/27075199.

2. Everett L. Worthington Jr. and Michael Scherer, "Forgiveness Is an Emotion-Focused Coping Strategy That Can Reduce
Health Risks and Promote Health Resilience: Theory, Review, and
Hypotheses," *Psychology and Health* 19, no. 3 (2004): 385–405, www
.tandfonline.com/doi/abs/10.1080/0887044042000196674.

3. This person's name has been changed for privacy.

8. The Power of Placebo

1. Robert Langreth, "Six Miracle Cancer Survivors," *Forbes,*
March 2009. www.forbes.com/2009/02/11/cancer-cure-experimental
-lifestyle-health_0212cancer.html#140bd28d6277.

2. S. M. Vaziri-Bozorg, A. R. Ghasemi-Esfe, O. Khalilzadeh, H.
Sotoudeh, H. Rokni-Yazdi, et al., "Antidepressant Effects of Magnetic
Resonance Imaging-Based Stimulation on Major Depressive Disorder:
A Double-Blind Randomized Clinical Trial," *Brain Imaging Behavior*
6, no. 1 (2012): 70–76, www.ncbi.nlm.nih.gov/pubmed/22069111.

3. William J. Cromie, "Depressed get a lift from MRI," *The
Harvard Gazette,* January 22, 2004. https://news.harvard.edu/gazette
/story/2004/01/depressed-get-a-lift-from-mri/.

4. Erwin Schrödinger, one of the founders of quantum mechanics, told a famous story about a cat. He did it to show how absurd quantum mechanics is, even though it's true. The cat, prior to
being observed, is both dead and alive at the same time until your
observation of it causes it to be either dead or alive. Observing the
cat dead creates a history of rigor mortis. Finding it alive creates its
history, for example, of hunger. Observation creates the past. (As a
psychiatrist, my first thought was that this means for my patients
that it's never too late to have a good childhood!)

9. Healing Your Identity

1. Faruk Tas, "Metastatic Behavior in Melanoma: Timing,
Pattern, Survival, and Influencing Factors," *Journal of Oncology,*

Volume 2012, Article ID 647684, http://dx.doi.org/10.1155/2012/647684.

2. K. A. Katz, E. Jonasch, F. S. Hodi, et al., "Melanoma of unknown primary: experience at Massachusetts general hospital and Dana-Farber Cancer Institute," *Melanoma Research*, vol. 15, no. 1, (2005): pp. 77–82.

3. G. Vijuk and A. S. Coates, "Survival of patients with visceral metastatic melanoma from an occult primary lesion: a retrospective matched cohort study," *Annals of Oncology*, vol. 9, no. 4, (1998): 419–422.

4. A good description can be found in Michael Pollan's *How to Change Your Mind* (New York: Penguin, 2018), 301.

5. "Dr. Vincent Felitti: Reflections on the Adverse Childhood Experiences (ACE) Study," YouTube video, 32:33, posted by National Congress of American Indians, June 23, 2016, www.youtube.com/watch?v=-ns8ko9-ljU.

10. You Are Not Your Illness

1. Harry McGurk and John MacDonald, "Hearing Lips and Seeing Voices," *Nature* 264, no. 5588 (1976): 746–748, www.nature.com/articles/264746a0.

2. A. J. Crum and E. J. Langer, "Mind-Set Matters: Exercise and the Placebo Effect," *Psychological Science* 18, no. 2 (2007): 165–171.

3. Becca R. Levy and Ellen Langer, "Aging Free From Negative Stereotypes: Successful Memory in China and Among the American Deaf," *Journal of Personality and Social Psychology* 66, no. 6 (1994): 989–997.

4. F. Pagnini, C. Cavalera, E. Volpato, B Comazzi, F. Vailati Riboni, C. Valota, K. Bercovitz, E. Molinari, P. Banfi, D. Phillips, and E. Langer, "Ageing as a mindset: a study protocol to rejuvenate older adults with a counterclockwise psychological intervention," *BMJ Open* 9, no. 7 (2019): e030411. www.ncbi.nlm.nih.gov/pubmed/31289097.

5. E. Smith, M. Desai, M. Slade, and B. Levy, "Positive Aging Views in the General Population Predict Better Long-Term

Cognition for Elders in Eight Countries," *Journal of Aging and Health*, July 24, 2018. https://doi.org/10.1177/0898264318784183.

6. Giovanni Pico della Miranola, *Oration on the Dignity of Man*, 1496.

7. J. E. Logan, E. N. Rampersaud, G. A. Sonn, K. Chamie, A. S. Belldegrun, et al., "Systemic Therapy for Metastatic Renal Cell Carcinoma: A Review and Update," *Reviews in Urology* 14, nos. 3–4 (2012): 65–78.

11. Healing Death

1. Lulu Wang. *This American Life,* "In Defense of Ignorance," Act One. Chicago Public Media, April 22, 2016.

2. Bernard Crettaz, *Cafés Mortels: Sortir la Mort du Silence* (Geneva, Switzerland: Labor et Fides, 2010).

3. Sophie Elmhirst, "Take Me to the Death Cafe," *Prospect,* January 22, 2015, www.prospectmagazine.co.uk/magazine/take-me -to-the-death-cafe.

12. Burn Your Boat

1. The story of Cortés and the boat burning, which may be apocryphal, is widely told, but I want to thank Tony Robbins for reminding me of this powerful old analogy.

2. D. Spiegel, J. R. Bloom, H. C. Kraemer, and E. Gottheil, "Effect of Psychosocial Treatment on Survival of Patients with Metastatic Breast Cancer," *Lancet* 2, no. 8668 (1989): 888–891, www .ncbi.nlm.nih.gov/pubmed/2571815.

3. A. J. Cunningham, C. V. Edmonds, C. Phillips, et al., "A Randomized Controlled Trial of the Effects on Survival of Group Psychological Therapy for Women with Metastatic Breast Cancer," *Psycho-Oncology* 7, no. 6 (1998): 508–517.

4. A. J. Cunningham, C. V. Edmonds, C. Phillips, K. I. Soots, D. Hedley, and G. A. Lockwood, "A Prospective, Longitudinal Study of the Relationship of Psychological Work to

Duration of Survival in Patients with Metastatic Cancer," *Psycho-Oncology* 9, no. 4 (2000): 323–339, www.ncbi.nlm.nih.gov/pubmed/10960930.

5. A. J. Cunningham, C. Phillips, J. Stephen, C. Edmonds, "Fighting for life: a qualitative analysis of the process of psychotherapy-assisted self-help in patients with metastatic cancer," *Integrative Cancer Therapies* 1, no. 2 (2002): 146–161.

6. A. J. Cunningham and K. Watson, "How Psychological Therapy May Prolong Survival in Cancer Patients," *Integrative Cancer Therapies* 3, no. 3 (2005): 214–229.

7. Marcia Angell, "Disease as a Reflection of the Psyche," *New England Journal of Medicine* 312, June 1985, 1570–1572, www.nejm.org/doi/full/10.1056/NEJM198506133122411.

8. Julia Belluz, "America's most famous back pain doctor said pain is in your head. Thousands think he's right." *Vox,* July 23, 2018. www.vox.com/science-and-health/2017/10/2/16338094/dr-john-sarno-healing-back-pain.

9. A. J. Burger, M. A. Lumley, J. N. Carty, D. V. Latsch, E. R. Thakur, M. E. Hyde-Nolan, A. M. Hijazi, and H. Schubiner, "The effects of a novel psychological attribution and emotional awareness and expression therapy for chronic musculoskeletal pain: A preliminary, uncontrolled trial." *Journal of Psychosomatic Research* 81 (February 2016): 1–8. www.ncbi.nlm.nih.gov/pubmed/26800632.

Conclusion

1. Peter H. Diamandis, Steven Kotler, *Abundance: The Future Is Better Than You Think* (New York: Free Press, 2012).

2. Rachael Donalds, "Digital Determinants of Health," filmed in New Bedford, CT. TEDx video, www.youtube.com/watch?v=89CjV6tqIAM.

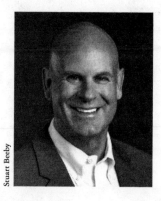

Stuart Beeby

Jeffrey D. Rediger, M.D., M.Div., is on the faculty at Harvard Medical School and is the medical director of McLean SouthEast Adult Psychiatry and of Community Affairs at McLean Hospital, one of the country's top psychiatric institutes and a leader in groundbreaking neuroscience research. A licensed physician and board-certified psychiatrist, he is also the chief of Behavioral Medicine at Good Samaritan Medical Center and has a master of divinity degree from Princeton Theological Seminary. Dr. Rediger has received numerous awards related to patient care and has been nominated for the National Bravewell Leadership Award, which recognizes physicians making significant contributions to the field of integrative medicine. His work has been featured on radio and television, including *Oprah Winfrey Show* and *Dr. Oz*.

www.drjeffreyrediger.com